Hormone Binding and Target Cell Activation in the Testis

CURRENT TOPICS IN MOLECULAR ENDOCRINOLOGY

Series Editors: Bert W. O'Malley and Anthony R. Means
Department of Cell Biology
Baylor College of Medicine
Houston, Texas

Volume 1:   *Hormone Binding and Target Cell Activation in the Testis*
Edited by Maria L. Dufau and Anthony R. Means

A Continuation Order Plan is available for this series. A continuation order will bring
delivery of each new volume immediately upon publication. Volumes are billed only upon
actual shipment. For further information please contact the publisher.

Hormone Binding and Target Cell Activation in the Testis

Edited by

Maria L. Dufau

Reproduction Research Branch
National Institute of Child Health and Human Development
National Institutes of Health
Bethesda, Maryland

and

Anthony R. Means

Department of Cell Biology
Baylor College of Medicine
Houston, Texas

SPRINGER SCIENCE+BUSINESS MEDIA, LLC

Library of Congress Cataloging in Publication Data

Main entry under title:

Hormone binding and target cell activation in the testis.

(Current topics in molecular endocrinology; v. 1)
"Proceedings of the workshop conference held at Baylor College of Medicine,
Houston, Texas, February 11-13, 1974, sponsored by the National Institute of Child
Health and Human Development and the Baylor Center for Population Research and
Reproductive Biology."
Includes bibliographical references and index.
1. Testicle—Congresses. 2. Hormones, Sex—Congresses. I. Dufau, Maria L.,
ed. II. Means, Anthony R., ed. III. United States. National Institute of Child
Health and Human Development. IV. Baylor University, Waco, Tex. College of
Medicine, Houston. Center for Population Research and Reproductive Biology.
V. Series. [DNLM: 1. Binding sites—Congresses. 2. Receptors, Hormone—
Congresses. 3. Testis—Metabolism—Congresses. W1 CU821 v. 1 1974 / WJ830
B612 1974]

QP255.B54   612.6'1   74-23709
ISBN 978-1-4684-2597-0   ISBN 978-1-4684-2595-6 (eBook)
DOI 10.1007/978-1-4684-2595-6

Proceedings of the Workshop Conference held at
Baylor College of Medicine, Houston, Texas, February 11-13, 1974
sponsored by the National Institute of Child Health and Human Development,
and the Baylor Center for Population Research and Reproductive Biology

© 1974 Springer Science+Business Media New York
Originally published by Plenum Press, New York in 1974
Softcover reprint of the hardcover 1st edition 1974

Foreword

It is curious that research in endocrinology has largely ignored the testis until quite recently. There were two important reasons for this neglect; first, methods of study were difficult, and second, spermatogenesis was considered to be the concern of the urologist or cell biologist but not the endocrinologist. Since it is now almost an ethical imperative that we develop a male contraceptive, and since a host of new techniques can be brought to bear on problems of testis function, research in male reproductive biology has effloresced. In fact, it has become possible to project a series of workshops on the testis, each dealing with discrete aspects of biochemistry, physiology and pathology.

It is fitting that this first Workshop should be on Binding and Activation, since this area is one of the frontiers in endocrinology. At our present rate of progress it is probable that each of the succeeding workshops will likewise bring together leaders in a rapidly developing area. The National Institute of Child Health and Human Development has the major Federal responsibility in reproductive biology, and has therefore agreed to sponsor this and succeeding workshops. On behalf of the Institute and for those members of the Committee who have organized this meeting, I welcome you. I am quite sure that this first Workshop on the Testis will initiate a series of important contributions to scientific thought in male reproductive biology.

Mortimer B. Lipsett, M.D.

February 1974

Preface

The Conference which this book represents would not have been possible without the support of Dr. Mortimer B. Lipsett and the NICHD. We are especially grateful to Dr. Lipsett for his central role in the organization and planning of the Conference. The format of this volume follows the order of presentations during the meeting, in which three basic areas are obvious. The first is concerned with the binding of LH and hCG to target tissues, and with some of the early metabolic actions of these gonadotropic hormones. The second area is concerned with generally similar information concerning the binding and actions of FSH. The final topics are concerned with the binding of steroid hormones within specific testicular cell types. This program and format resulted from the recommendations of an organizing committee which consisted of several of the scientists who served as the chairpersons of the various sessions during the Conference. For their services we are most appreciative.

The editors also wish to express their sincere thanks to the secretarial staff of the Department of Cell Biology for making our stay in Houston a pleasant one. The participants themselves must be commended for their timely and valuable contributions which made possible both the conference and this book. Finally, we owe a debt of gratitude to Ms. Terri Sellner for the preparation and typing of the manuscripts, and to Plenum Press for maintaining a high priority for the volume in regard to the time of publication.

Anthony R. Means, Ph.D.
Maria L. Dufau, M.D.

August 1974

Contents

GONADOTROPIN BINDING AND ACTIVATION OF THE

INTERSTITIAL CELLS OF THE TESTIS

K. J. Catt, T. Tsuruhara, C. Mendelson,
J-M. Ketelslegers and M. L. Dufau

Section on Hormonal Regulation
Reproduction Research Branch
National Institute of Child Health and Human Development
National Institutes of Health
Bethesda, Maryland 20014

Tissue receptor sites with high affinity for luteinizing hormone (LH) and human chorionic gonadotropin (hCG) have been defined in the interstitial cells of the testis, and also in the normal and gonadotropin-luteinized rat ovary (1-8). Comparable binding sites have also been demonstrated in the bovine corpus luteum, and in porcine granulosa cells during maturation in vivo and in vitro (9). The common receptor site for LH and hCG in these tissues is highly specific, with binding affinity only for molecules with the conformation characteristics of LH and chorionic gonadotropin. The biological specificity of hormone binding is demonstrable with LH from a wide variety of species, and with the placental gonadotropins of man, primates and the horse (2). The properties of the testis LH/hCG receptors, and their applications to radioligand-receptor assay, have been previously described in detail (2). In this chapter, the characteristics and application of gonadotropin receptors will be briefly reviewed, and more recent studies on the analysis of hormone-receptor interactions and the target cell responses to gonadotropins will be described.

(A) Methods of Study

(1) Tissue preparations

For binding studies, homogenates of the adult rat testis are prepared in phosphate-buffered saline by Teflon-glass homogenization, or more conveniently by dispersion in a Waring blender for one to two minutes. The testis fragments are centrifuged

1

at 1500 g to isolate the major binding fraction, which includes more than 80% of the gonadotropin binding sites when centrifugation is performed in physiological salt solutions. In the presence of 5% sucrose, a much wider dispersal of binding fragments is obtained, and centrifugation at 10,000 g is necessary to sediment the majority of the gonadotropin binding sites. For binding studies in which separation of bound and free tracer is to be performed by centrifugation, the original binding fraction should be prepared by centrifugation at the appropriate force (e.g. 1500 g) to be used subsequently for isolation of the bound hormone. If this simple step is not performed during preparation of the binding fraction, a significant amount of bound hormone will remain in the 1500 g supernatant when centrifugation is performed at the completion of incubation, and will be included with the 'free' hormone component. Such misclassification can invalidate the calculated values for bound/free ratio, and may introduce errors into the results of computation procedures for derivation of the association constant and binding capacity of the receptor sites.

Separation of bound and free hormone can also be effected by filtration through albumin-soaked glass-fiber or millipore filters. In this case, less voluminous binding fractions are prepared by subjecting the testis homogenate to preliminary centrifugation at 120 g, followed by centrifugation of the supernatant solution at 20,000 g to sediment particulate binding activity. For binding preparations of high activity:protein ratio, this sequence of centrifugation steps is applied to the fragmented interstitial fraction prepared by teasing apart the testis tubules as previously described (1). Such preparations are enriched in interstitial cell membrane fragments, and are particularly useful for binding studies in which incubation with labeled LH or hCG is followed by filtration to isolate the bound hormone. The filtration method is also of value when sensitive radioligand-receptor assays using very small quantities of testis homogenate are performed, as described below.

(2) Labeled Gonadotropins

The most convenient gonadotropin tracer for binding studies with interstitial cell receptors is prepared by iodination of hCG with ^{125}I, to a ratio of approximately one atom per molecule (40 μCi/μg). Iodination is performed by a modification of the Chloramine T procedure, employing minimal oxidant concentration, low temperature and short reaction time as previously described (1). Labeling can also be performed by the lactoperoxidase procedure, with relatively little detectable difference between the binding properties of hCG tracer prepared by either method. However, human and sheep LH appear to be more readily damaged by the Chloramine T method, and like FSH and prolactin, are more satisfactorily labeled by the lactoperoxidase method.

Purification of the labeled hormone can be performed by cellulose adsorption chromatography, or by gel filtration on Sephadex G-100 or Biogel P60. Our preference is for the "group-specific" affinity chromatography procedure based upon adsorption to Sepharose-Concanavalin A, followed by elution of the labeled hormone by 0.2 M methyl-mannopyranoside (10). This method has also been of considerable value for purification of ^{125}I-labeled human FSH for receptor binding studies, after iodination by the lactoperoxidase procedure.

The labeled tracer should be evaluated after purification by determination of its biological specific activity (11), and of the ability to bind to excess receptor sites. Specific activity can be determined by self-displacement in a radioimmunoassay for hCG, but the most appropriate estimate is derived from measurement by in vitro bioassay or by self-displacement assay in the radio-ligand-receptor assay system. In general, the specific activity determined by receptor assay is somewhat higher than that measured by radioimmunoassay, and represents a more biologic-ally relevant estimate of radioactivity in terms of hormonal activity.

Measurement of the extent to which labeled hormone can be bound by excess receptor sites also provides a useful procedure for correction of the 'true' free hormone concentration during binding studies (12). This is determined by measuring the maxi-mum proportion of tracer which can be bound by increasing con-centrations of the receptor fraction, and should logically reflect the biologically active fraction of the tracer preparations. Such an estimate can obviously be valid and useful if determined under appropriate conditions to minimize hormone and receptor degra-dation, both of which can influence the maximum binding activity of the tracer preparation. In some studies, increasing receptor concentration has been accompanied by increasing, and then decreasing, levels of tracer binding, a phenomenon attributable to effect of increasing hormone degradation activity in the par-ticulate binding fraction. In the testis binding system, incuba-tion at 25° C for 16 hours has been shown to be accompanied by minimal hormone degradation, and can be employed for measure-ment of the maximum binding activity of labeled gonadotropin. In most tracer preparations, the maximum level of bound ^{125}I-hCG reaches a plateau in the region of 60%, a value commen-surate with the biological activity of the hormone preparation (10-12,000 IU/mg) in relation to the reported maximum attain-able activity of purified hCG (15-18,000 IU/mg). In contrast to the free tracer, which includes a proportion of inactive labeled hormone, the specific receptor-bound tracer can be considered to be fully active, and represents hormone of maximum biological activity.

Application of such corrections is not necessary when the particulate receptors are employed for radioligand-receptor assay and comparative binding-inhibition studies with modified gonadotropin preparations. However, the corrections should be made during quantitative binding studies for the determination of rate constants and equilibrium constants, in order to obtain the most accurate and absolute measurement of these quantities (13).

(B) General Properties of Gonadotropin Receptors

Unlike certain other peptide hormones, including insulin, growth hormone and prolactin, the receptor sites for LH and hCG appear to be confined to the obvious target cells in the testis and ovary. Specific binding of labeled hCG is not demonstrable in tissues of the male rat other than the testis, where binding is confined to the interstitial cell compartment (Fig. 1). No significant binding of labeled LH or hCG to tubule elements is demonstrable, and conversely FSH binding has been shown to be confined to the tubules with no uptake by the interstitial cells.

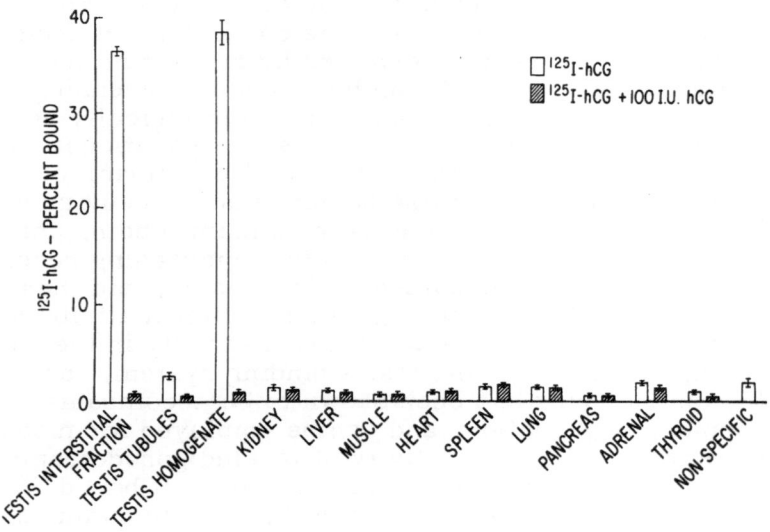

Figure 1. Specificity of ^{125}I-hCG binding to gonadal compartments and various tissues of the rat. In each case, the 1500 g fraction of the tissue homogenate was incubated with 50,000 cpm of ^{125}I-hCG, in the absence and presence of excess unlabeled hCG.

A small and variable uptake by liver and kidney homogenates is sometimes seen, an in vitro effect which may be consistent with the accumulation of labeled hormone in these tissues after injection in vivo (14). However, this binding is not of the specific, high-affinity type which is characteristic of the gonadal receptors. Many labeled hormones are concentrated by the proximal renal tubules, and rapid hepatic uptake of desialylated glycoproteins is a well-documented phenomenon (15). Whether the latter mechanism represents a normal step in the metabolism of glycprotein hormones is less certain, since rapid hepatic uptake of desialylated gonadotropins has only been demonstrated with hormones subjected to enzymatic desialylation in vitro and subsequently administered to the experimental animal.

The binding of LH and hCG to testicular receptors has been shown to be a temperature-dependent saturable process, with relatively high equilibrium association constant in the range of $2\text{-}6 \times 10^{10}$ M^{-1} (1-3). Binding occurs rapidly at 37° C, depending upon the relative concentrations of hormone and receptor sites, and can be analyzed by computer programs based upon the second-order bimolecular reaction equation (Fig. 2). Both

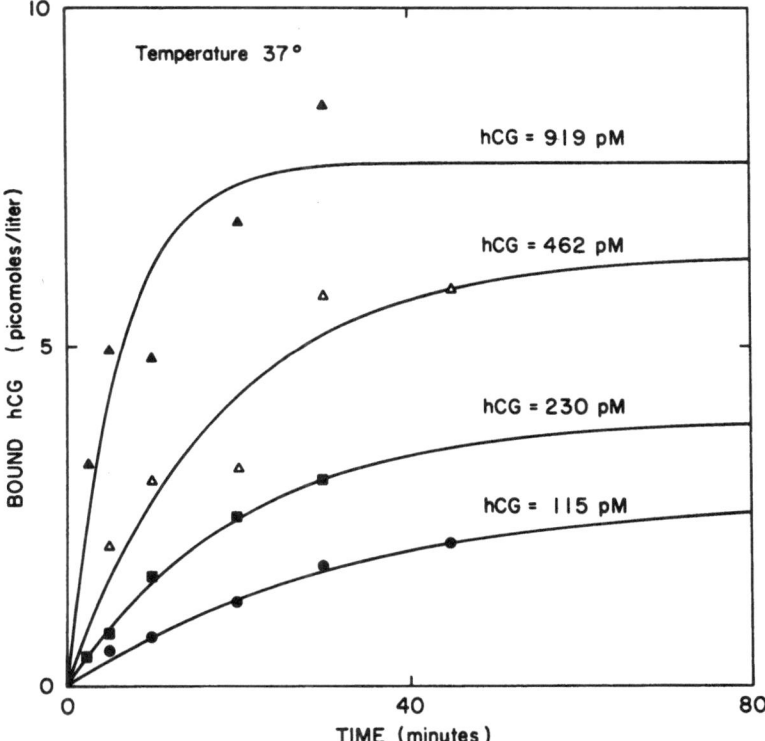

Figure 2. Time course of gonadotropin binding by testis

receptors at 37° C, in the presence of several concentrations of ^{125}I-hCG. The continuous lines were generated by computer analysis of the binding data according to the second-order rate equation as described by Ketelslegers et al (13).

hormones interact with a common receptor site in the interstitial cell, which appears to have a higher avidity for hCG than for LH. This difference could be due to the more complete retention of biological activity of radiiodinated hCG, rather than to a true difference in binding affinity of the receptor sites for the native hormone. However, the consistent differences in slope between binding-inhibition curves for human hormones, both LH and hCG, and LH from other species (2), indicates that the rat testis receptors may possess higher affinity for the human hormones. The LH/hCG receptors of the rat testis have been found to be associated with vesicular membranous material after sucrose density gradient centrifugation of fragmented interstitial cells (4). The distribution of ^{125}I-hCG binding activity in a 5-40% sucrose gradient is shown in Figure 3. The peak of binding activity occurs at a

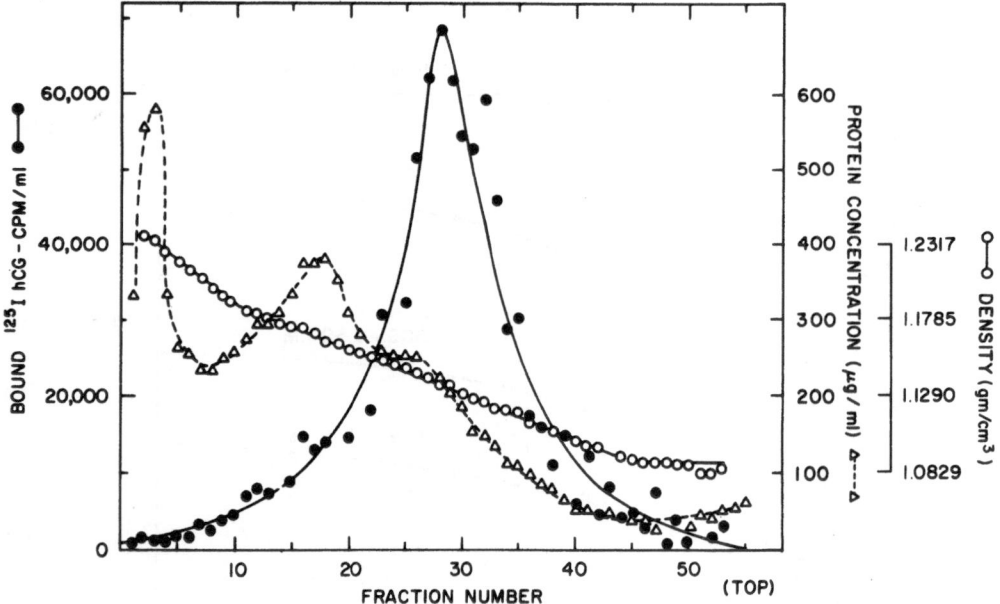

Figure 3. Distribution of gonadotropin binding activity after continuous density gradient centrifugation of testis particles in 5-40% sucrose.

density of 1.13, and is coincident with the peak activity of plasma membrane marker enzymes, such as 5' nucleotidase, as illustrated in Figure 4.

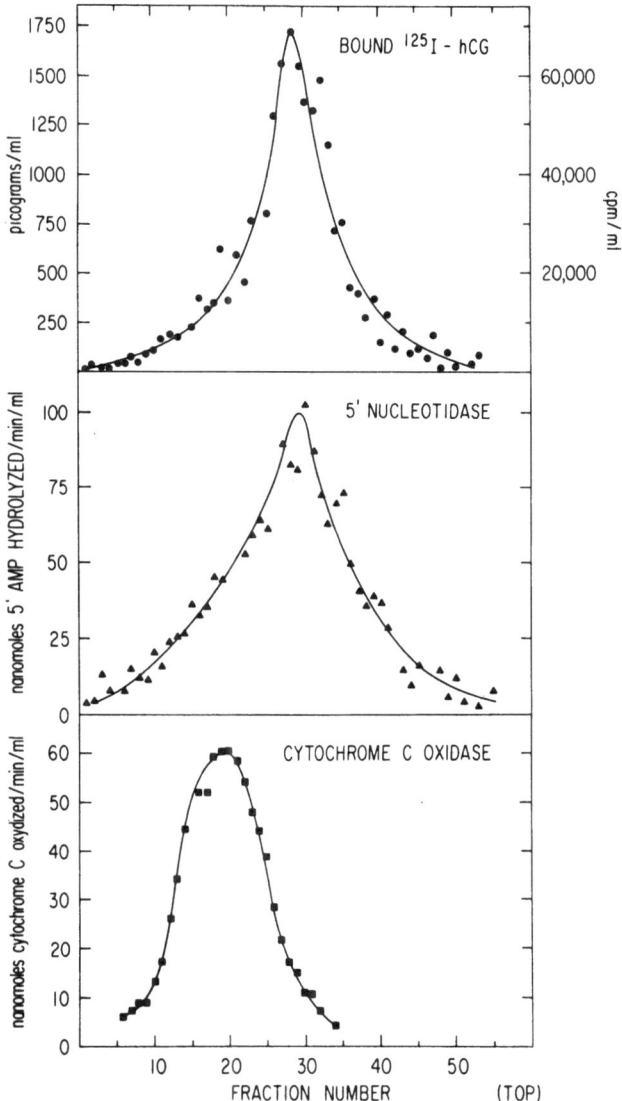

Figure 4.   Comparison of the sedimentation profile of testis binding particles in 5-40% sucrose with the positions of marker enzymes for plasma membrane (5' nucleotidase) and mitochondria (cytochrome C oxidase).

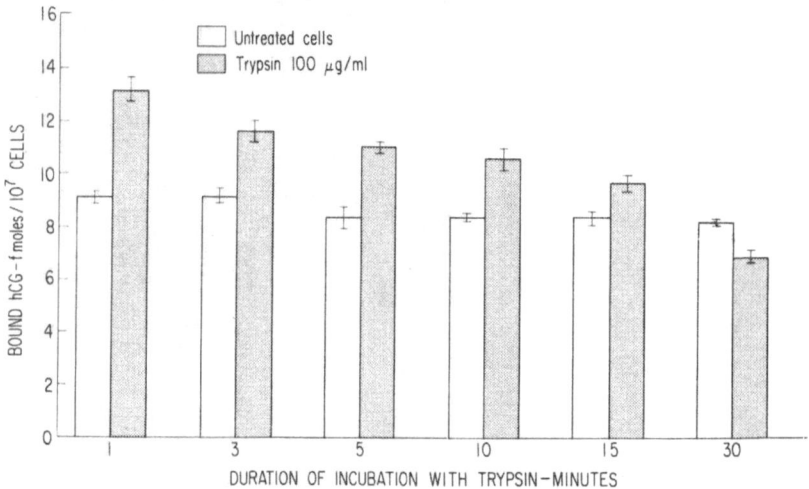

Figure 5. Enhancement of ^{125}I-hCG binding by dispersed Leydig cells after exposure of the cell preparation to trypsin (100 μg/ml).

The plasma membrane location of gonadotropin receptors is indirectly supported by the ability of sepharose-coupled LH to activate testicular steroidogenesis in vitro (16), and by the substantial recovery of cell-bound hCG from testicular tissues following exposure to low pH (16). Also, brief digestion of dispersed Leydig cells with proteolytic enzymes causes alterations in subsequent binding of ^{125}I-hCG, initially with increased uptake and after more prolonged exposure with loss of binding capacity (Figure 5). Enhanced uptake of labeled insulin by adipocytes and liver cells has previously been demonstrated after brief exposure to trypsin and phospholipase C (17, 18), and may reflect exposure of receptors and greater accessibility to hormone in the surrounding medium. The abolition of hormone binding caused by more extensive proteolytic digestion doubtless reflects the predominantly peptide nature of the receptors. Of other enzymes tested, phospholipase A also markedly reduced binding of hCG to particulate testis receptors, while phospholipase C and neuraminidase have no significant effect (Figure 6).

(C) Application of Testis Receptors to Radioligand-Receptor Assay of LH and hCG

Radioligand-receptor assays for LH and hCG have been established with homogenates of rat testis and ovary (1, 2),

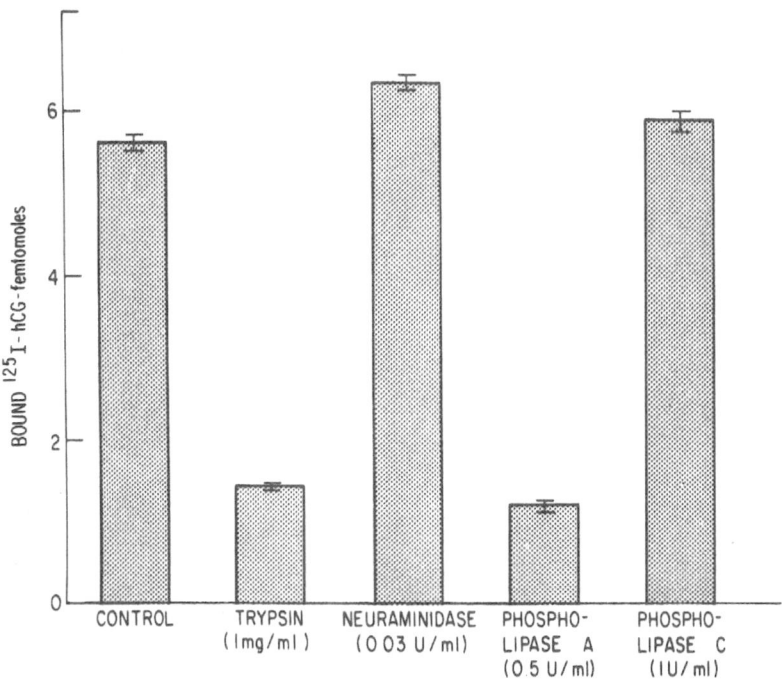

Figure 6. Effect of enzyme treatment upon the gonadotropin
binding activity of testis particles. Specific binding of ^{125}I-hCG
is largely abolished by exposure to phospholipase A and trypsin
(1 mg/ml), and is not affected by phospholipase C and neuraminidase.

and have proven to be of value for in vitro bioassay of these
hormones in tissue extracts, pregnancy plasma and hormone
preparations. Assays have been usually performed in a total
volume of 1 ml, containing 0.5 ml of an appropriately diluted rat
testis homogenate. As shown in Figure 7, adequate binding of
^{125}I-hCG is obtained after dilution as far as one testis per 40
ml, when each assay vial contains the equivalent of one eightieth
of a testis.

Relatively high binding of ^{125}I-hCG can also be obtained with
testis homogenates from other species, particularly with pig testis homogenate as shown in Figure 8. The binding activity of
fresh rat testis homogenates is usually higher than that of frozen
testes, but adequate binding curves can be obtained with testes

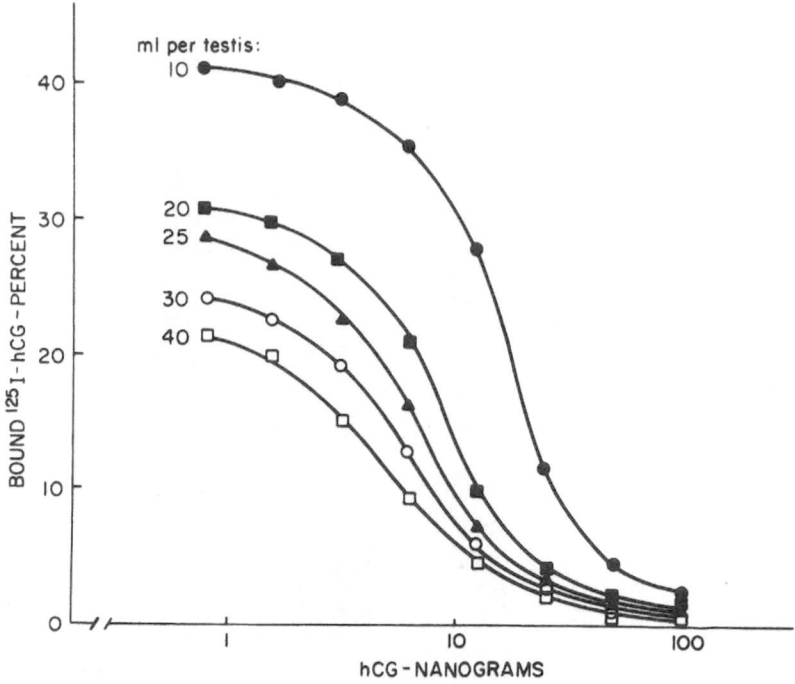

Figure 7. Radioligand-receptor assay standard curves obtained with increasing dilutions of rat testis homogenate.

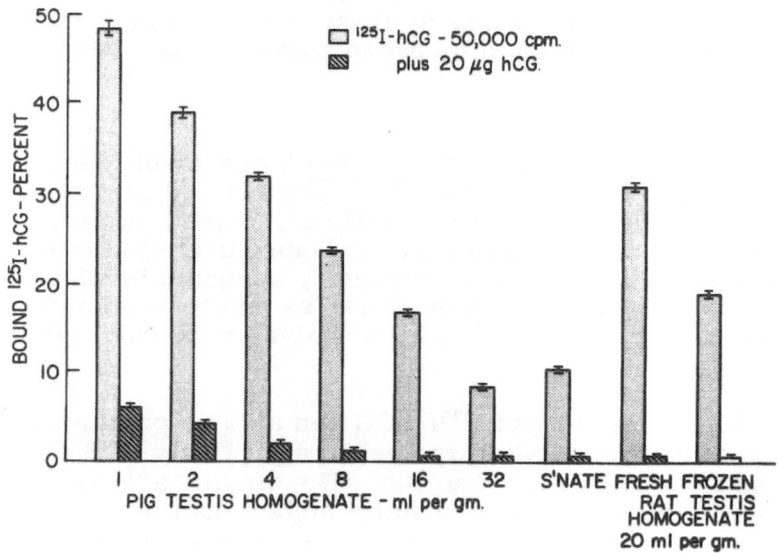

obtained in bulk (e.g., from Pelfreeze, Ark.) and stored frozen for several months at -60° C. Activity is lost more rapidly when tissue is stored at -15° C, but homogenates once prepared can be stored on ice for several days without significant loss of binding affinity. The relative potencies of hormone preparations are similar when assayed by the radioligand-receptor method employing either pig or rat testis homogenate, as demonstrated in Figure 9.

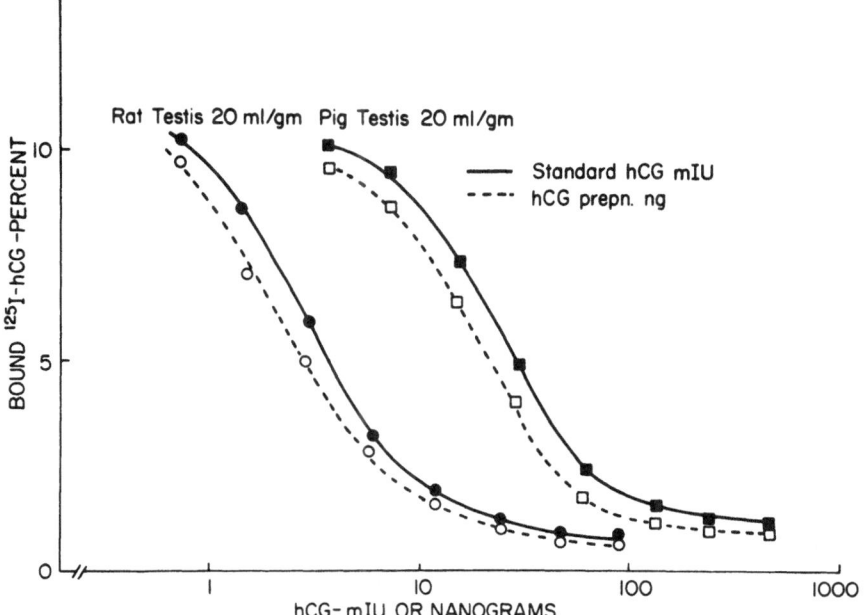

Figure 9. Radioligand-receptor assay of hCG in the presence of the 1500 g binding fraction prepared from homogenized pig and rat testis.

Figure 8. Comparison of ^{125}I-hCG binding to homogenates of the pig and rat testis. Although Leydig cells comprise a much greater proportion of the testis in the pig, binding activity was usually higher in rat testis homogenate at comparable degrees of dilution.

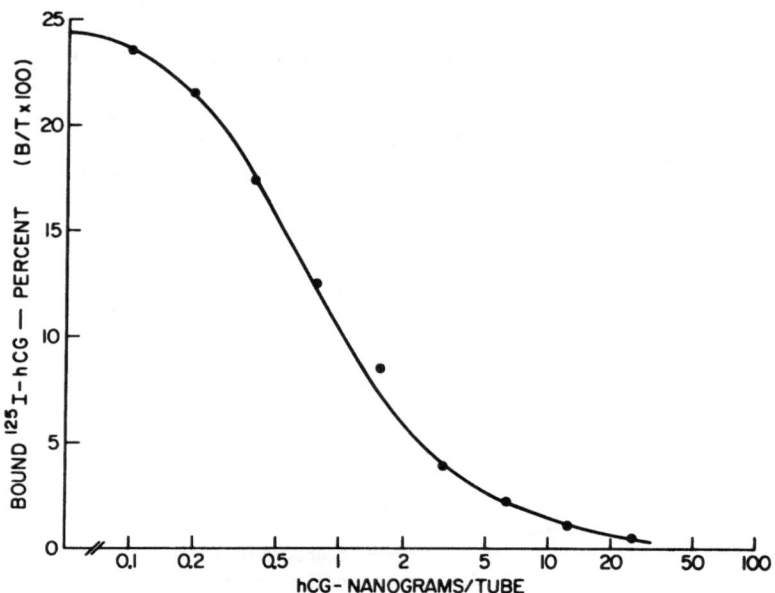

Figure 10. Increased sensitivity of the radioligand-receptor assay, performed in an incubation volume of 0.2 ml with binding particles equivalent to 1/100 of a testis.

The sensitivity of the assay system can be significantly increased by reducing the volume of the reaction of 0.2 ml, as shown in Figure 10. Under these conditions, the sensitivity of the procedure is increased to 50 pg (0.5 mIU) of hCG, with 50% displacement by 1 ng hCG. This version of the assay approaches the sensitivity of radioimmunoassay, but is still susceptible to non-specific interference by plasma proteins, which prevents accurate measurement of hCG in plasma below levels of about 5-10 nanograms per ml. Such interference can be avoided by preliminary extraction of plasma gonadotropins by adsorption to Sepharose-Concanavalin A, as previously described (10). For pregnancy plasma, serial dilutions give binding-inhibition with slopes parallel to that of the hCG standard (Fig. 11), and permit accurate quantitation of circulating hCG soon after implantation. In our experience, it is definitely not possible to detect gonadotropin in plasma prior to the rise which has been demonstrated by radioimmunoassay to occur about 10-12 days after conception. The radioligand-receptor assay can also be applied to measurement of chorionic gonadotropin in other species. In the rhesus monkey, binding-inhibition curves obtained with pregnancy plasma are parallel to those of hCG and partially purified monkey chorionic gonadotropin (Fig. 12). The equine pregnancy

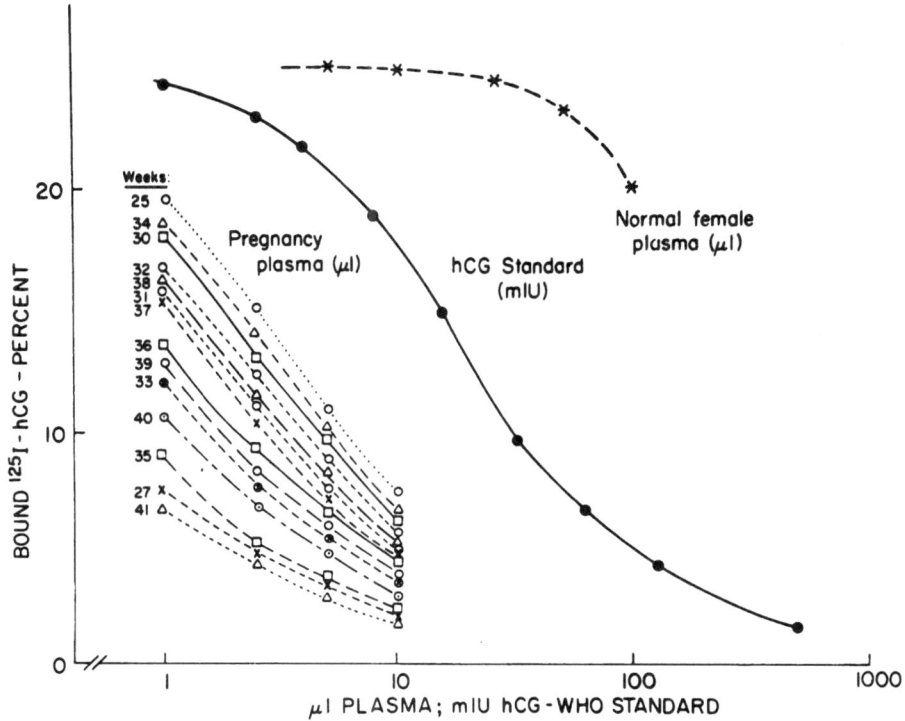

Figure 11. Radioligand-receptor assay of hCG in a series of plasma samples from pregnant subjects, by comparison with plasma from a non-pregnant female.

gonadotropin can also be measured by radioligand-receptor assay; PMSG gives binding-inhibition curves which are less steep than those of the human and primate hormones, and of similar slope to those of ovine, bovine, porcine and murine luteinizing hormone.

Determination of the LH content of various hormone preparations by radioligand assays gives values which are usually consistent with those derived by conventional bioassay. When measurements are performed upon hormones characterized by a short plasma half-life in vivo, the values determined by radioligand-receptor assay are frequently higher than those obtained by conventional bioassays. This is a particularly notable feature of desialylated hormones, and has been observed with both hLH and hCG after removal of neuraminic acid residues (4,19,20). The biological activity of ovine LH, which contains no sialic acid and has a relatively short plasma half-life, is also considerably higher in vitro than in vivo when assayed against standards of considerably longer half-life (e.g., the 2nd IRP hMG).

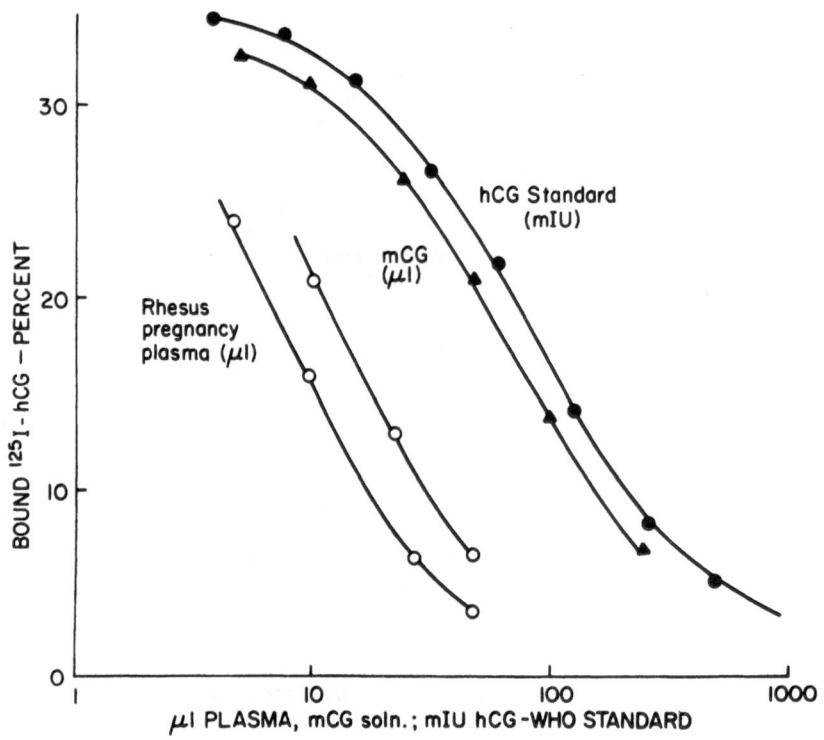

Figure 12. Binding-inhibition curves for semi-purified mCG
(Dr. G. Hodgen) and plasma of pregnant rhesus monkeys, in
the radioligand-receptor assay employing testis particles and
^{125}I-hCG.

Application of the radioligand-receptor assay to comparison
of a number of standard hormone preparations is illustrated in
Figure 13. In this case, several gonadotropin preparations from
the MRC series, including pituitary LH (68/40), FSH (68/39)
and LH/FSH (69/104), were assayed simultaneously with 2nd IRP
hMG (urinary LH/FSH), LER 907 (pituitary LH/FSH, the source
of MRC 69/104), purified urinary FSH (Serono), pituitary TSH
(MRC 68/38, with substantial LH contamination) and pituitary
GH. The absence of LH activity in the purified urinary FSH and
pituitary GH preparations is clearly apparent. The LH activity
observed in the MRC preparations of TSH and FSH is consistent
with the LH contamination measured by bioassay in these standards. The LER 907 and MRC 69/104 are almost equipotent on
a weight basis though widely separated in the figure by comparison of nanograms of LER 907 with microliters of a more concentrated solution of the 69/104 standard. All preparations

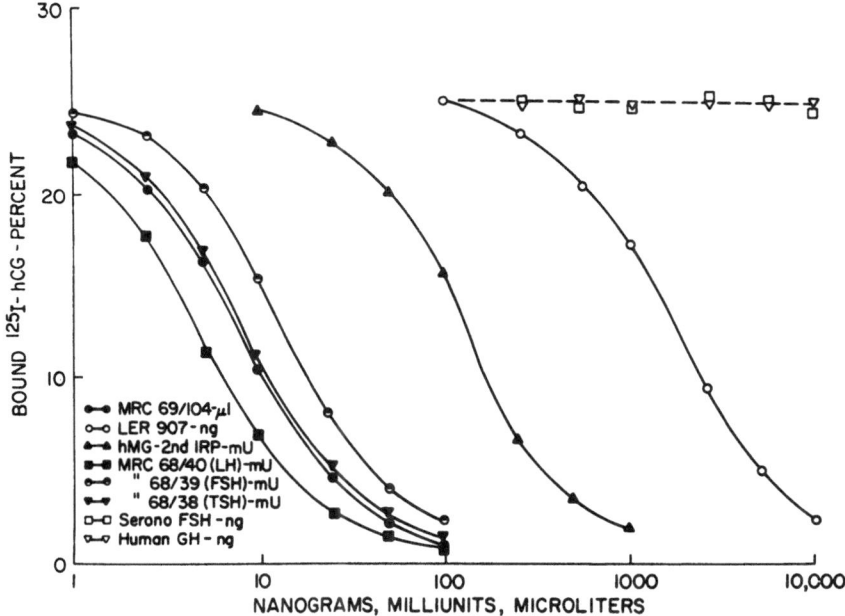

Figure 13. Comparative LH activities of a number of pituitary hormone preparations as shown by binding-inhibition potency in the radioligand-receptor assay. No activity was detected in hGH and urinary FSH. The LH activity determined in the other preparations were similar to those measured by conventional bioassay.

containing LH give parallel slopes in the assay, and derivation of potency estimates can be performed with high precision (less than 0.05) by computer programs for analysis of parallel-line bioassay data. Because the spread of data points covers a much wider range than obtained with conventional bioassays, programs devised for linearization, weighted least-squares regression analysis and comparison of radioimmunoassay binding inhibition curves are particularly useful for analysis of radioligand-receptor assay data.

In addition to measurement of LH and hCG concentrations in body fluids and/or tissue extracts and hormone preparations, the radioligand-receptor system is of considerable value for studies on the structure-function relations of gonadotropins in vitro. By this method, a single aspect of hormonal activity, that of binding to the specific receptor sites, can be evaluated quite separately from other aspects, such as metabolic clearance and target cell activation. The characteristic subunit structure and glycoprotein

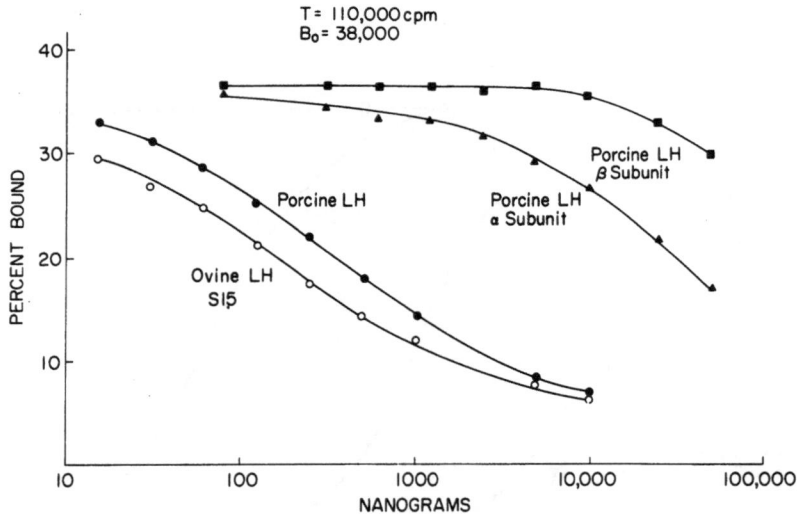

Figure 14. Comparative binding-inhibition potencies of ovine and porcine LH, and porcine LH subunits. The porcine LH preparations were provided by Dr. G. Hennen.

nature of the gonadotropins has obvious implications for the possible structural basis of hormonal specificity. Thus, the ß subunits of glycoprotein hormones are known to be the determinants of the specific biological actions of the individual hormones. After dissociation, the α and ß subunits of ovine LH, bovine LH and hCG are virtually devoid of binding-inhibition activity in the radioligand-receptor assay (21). The small amount of activity present in some subunit preparations can be accounted for by contamination with traces of the native hormone. The binding-inhibition activity of porcine LH subunits is also extremely low (Fig. 14). By comparison with the intact hormone, the activities of the α and ß subunits of porcine LH are only 1% and 0.1%, respectively, by weight. On a molar basis, these activities would be even further reduced by a factor of approximately 0.5.

The biological activities of the α and ß subunits of porcine LH in terms of target cell activation are also extremely low, in keeping with their low binding activity in the radioligand assay. Stimulation of cyclic AMP formation and testosterone production by the rat testis in vitro is shown in Figure 15, by comparison with the effects of intact porcine LH and ovine LH. For comparable stimulation of testosterone production, about 100 times as much of the subunits is required. It is also notable that although testosterone formation is induced by high concentrations of the subunits, no accompanying

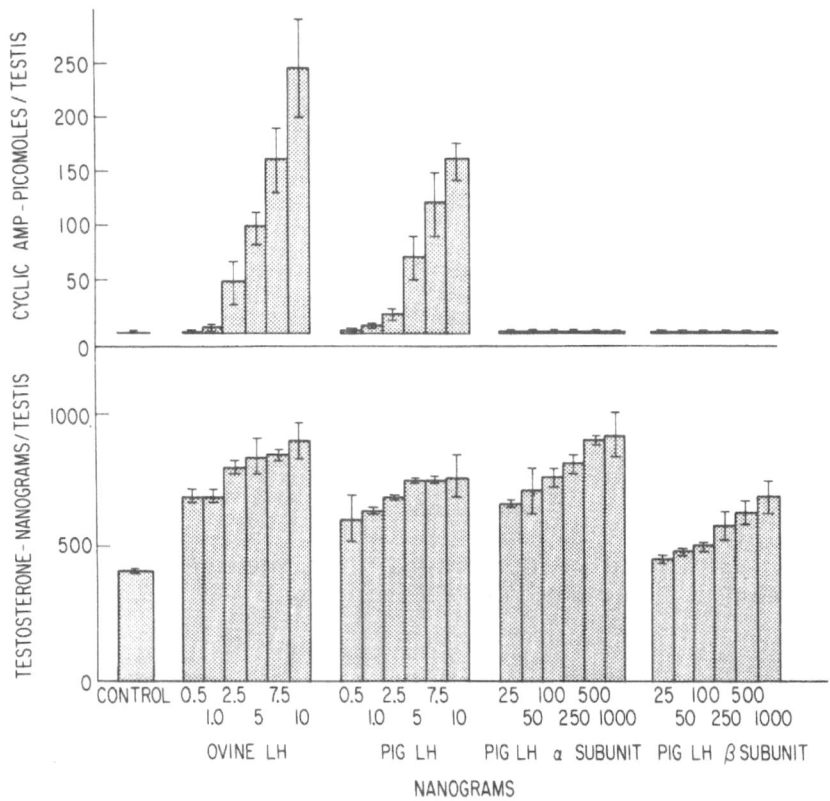

Figure 15. Stimulation of cyclic AMP production (above) and testos-terone synthesis (below) by ovine and porcine LH and porcine LH subunits.

stimulation of cyclic AMP formation is detectable. This dissociation between steroid synthesis and cyclic AMP formation is a character-istic feature of the Leydig cell response to low concentrations of gonadotropin, as described below. In this case, the phenomenon is observed during stimulation by high concentrations of gonadotropin subunits which are of low efficacy, or are contaminated with low levels of the intact hormone. These results are commensurate with the view that gonadotropin subunits possess little or no intrinsic biological activity in the dissociated state. Following recombination of subunits, substantial recovery of biological activity has been des-cribed in several assay systems, and is shown for the binding activity of ovine LH subunits in Figure 16.

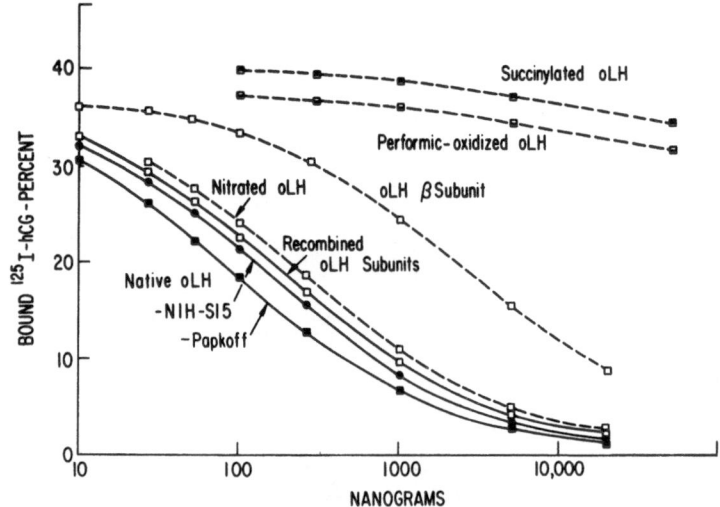

Figure 16. Radioligand-receptor assay of ovine LH, LH. subunits and chemically modified derivatives prepared by Dr. H. Papkoff.

The effects of a variety of chemical modifications of the gonadotropin molecule upon receptor binding are also shown in Figure 16. After nitration, about one-third of the original hormonal activity is retained by the mono-nitro derivative. Oxidation of sulfhydryl groups with performic acid, and succinylation of carboxyl side chains, are both accompanied by almost complete loss of binding activity. The importance of disulfide bonds for hormonal activity has also been indicated by the major loss of binding potency which follows exposure of hCG to dithiothreitol and other reducing agents (22, 23). Elsewhere in this volume, quantitative studies on the effects of nitration, succinylation and maleilyation are described by Ward et al. Such experiments have begun to provide information about the conformational and charge requirements for the biological activity of LH and hCG at the receptor site, and are most conveniently monitored by binding-inhibition activity in the radioligand-receptor assay system.

In addition to changes in the protein component of glycoprotein hormones, modification of the carbohydrate side chains has also been shown to influence the biological activity of LH and hCG. Previous studies have demonstrated that removal of sialic acid and galactose residues from hCG did not reduce binding affinity for the testis receptors (19, 20). Although activation of testosterone synthesis was moderately reduced, the residual in vitro biological activity was still very much higher than that observed by conventional bioassay. The very low activity values obtained

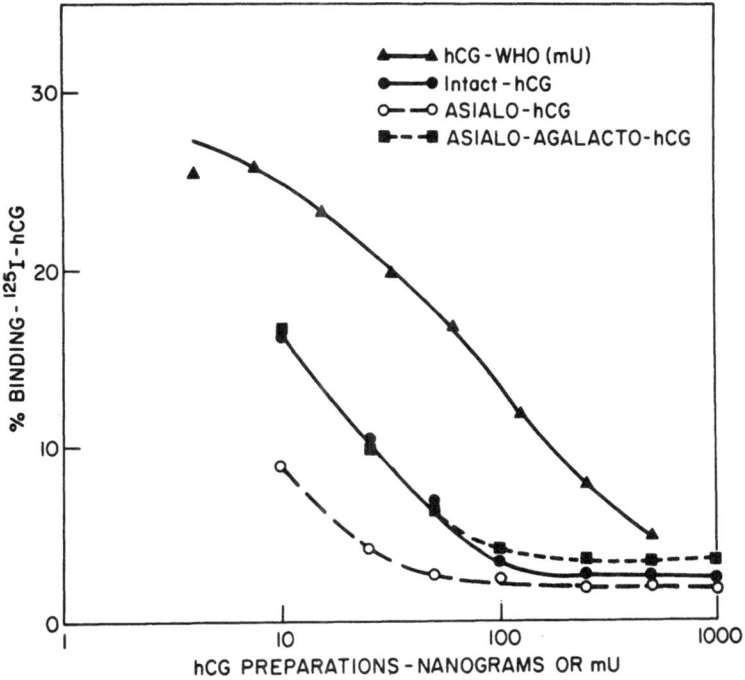

Figure 17. Binding-inhibition activity of intact, asialo- and asialo-agalacto-hCG in the radioligand-receptor assay. Asialo-hCG exhibits higher affinity for testis receptors than the intact hormone.

in the latter assays are due to rapid plasma clearance of the modified glycoproteins, and do not reflect the intrinsic activity at the target cell level. Removal of sialic acid residues from hCG is often accompanied by an increase in binding activity, attributable to reduction of the charge of the modified hormone (Fig. 17). Additional removal of galactose residues results in a return ot the original level of binding activity on a weight basis, which would be equivalent to an approximately 25% increase in activity on a molar basis. The reduction in Leydig cell stimulation by asialo-hCG and asialo-agalacto-hCG has been previously described (20), with testosterone responses equivalent to molar potency ratios of about 50% and 15% in comparison to the intact hormone. The ability of the modified glycoproteins to stimulate cyclic AMP formation in the testis is also substantially reduced, particularly for the asialo-agalacto-preparation (Fig. 18). These results indicate that the reduced steroidogenic potency after removal of carbohydrate residues is accompanied by less extensive activation of cyclic AMP formation in the Leydig cell. Thus, the modified glycoprotein hormones appear to have reduced efficacy, in the sense applied to drug action

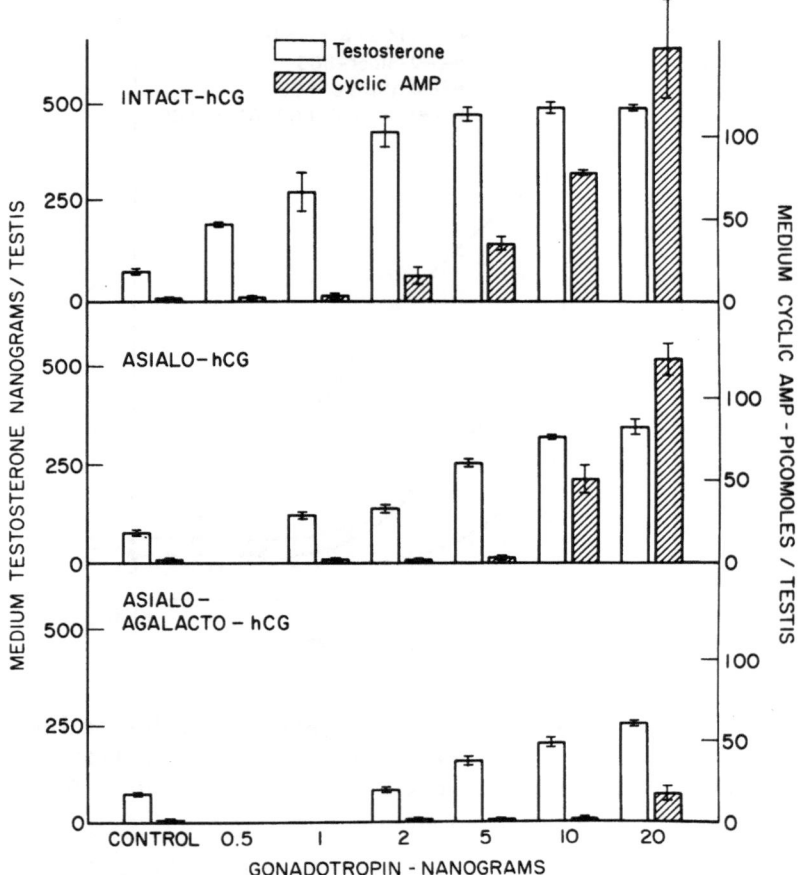

Figure 18. Stimulation of cyclic AMP and testosterone production
by the rat testis in vitro, in the presence of intact hCG, asialo-
hCG and asialo-agalacto-hCG. In this and succeeding figures,
cyclic AMP and testosterone were measured by radioimmunoassay
(27).

by Stephenson (24), so that relatively more receptor sites must be
occupied to evoke an equivalent hormonal response in terms of
cyclic AMP and testosterone synthesis.

The possibility that the reduced activity of the modified glycoproteins is caused by associated alterations of the protein component of the molecule should also be considered. The extent to which
such changes may occur during the sequential digestions with

enzymes to remove sugar residues must be carefully evaluated before the results of such treatment are attributed solely to changes
in the carbohydrate components of the molecule. Whatever the
mechanism for these changes, the retention of receptor binding
activity in the presence of reduced biological activity in vitro are
features which are characteristic of partial agonists, as originally
defined by Stephenson (24). Since partial agonists are also competitive antagonists under appropriate conditions, it is likely that
further analysis of the role of carbohydrate residues in gonadotropin
function will lead to the development of inhibitors of gonadotropin
action at the target cell. Such inhibitors would be unlikely to be
effective in vivo, due to the rapid metabolism of the modified glcyo-
proteins, but may be of value as in vitro antagonists of LH and hCG.
Evidence for the possible antagonist action of such derivatives is
described elsewhere in this volume by Bahl and colleagues, together
with studies which suggest a functional role for more deeply situated
sugar residues in hormone binding to the receptor site.

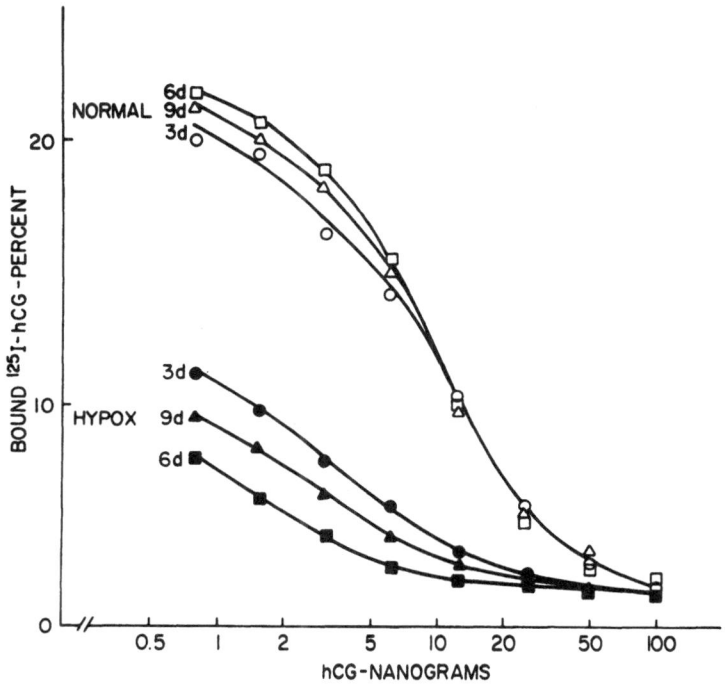

Figure 19. Binding of ^{125}I-hCG and inhibition by unlabeled gonadotropin, in homogenates of testes from normal and hypophysectomized
rats. Testes were obtained from control and treated animals at
intervals of 3 days following hypophysectomy.

The effects of hypophysectomy upon gonadotropin binding and target cell responses were studied in mature Sprague-Dawley rats. After hypophysectomy, the hCG binding activity of testis homogenates was markedly reduced within three days, and remained low at six and nine days (Fig. 19). Treatment of hypophysectomized rats with various combinations of LH, FSH and prolactin did not restore hCG binding activity; however, the levels of LH employed (100 μg daily) may have been large enough to cause partial occupancy of LH receptors in vivo, with subsequent reduction of binding capacity for labeled hCG in vitro. The loss of binding activity in homogenates prepared soon after hypophysectomy suggests that the receptor population must be continually replenished by pituitary-dependent stimulating factors. Conversely, alteration of the properties of the Leydig cell membrane following hypophysectomy may cause a relative loss of membrane fragments from the 1500 g fraction, leading to an apparent loss of binding activity during in vitro uptake of ^{125}I-hCG. The latter possibility is supported by simultaneous studies of ^{125}I-hCG binding to testis homogenate and whole testis, as well as testosterone production in response to hCG following hypophysectomy (Fig. 20). These experiments confirm the loss of binding capacity of testis homogenates from 3-9 days post-hypophysectomy, yet show no significant change in specific binding by the intact tissue during incubation of intact testis in vitro. By contrast, the dose-response relation between testosterone formation and hCG concentration shows a fall in the sensitivity of the testis to gonadotropin which is most marked at 3 days, with partial recovery of response at 9 days. These results suggest that the intact testis retains binding capacity for hCG but loses responsiveness to gonadotropin in the days following hypophysectomy. The loss of binding capacity in testis homogenates after hypophysectomy is not accompanied by a demonstrable change in affinity of the receptor sites, and may reflect an altered state of the cell membranes with resultant change in the sedimentation properties of the fragmented interstitial cell particles.

(D) Activation of Leydig Cell Functions by Gonadotropin

In addition to binding studies with testis homogenates described above, the properties of gonadotropin receptors have also been evaluated in intact Leydig cells, and correlated with metabolic responses such as cyclic AMP formation and testosterone synthesis. Initial studies in the decapsulated intact rat testis showed that subnanogram levels of hCG markedly stimulated testosterone production and release in vitro (16,25) and that cyclic AMP formation and release was stimulated by higher gonadotropin concentrations (26,27). Correlation of ^{125}I-hCG binding with such gonadotropin-induced responses revealed that hormone binding is initially accompanied by increasing stimulation of testosterone synthesis, which

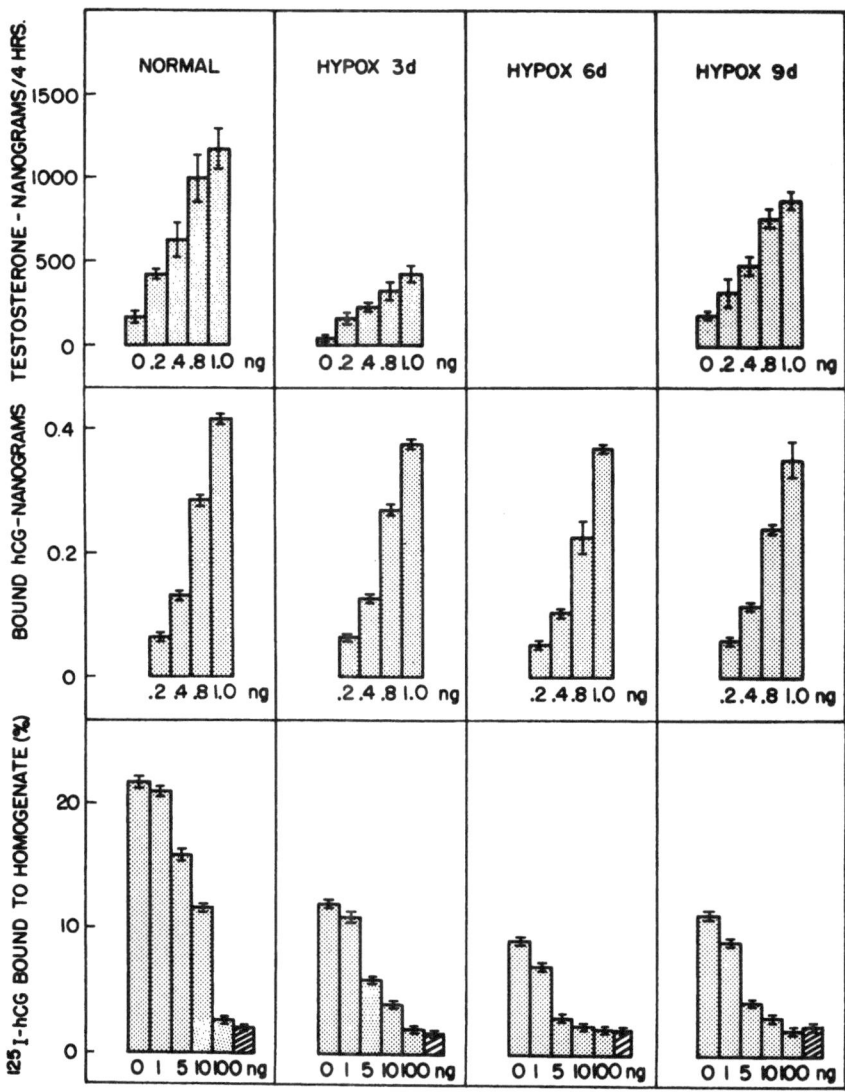

Figure 20. Binding of ^{125}I-hCG to testis homogenate (lower), and intact testis (middle) in normal and hypophysectomized rats. The accompanying stimulation of testosterone synthesis is shown in the upper panel.

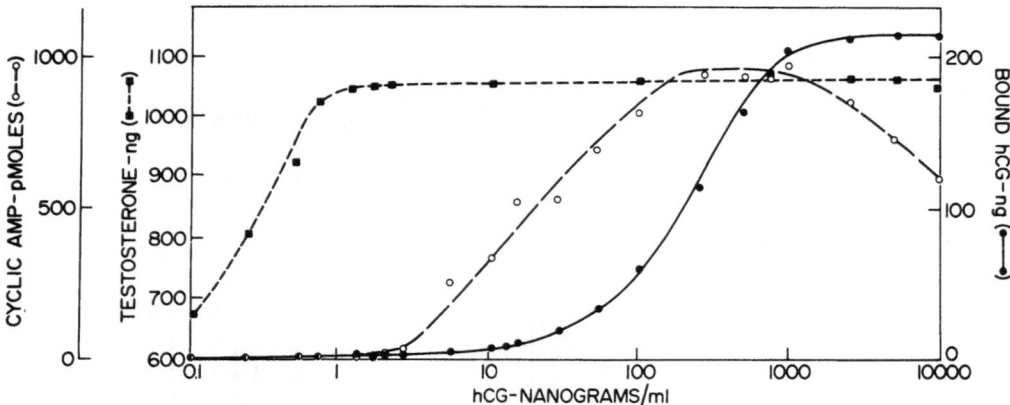

Figure 21. Correlation between hCG binding and activation of
cyclic AMP and testosterone synthesis in the rat testis, at
various concentrations of hCG in the incubation medium.

reaches a plateau when only a small proportion ($< 1\%$) of the total
binding sites are occupied. Formation of cyclic AMP is not
detectable until testosterone production is almost maximal; synthesis and release of the nucleotide then proceeds in parallel with
hormone binding. These relationships are illustrated by the data
in Figure 21, and have been found to occur in dispersed Leydig
cells (5) as well as in the intact testis (28). Such studies have
therefore revealed two distinct aspects of the testis response to
gonadotropins. First, that the Leydig cell appears to contain a
large excess of receptors above the number which must be occupied
to elicit a maximum steroidogenic response. Such 'spare' receptors
have also been described in other drug and hormone-sensitive tissues (17, 24, 29, 30) and may represent a mechanism for enhancing
the sensitivity of end-organs to low levels of circulating trophic
factors.

Second, the initial stages of stimulation by gonadotropins,
resulting in maximum activation of steroidogenesis, are not
accompanied by a detectable change in cyclic AMP concentration.
The latter observations have also been made in certain other
hormone-sensitive tissues, raising a question about the supposed
intermediate role of cyclic AMP in all phases of peptide hormone
action. However, the absence of a detectable change in cAMP
levels during stimulation of steroidogenesis with low concentration
of trophic hormone could result from an initial rise or translocation of cyclic AMP in a small intracellular compartment. At
higher hormone concentrations, cyclic AMP production becomes
detectable and is accompanied by extensive release of nucleotide

into the incubation medium. The stimulation of testosterone production by low hCG levels is significantly enhanced in the presence of phosphodiesterase inhibitors such as theophylline or methyl-isobutyl xanthine (MIX). The quantity of cyclic AMP produced during gonadotropin stimulation is always considerably increased in the presence of the theophylline or MIX, but again there is no detectable change in cyclic AMP levels in the presence of low hCG concentrations which maximally stimulate steroidogeneis (Fig. 22).

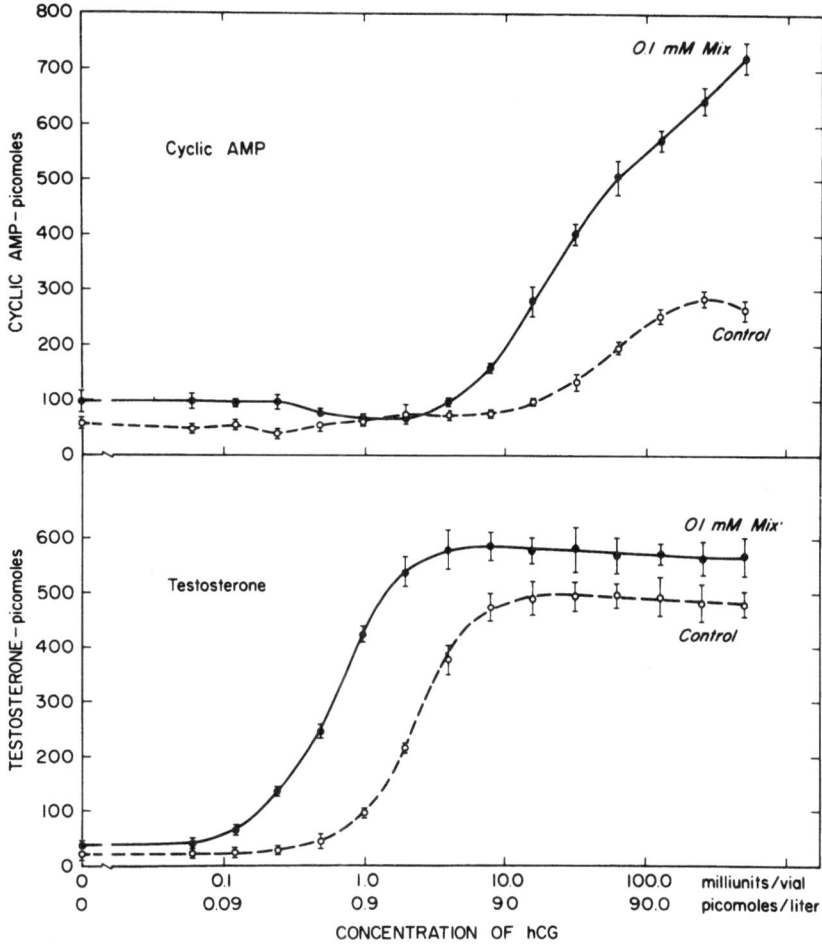

Figure 22. Effect of phosphodiesterase inhibition by 0.1 mM MIX upon the cyclic AMP and testosterone responses to hCG, in collagenase-dispersed Leydig cells.

Such effects of phosphodiesterase inhibition support the established view regarding the role of cyclic AMP in peptide hormone action, albeit at extremely low concentration. Also, changes in a critical 'active' nucleotide pool may not be detectable against the total intracellular concentration of cyclic AMP, most of which is in a metabolically inactive form.

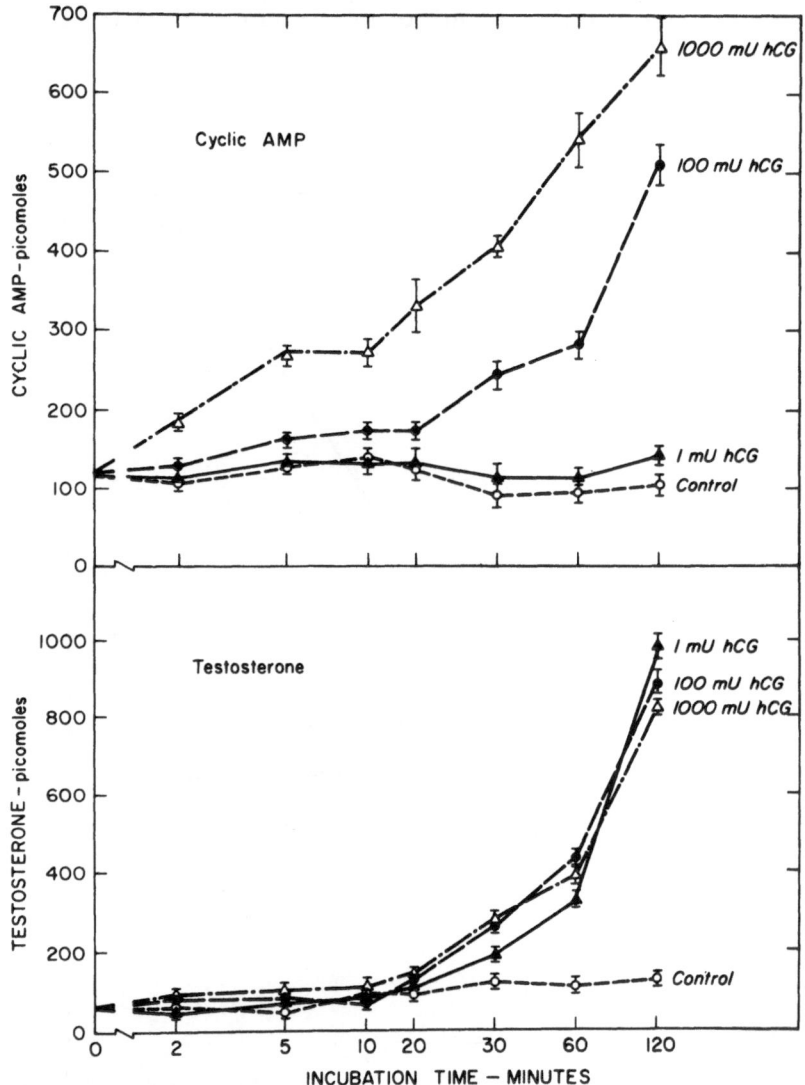

Figure 23. The time course of cyclic AMP formation and testosterone synthesis by dispersed Leydig cells in response to increasing concentrations of hCG. The lowest concentration of hCG (1 mU per vial) induced maximal stimulation of testosterone synthesis, with no change in the levels of cyclic AMP at any time.

The time course of stimulation of cyclic AMP and testosterone in the presence of increasing gonadotropin concentrations is also of interest in regard to the relations between nucleotide production and steroidogenesis. As illustrated in Figure 23, testosterone synthesis is maximally stimulated by 1 mU (100 pg) of hCG, and no further increase in the extent or the onset of testosterone formation is apparent at higher gonadotropin concentrations (lower panel). Under no circumstances are testosterone levels increased before 15-20 minutes following addition of gonadotropin, implying that several relatively slow metabolic steps must occur during this period. By contrast, the formation of cyclic AMP is markedly enhanced in extent and rapidity of onset in the presence of high gonadotropin concentrations (Fig. 23, upper panel). Under these circumstances, detectable increases in cyclic AMP formation occur as soon as one minute after addition of gonadotropin (27) while the synthesis of testosterone does not rise until 15-20 minutes later. Such a rapid and extensive rise of cyclic AMP production is consistent with the rapid saturation of the Leydig cell receptors at high gonadotropin concentrations, with immediate activation of adenylate cyclase. Most of the 'spare' receptors are probably coupled to adenylate cyclase, resulting in marked enhancement of cyclic AMP during more extensive receptor occupancy in the presence of high gonadotropin concentrations.

The period of delay between receptor binding and testosterone synthesis suggests that a complex series of metabolic events may occur before enhancement of steroidogenesis becomes apparent. The specific events which follow protein kinase activation in the Leydig cell have not been defined, but appear to depend upon RNA and protein synthesis. In the presence of Actinomycin D or cycloheximide, the effect of hCG upon steroid synthesis is abolished, while there is no significant change in cyclic AMP formation (Figure 24). The relationship of the synthesis of messenger RNA and protein to gonadotropin stimulation of testosterone synthesis in the Leydig cell is currently being investigated. In operating through an apparently obligatory effect upon transcription, the mechanism of action of gonadotropins may differ from that of ACTH upon the adrenal, in which the requirement for protein synthesis appears to be met by translation of existing mRNA molecules (31).

The high sensitivity of testis tissue and dispersed Leydig cells has been applied to the development of an in vitro bioassay for LH and hCG (32). Recently, the dispersed Leydig cell assay has been further improved in sensitivity by incubation in the presence of 0.1 mM MIX. Under these conditions, the production of testosterone by collagenase-dispersed Leydig cells in vitro gives a dose-response curve with added hCG over the range from 2 pg to 100 pg hCG. The corresponding sensitivity for human LH in terms of 2nd IRP-hMG is about 0.05 mU per vial, with working range up to

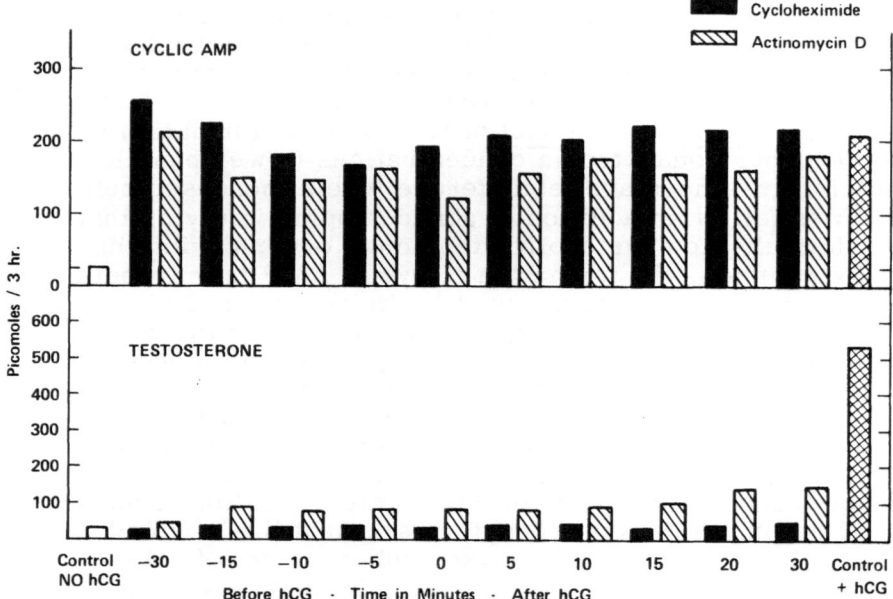

Figure 24.   Effects of cycloheximide (10 µg/ml) and actinomycin D (10 µg/ml) upon the production of cyclic AMP (above) and testosterone (below) by dispersed Leydig cells.   Incubations were performed in the presence of 10 ng hCG to induce maximum steroidogenesis. Addition of cycloheximide abolished the subsequent testosterone response, with no significant effect upon cyclic AMP formation.   Actinomycin D markedly reduced the testosterone response, and caused a small but consistent reduction in cyclic AMP formation.

about 4 mU per vial.   The precision of the assay is quite high, with index of precision (λ) of less than 0.04, and Finney's 'g' of 0.025. The high sensitivity of the <u>in vitro</u> bioassay permits determination of LH and hCG in unextracted plasma (31) and provides for the first time a method suitable for measurement of the biologically active circulating gonadotropin levels.

Acknowledgements

We are grateful to Dr. G. Hennen for providing purified porcine LH and subunits, and to Dr. H. Papkoff for providing highly purified ovine LH, subunits and chemically modified derivatives of ovine LH. The purified hCG employed for these studies was generously donated by Dr. R. Canfield.

References

1. Catt, K. J., Dufau, M. L. and Tsuruhara, T., J. Clin. Endocr. 32: 860, 1971.

2. Catt, K. J., Dufau, M. L. and Tsuruhara, T., J. Clin. Endocr. 34: 123, 1972.

3. Catt, K. J., Tsuruhara, T. and Dufau, M. L., Biochim. Biophys. Acta 279: 194, 1972.

4. Tsuruhara, T., Van Hall, E. V., Dufau, M. L., and Catt, K. J., Endocrinology 91: 463, 1972.

5. Catt, K. J., and Dufau, M. L., Adv. Expt. Med. Biol. 36: 379, 1973.

6. Lee, C. Y., and Ryan, R. J., Endocrinology 89: 1515, 1971.

7. Gospodarowicz, D., J. Biol. Chem. 248: 5042, 1973.

8. Danzo, B., Biochim. Biophys. Acta 304: 560, 1973.

9. Channing, C. P. and Kammerman, S., Biol. Reprod. 10: 179, 1974.

10. Dufau, M. L., Tsuruhara, T., and Catt, K. J., Biochim. Biophys. Acta 278: 281, 1972.

11. Dufau, M. L., Catt, K. J. and Tsuruhara, T., Proc. Nat. Acad. Sci. USA 69: 2414, 1972.

12. Midgley, A. R., In International Congress on Gonadotropins, Bangalore, India, 1973 (in press).

13. Ketelslegers, J-M., Knott, G., and Catt, K. J., This volume, p. 31.

14. deKretser, D. M,., Catt, K. J., and Paulsen, C. A., Endocrinology 88: 332, 1971.

15. Ashwell, G., and Morell, A. G., In Glycoproteins of Blood Cells and Plasma, Greenwalt, T. J. (ed.), Lippincott, Philadelphia, 1971, p. 173.

16. Dufau, M. L., Catt, K. J., and Tsuruhara, T., Biochim. Biophys. Acta 252: 574, 1971.

17. Kono, T., and Barham, T. W., J. Biol. Chem. 246: 6210, 1971.

18.   Cuatrecasas, P., J. Biol. Chem. <u>246</u>: 6532, 1971.

19.   Dufau, M. L., Catt, K. J., and Tsuruhara, T., Biochem. Biophys. Res. Comm. <u>44</u>: 1022, 1971.

20.   Tsuruhara, T., Dufau, M. L., Hickman, J., and Catt, K. J., Endocrinology <u>91</u>: 296, 1972.

21.   Catt, K. J., Dufau, M. L., and Tsuruhara, T., J. Clin. Endocr. <u>36</u>: 73, 1973.

22.   Dufau, M. L., Charreau, E., and Catt, K. J., J. Biol. Chem. <u>248</u>: 6973, 1973.

23.   Dufau, M. L., Ryan, D. and Catt, K. J., Biochim. Biophys. Acta, in press.

24.   Stephenson, R. P., Brit. J. Pharmacol. <u>11</u>: 379, 1956.

25.   Dufau, M. L., Watanabe, K., and Catt, K. J. Endocrinology <u>92</u>: 6, 1973.

26.   Dufau, M. L., Catt, K. J., Tsuruhara, T., Endocrinology <u>90</u>: 1032, 1972.

27.   Catt, K. J., Watanabe, K., and Dufau, M. L., Nature <u>239</u>: 280, 1972.

28.   Catt, K. J., and Dufau, M. L., Nature New Biol. <u>242</u>: 246, 1973.

29.   Eggena, P., Schwartz, I. L., and Walter, W., J. General Physiol. <u>56</u>: 250, 1971.

30.   Beall, R. J. and Sayers, G., Arch. Biochem. Biophys. <u>148</u>: 70, 1972.

31.   Garren, L. D., Gill, G. N., Masui, H., and Walton, G. M., Recent Progr. Hormone Res. <u>27</u>: 433, 1971.

32.   Dufau, M. L., Mendelson, C. and Catt, K. J., J. Clin. Endocr. Metab., in press.

COMPUTER ANALYSIS OF THE BINDING REACTION BETWEEN hCG AND GONADOTROPIN RECEPTORS OF THE RAT TESTIS

J. M. Ketelslegers, G. D. Knott and K. J. Catt

Section on Hormonal Regulation
National Institute of Child Health and Human Developmen

and

Division of Computer Research

National Institutes of Health
Bethesda, Maryland

The presence of specific high-affinity binding sites for luteinizng hormone (LH) and human chorionic gonadotropin (hCG) has been established in the Leydig cells of the rat testis (1-3). The binding of hCG to these receptors has been demonstrated to be a saturable process, and the velocity of binding shows marked temperature dependence (3). Analysis of gonadotropin binding data by Scatchard plots previously indicated the presence of a single class of binding sites (3). To define more accurately the association constant and the rate constants of this hormone-receptor interaction, more detailed equilibrium and kinetic experiments were performed, and the data analyzed with an interactive non-linear curve fitting program. This analytical system (MLAB) has been previously described (4, 5), and runs on a PDP-10 digital time-sharing computer. This approach has the advantage of permitting the use of complex models while performing simultaneous fits to multiple sets of data, without a significant increase in the complexity of the computation procedure. In particular, data expressing the total bound hormone and the non-specifically bound hormone as functions of the initial hormone concentration could be analyzed simultaneously, with computation of specific binding from the results of the simultaneous fitting process.

Experimental Procedures

Gonadotropin Preparations

Highly purified hCG with biological activity of 10,000-12,000 IU/mg as measured by the ventral prostate weight assay (6), steroidogenesis in the isolated rat testis (7) and radioligand-receptor assay (8) was obtained from Dr. Canfield. All calculations of hCG molar concentrations were corrected for the biological activity of the preparation (to the expected potency of 15,000 IU/mg for fully active hCG) and were based on a molecular weight of 38,000 (9,10).

Preparation of ^{125}I-hCG

Biologically active ^{125}I-hCG with specific activity of 10-25 μCi/μg as determined by radioimmunoassay (11) was prepared using a modification of the chloramine-T method as previously described (2,12), the labeled hormone being isolated by elution from Sepharose-concanavalin A (12). Various ratios of ^{125}I-hCG and unlabeled hCG were employed to obtain the required ranges of hormone concentration.

Rat Testis Homogenate Preparations

All experiments were performed with the 1500 g pellet from homogenates of the adult rat testis; this preparation has been previously shown to contain 80% of the binding activity present in the total homogenate (3). The pellets were resuspended in 10-50 ml of 0.01 M phosphate buffer containing 150 mM NaCl and 2.5 mM CaCl$_2$, pH 7.4 (PBS). The concentration of receptor sites in each preparation was determined by equilibrium binding studies performed at 24°.

Separation of Bound and Free Hormone

Receptor-bound and free hormone were separated by filtration of the incubation mixtures through 2.4 cm Whatman GF/C glass fiber filters after dilution of the 1 ml samples with 3 ml of ice-cold PBS containing 0.1% bovine gamma globulin. Each filter was then washed with 6 ml of PBS containing 0.1% of bovine serum albumin and the bound radioactivity determined in a Packard automatic gamma-spectrometer.

Equilibrium Experiments

Equilibrium studies were performed at 24° by incubation with continuous shaking (150 cycles/min) for 22 hours; in all experiments, 0.5 ml of testis homogenate was mixed with 0.5 ml of the tracer solutions containing increasing concentrations of ^{125}I-hCG. Non-specific binding was determined for each ^{125}I-hCG concentration, in the presence of an excess of unlabeled hCG (Pregnyl-Organon, 100 IU/ml).

Kinetic Experiments

(a) Association experiments

Equal volumes of the testis homogenate and hCG solutions were mixed and incubated at 24° or 37°, with continuous shaking (150 cycles/min) as individual aliquots of 1 ml or as bulk suspensions of 40 ml. At successive time intervals, 1 ml samples were withdrawn and filtered; non-specific binding was determined for each point, in the presence of an excess of unlabeled hCG.

(b) Dissociation experiments

The dissociation rate of ^{125}I-hCG bound to the receptors was studied after an excess of unlabeled hCG (Pregnyl-Organon, 100 IU/ml) was added to the incubation mixture.

Mathematical Models

The hormone-receptor interaction was treated as a simple reversible bi-molecular reaction

$$P \; + \; Q \; \underset{k_2}{\overset{k_1}{\rightleftarrows}} \; B$$

where
P = concentration of free hCG
Q = concentration of free receptor
B = concentration of hormone-receptor complex
k_1 = association rate constant (M^{-1} min^{-1})
k_2 = dissociation rate constant (min^{-1})

   The kinetics of this reaction are expressed by the second-order chemical kinetic differential equation:

$$dB(t)/dt = k_1 P(t)Q(t) - k_2 B(t); \quad B(0) = B_0 \qquad (1)$$

where,
t   = time (minutes)
$B(t)$ = concentration of hormone-receptor complex at time t
$P(t)$ = concentration of free hCG at time t
$Q(t)$ = concentration of free receptor at time t
$B(0)$ = amount of hormone-receptor complex at time 0.

   In the case of an association experiment, $B_0 = 0$. In the case of a dissociation experiment, in which the association of ^{125}I-hCG is stopped by the addition of an "infinitely" large excess of unlabeled hCG, $k_1 = 0$, and B_0 is the concentration of hormone-receptor complex mesured at the moment when the association process is interrupted. In this latter form, the function expresses a first-order kinetic process.

   When no hormone or receptor degradation occurs, $P(t)$ and $Q(t)$ of (1) can respectively be expressed as follows:

$$P(t) = P_0 - B(t)$$
$$Q(t) = Q_0 - B(t)$$

where
P_0 = initial concentration of free hCG
Q_0 = initial concentration of free binding sites.

   $P(t)$ and $Q(t)$ can also be defined by more complex expressions, including terms for hormone and receptor degradation. These models, to be described in a more detailed study (19), have enabled us to establish that degradation of the free hormone and free receptor at 24° has little significant effect on the determination of k_1 from the association experiments.

   In the present paper, the reported values for k_1 were determined from association experiments by curve fitting, using equation (1) as model, without modifications for hormone or receptor degradation; the k_2 parameter was held constant at a value determined independently from dissociation experiments.

   Equilibrium can be defined as the state at which the rate of change of the hormone-receptor complex concentration equals zero, i.e., $dB(t)/dt = 0$.

Equation (1) then becomes:

$$k_1(P_0 - B(t_e))(Q_0 - B(t_e)) - k_2 B(t_e) = 0 \qquad (2)$$

where t_e is the time required to reach equilibrium, and $B(t_e)$ the concentration of hormone-receptor complex at equilibrium.

Solving (2) for $B(t_e)$, the function (3) is obtained

$$B(t_e) = 0.5[(P_0 + Q_0 + 1/K_a) - \sqrt{(P_0 + Q_0 + 1/K_a)^2 - 4P_0 Q_0}] \qquad (3)$$

where

$$K_a = k_1/k_2 \qquad (M^{-1})$$

Experimental evidence, derived during saturation studies performed by adding increasing amounts of labeled hormone to a fixed quantity of receptors, has demonstrated that the non-specifically bound radioactivity is linearly related to the total radioactivity. This is expressed by

$$B_{ns} = A P_0 + I \qquad (4)$$

where

B_{ns} = concentration of non-specifically bound ^{125}I-hCG
A = slope of the line expressing B_{ns} as a function of P_0
I = intercept of this line, representing the value of the counter background if this is not subtracted from the experimental data points.

For a given experiment, the total bound ^{125}I-hCG can be expressed by the sum of (3) and (4).

$$B_t = B_s + B_{ns} \qquad (5)$$

where
B_t = concentration of total bound ^{125}I-hCG as a function of P_0
B_s = concentration of specifically bound ^{125}I-hCG as defined in (3)
B_{ns} = concentration of non-specifically bound ^{125}I-hCG as defined in (4)

In the present study, the values of Q_0, K_a, and A were determined by fitting simultaneously the data expressing the total and non-specifically bound ^{125}I-hCG at equilibrium as functions of P_0 respectively to (5) and (4).

BOUND HCG (PICOMOLES/LITER)

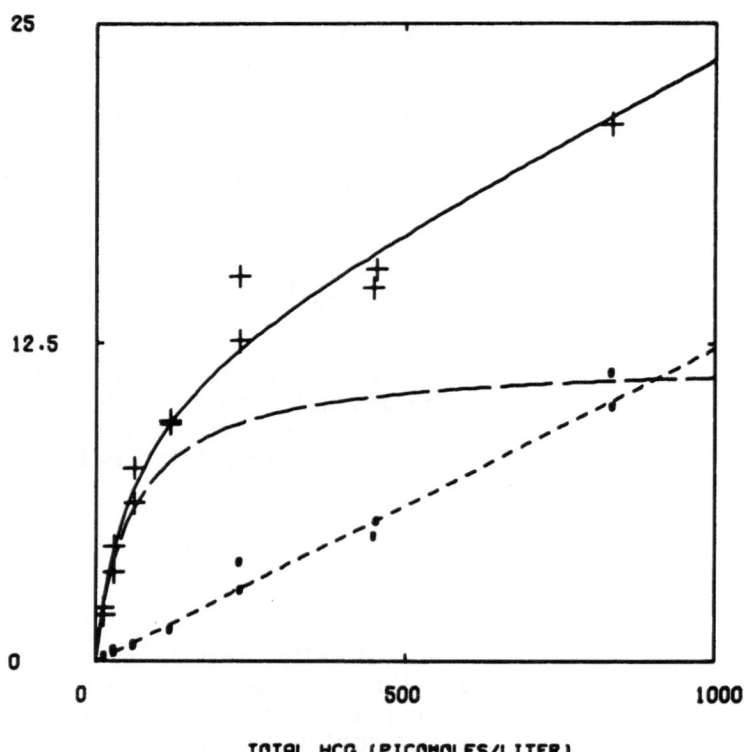

TOTAL HCG (PICOMOLES/LITER)

Figure 1. Saturation curve obtained by adding increasing amounts of ^{125}I-hCG to constant aliquots of testis homogenate, equivalent to one-fortieth of a testis. Total bound (+——+) and non-specifically bound (o---o) hCG were simultaneously analyzed by curve-fitting as described in Mathematical Models. The solid and dotted lines represent the best fits of equation (5) with the total bound hormone concentration and of equation (4) with the non-specifically bound hormone, both measurements being expressed as a function of the total hormone concentration. The dashed line (- - -) is the theoretical curve generated by using equation (3) as model, the values of K_a and Q_0 having been defined by fitting simultaneously the total and non-specifically bound hormone data as described; it represents the specifically bound ^{125}I-hCG as a function of the total hormone concentration.

Results

A saturation curve obtained by incubation of testis homogenate with increasing concentrations of ^{125}I-hCG is shown in Figure 1. The total bound and non-specific bound ^{125}I-hCG concentrations are plotted as functions of the total ^{125}I-hCG concentration. The theoretical curves obtained by simultaneous use of both equations (4) and (5) as the model for curve fitting, corresponded closely to the two sets of experimental data. The values of K_a and Q_0 so obtained were respectively 2.03×10^{10} M^{-1} and 1.15×10^{-11} M. Using these values in equation (3), the theoretical saturation curve could be computed; the specific binding of ^{125}I-hCG appeared to be a saturable process, while the non-specific binding was linearly related to the total hormone concentration over the entire range of concentrations used in the experiment. As shown in Figure 2, a Hill plot of the equilibrium

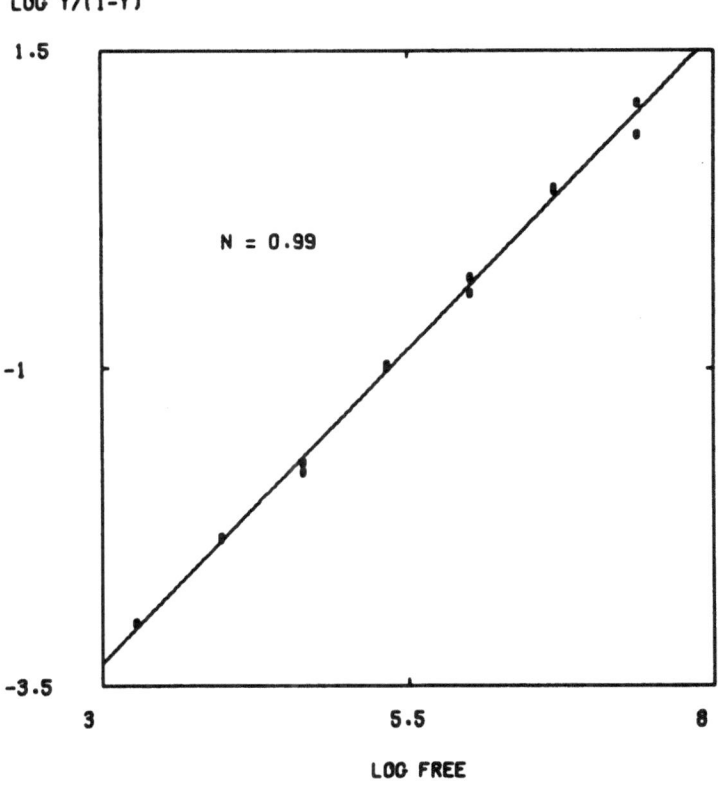

LOG Y/(1-Y)

N = 0.99

LOG FREE

Figure 2. Hill plot of equilibrium data. The fractional saturation, y, was calculated from the total sites, Q_0, determined as in Figure 1. A straight line was obtained; the Hill coefficient was 0.99 ± 0.02.

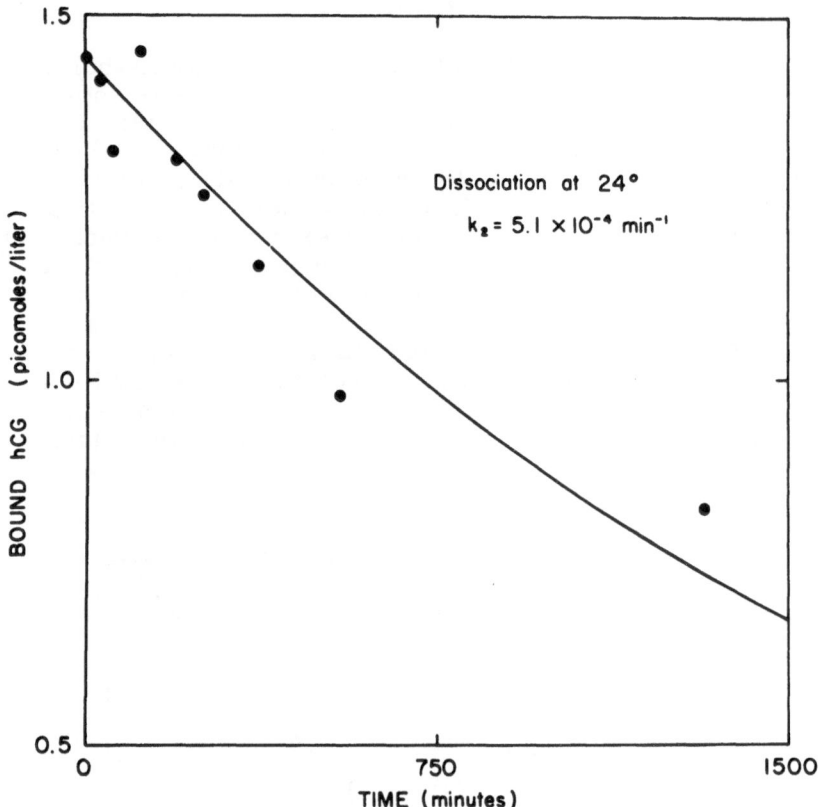

Figure 3. Time course of the dissociation of ^{125}I-hCG from its binding sites at 24°. The solid line represents the theoretical curve obtained by using equation (1) as model. The value of zero was assigned to k_1, and k_2 was adjusted by the curve-fitting process to the value giving the best fit of the model with the experimental data.

data gives a straight line with slope of 0.99 ± 0.02.

At 24°, the dissociation rate of hCG from its binding sites was observed to follow a single exponential model, indicating first-order kinetics (Figure 3). The value of k_2 obtained from this data was 5.1×10^{-4} min^{-1}. At 37° the dissociation rate was significantly higher.

The time course of the binding of hCG to its receptors could be fitted completely, from zero time until arrival at equilibrium, by using as model the second-order chemical kinetic differential equation (Figure 4). As expected, the initial binding velocity and the time required to reach equilibrium were dependent on the

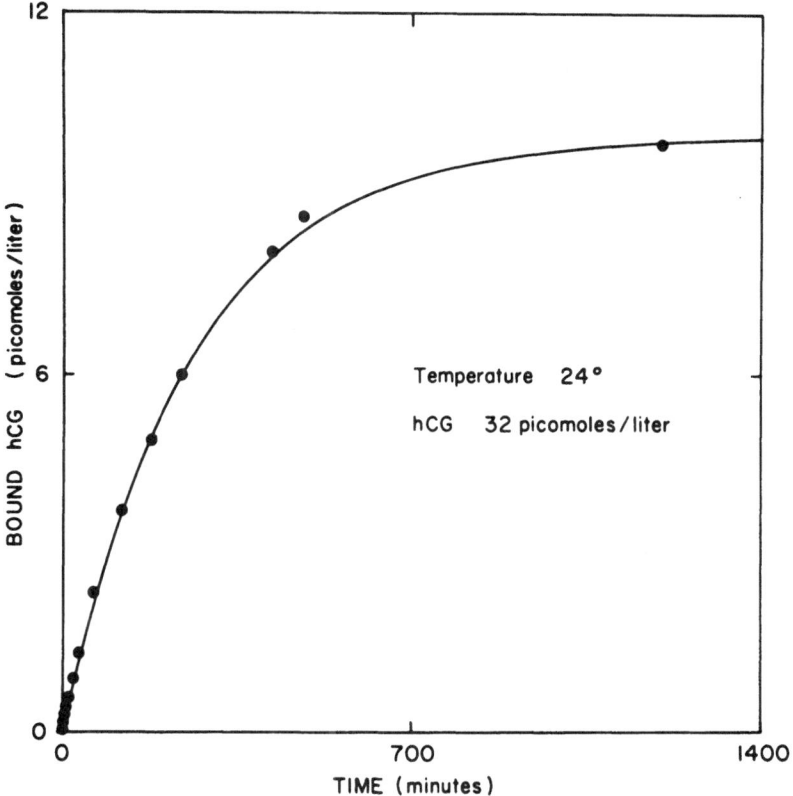

Figure 4. Time course of the association of ^{125}I-hCG with its receptors in the rat testis at 24°; the experiment was continued until equilibrium was reached. The binding capacity of the testis homogenate was 40 picomoles/liter. The solid line represents the best fit of the data with the differential equation for second-order chemical kinetics (1).

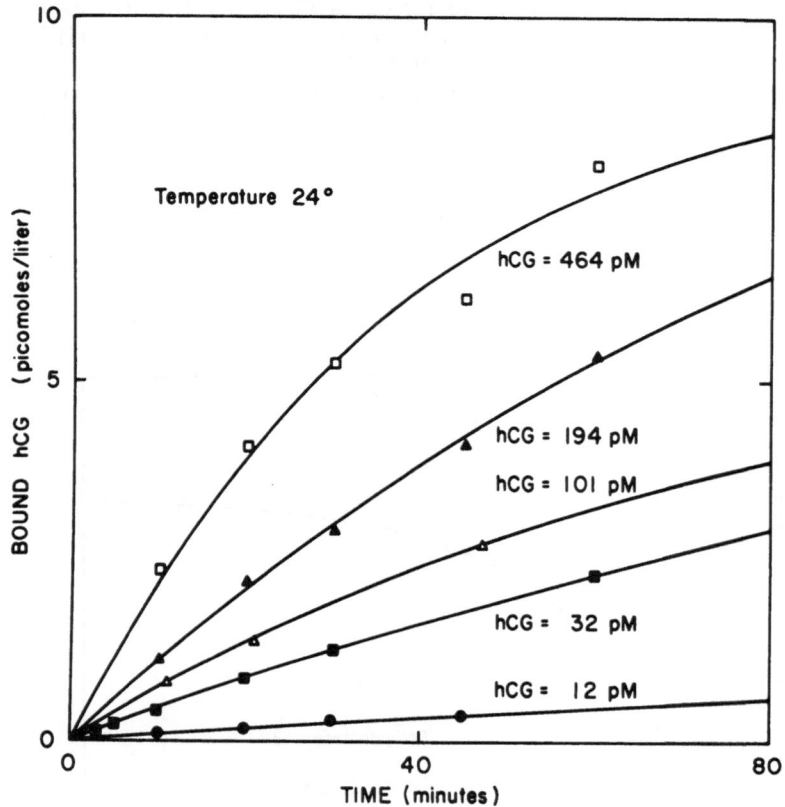

Figure 5. Effect of the initial hCG concentration on the binding velocity of the hormone with its receptors in the rat testis, at 24°. The binding capacities of the different incubation mixtures were respectively 20 picomoles/liter (●—●, △—△), 22 picomoles/liter (▲—▲, □—□) and 41 picomoles per liter (■—■). The solid lines represent the best fits of the data with the second-order chemical kinetics differential equation (1).

hormone concentration in the medium (Figure 5), and the initial binding velocities were higher at 37° than at 24°.

Table 1 summarizes the values of k_1 determined by curve fitting from association experiments performed at 24°. The mean of nine independent determinations was 3.11 + 0.31 (SE) x 10^7 M^{-1} min⁻¹. Over a wide range of hCG and binding site concentrations, there was no significant relation between

Table 1

Values of k_1 Derived from Association Data at

24ºC. $k_2 = 5.1 \times 10^{-4}$ min^{-1}

Concentration of hCG	Concentration of binding sites	k_1
(M · 10^{-12})	(M · 10^{-12})	(10^7·M^{-1}·min^{-1})
2	20	3.78
12	20	3.25
20	4	4.38
32	41	3.22
34	15	1.86
98	4	4.14
101	20	3.24
194	22	2.43
464	22	1.72
MEAN ± SE		3.11 ± 0.31

the estimates of k_1 and the individual reactant concentrations. That is, the value derived from the association rate constant was independent of the concentrations of hormone and receptor. Similar observations were obtained at 37°; at that temperature, the mean value for k_1 was 5.51 ± 0.14 (SE) $\times 10^7$ M^{-1} min^{-1}.

Discussion

The use of an interactive non-linear curve fitting program, with differential equation solving abilities and a convenient communication language, has enabled us to perform an accurate and precise analysis of the interaction of hCG with specific gonadotropin receptors in the rat testis. The results of the analysis of kinetic and equilibrium data have demonstrated that the interaction of hCG with its binding sites is consistent with a single reversible bimolecular reaction.

In most of the usual expressions employed to analyze equilibrium binding data, the specifically bound hormone concentrations are related to the free hormone concentrations.

This is the case in the Michaelis-Menten and the Scatchard (13) expressions. In most experimental binding systems, the free hormone concentrations are not directly measured, but derived by subtracting the bound from the total hormone concentrations over the range of experimental data points. This practice cumulates the errors of measurement of both the bound and the total hormone concentrations. The total hormone concentration can be measured independently and with high precision, in contrast to the inherently greater error which accompanies computation of the free hormone concentration. Therefore, we have derived from the second-order chemical kinetics equation, the relation between the concentrations of hormone-receptor complex at equilibrium and the total concentration of hormone. Based on that equation, a model was developed for determination of the equilibrium constant and the binding capacity of a receptor preparation by simultaneous curve fitting to the two sets of data obtained when increasing amounts of ^{125}I-hCG are added to a fixed amount of receptor preparation: the total bound and the non-specifically bound hormone expressed as functions of the total hormone concentration. Analysis of our equilibrium binding studies with this model confirmed the apparent homogeneity of the binding sites for hCG in the adult rat testis, and gave values of K_a which were closely related to those obtained by kinetic experiments.

Direct dissociation experiments showed that the dissociation process was consistent with first-order kinetics. Moreover, a good fit of the experimental association data with the theoretical curves calculated using the second-order chemical kinetics differential equation was obtained over a wide range of hormone and receptor concentrations. There was no systematic relationship between k_1 and these parameters. Such relative independence of k_1 from the reactant concentrations is an essential criterion for the validity of the application of the second-order kinetic models. Both k_1 and k_2 were higher at 37° than at 24°, confirming the temperature dependency of the interaction between hCG and its receptors (3).

The value of k_1 derived from our data at 24° is approximately 5 times lower than the association rate constant reported for the binding of ovine LH to plasma membranes of the bovine corpus luteum at 23° (14) and about 10 times lower than the value reported for the binding of hCG at 25° to a 2000 g subcellular fraction of pseudopregnant rat ovaries (15). Also, the slow dissociation rate of the hormone-receptor complex in the rat testis contrasts with the rapid dissociation of ovine LH from bovine corpus luteum plasma membranes. However, the dissociation process of hCG from rat ovaries was observed to be biphasic (15), with a slow component of the same order of magnitude as the dissociation rate of hCG from the rat testis receptor.

Differences in the nature of the particulate receptor preparations, the methods used to label the hormones, the stability
of the labeled hormones, and the nature of the gonadotropins used
as tracer, could account for discrepancies between the values
observed by different laboratories. In addition, the intrinsic
rate constants of gonadotropin receptors in the testis and ovary
may not be identical, though there is no significant difference in
the equilibrium association constants of testis and ovarian receptors as determined by binding studies with labeled hCG (16, 17).

For optimal determination of the binding constants of gonadotropin and other hormone-receptor interactions, it is essential
that the labeled peptides be carefully characterized in terms of
specific activity and retention of biological activity. Because
gonadotropins employed for iodination are not usually of maximum
attainable biological activity, the labeled preparations commonly
contain a proportion of inactive molecules, for which correction
must be made during calculation of binding constants. This
factor can be evaluated by determining the proportion of labeled
hormone which can be bound by incubation with an excess of receptor sites (18). Thus, if only 60% of the tracer can be bound by
excess receptors, then 40% of the total radioactivity will be present as inactive tracer in the free fraction, which should be
corrected accordingly. This method has proven to be of value
during more extensive studies on LH and hCG binding to gonadal
receptors (19). However, such procedures require individual
validation before application to other labeled gonadotropins, since
exposure of certain peptides to high concentrations of cell membranes or homogenates may cause significant hormone degradation. This would result in a falsely low value for the content of
biologically active hormone present in the labeled preparation.

Determination of specific activity of labeled tracer hormone
should be performed by quantitation in terms of the unlabeled
gonadotropin in a suitable assay system. Measurements of
tracer mass, by self-displacement in a radioimmunoassay or
radioligand-receptor assay, are minimum requirements if the
binding data is to be employed for calculation of valid kinetic
and equilibrium constants. In vivo bioassay of labeled gonadotropin by conventional methods has been described (16), but
is much more conveniently performed in vitro by sensitive bioassays which employ the steroidogenic response of dispersed
testis or ovarian target cells. The application of these correction factors to ^{125}I-hCG binding data has a significant but
relatively small effect upon the derivation of gonadotropin binding constants, as will be described in more detail elsewhere
(19). The useful effects of such procedures are most evident
during computation of binding data derived from saturation
experiments based upon the use of varying ratios of labeled and
unlabeled gonadotropins.

References

1. DeKretser, D. M., Catt, K. J., Burger, H. G. and Smith, G. C., J. Endocr. 43: 105, 1969.

2. Catt, K. J., Dufau, M. L. and Tsuruhara, T., J. Clin. Endocr. 32: 860, 1971.

3. Catt, K. J., Tsuruhara, T., and Dufau, M. L., Biochim. Biophys. Acta 279: 194, 1972.

4. Knott, G. D. and Reece, D. K., in Proceedings of the ONLINE '72 International Conference, Vol. 1, pp. 497-526, Brunel University, England, Sept. 1972.

5. Knott, G. D. and Shrager, R. I., In Computer Graphics: Proceedings of the SIGGRAPH Computers in Medicine Symposium, Vol. 6, No. 4, pp. 138-141, ACM, SIGGRAPH Notices, Winter 1972.

6. MacArthur, J. W., Endocrinology 50: 304, 1952.

7. Dufau, M. L., Catt, K. J., and Tsuruhara, T., Biochim. Biophys. Acta 252: 574, 1971.

8. Catt, K. J., Dufau, M. L., and Tsuruhara, T., J. Clin. Endocr. 34: 123, 1972.

9   Bellisario, R., Carlsen, R. B. and Bahl, O. P., J. Biol. Chem. 248: 6796, 1973.

10. Carlsen, R. B., Bahl, O. P., and Swaminathan, N., J. Biol. Chem. 248: 6810, 1973.

11. Catt, K. J., Acta Endocrinol. (Kbh) 63, Suppl. 142: 222, 1969.

12. Dufau, M. L., Catt, K. J., and Tsuruhara, T., Proc. Natl. Acad. Sci. USA, 69: 2414, 1972.

13. Scatchard, G., Ann. N. Y. Acad. Sci. 51: 660, 1949.

14. Gospodarowicz, D., J. Biol. Chem. 248: 5042, 1973.

15. Lee, C. Y., and Ryan, R. J., Biochemistry 12: 4609, 1973.

16. Tsuruhara, T., Van Hall, E. V., Dufau, M. L., and Catt, K. J., Endocrinology 91: 463, 1972.

17. Dufau, M. L., Charreau, E. H., Ryan, D., and Catt, K. J., F.E.B.S. Letters 39: 149, 1974.

18. Midgley, A. R., In International Congress on Gonado-tropins, Bangalore, India, 1973 (in press).

19. Ketelslegers, J. M., Knott, G., and Catt, K. J., unpublished observations.

CHARACTERISTICS OF SOLUBLE GONADOTROPIN
RECEPTORS FOR LH AND HCG

Maria L. Dufau, E. Charreau, D. Ryan and K. J. Catt

Reproduction Research Branch
National Institute of Child Health and Human Development
National Institutes of Health
Bethesda, Maryland 20014

In order initiate studies on the molecular properties of the gonadotropin receptor sites for luteinizing hormone, subcellular fractions of testis and ovarian homogenates with specific binding affinity for LH and hCG have been treated with non-ionic detergents such as 'Triton X-100' and 'Lubrol' to obtain "solubilized" receptor preparations which are suitable for binding studies and physico-chemical characterization (1-3).

Extraction and Binding Studies

The gonadotropin receptors of rat testis and ovary were solubilized by detergent extraction of the 120-27,000 g binding fraction of fragmented interstitial cells, or ovarian homogenates prepared from the gonads of PMS/hCG treated immature female rats. The 27,000 g pellets were dispersed in 1% Triton X-100 for 30 minutes at 4°C, and the majority of the gonadotropin binding activity was recovered in the supernatant fraction of the detergent-extracted particles after centrifugation of the solubilized preparation at 360,000 g for 2 hours. Binding activity of the soluble receptor preparation was determined by equilibration with ^{125}I-hCG tracer (4) for 16 hours at 4°C. Separation of bound and free tracer hormone was performed by a double precipitation of the bound complex with polyethylene glycol (1), followed by counting of the bound radioactivity in an automatic gamma spectrometer. The effect of increasing polyethylene glycol concentration upon precipitation of the soluble receptor-hormone complex showed that optimal separation was obtained at 12%

47

polyethylene glycol, higher concentrations causing increasing
precipitation of the free hormone. By this method, specific
binding of up to 40% of the added ^{125}I-hCG tracer was demonstrable, and the non-specific radioactivity precipitated was less than
1% of the added tracer hormone (Figure 1).

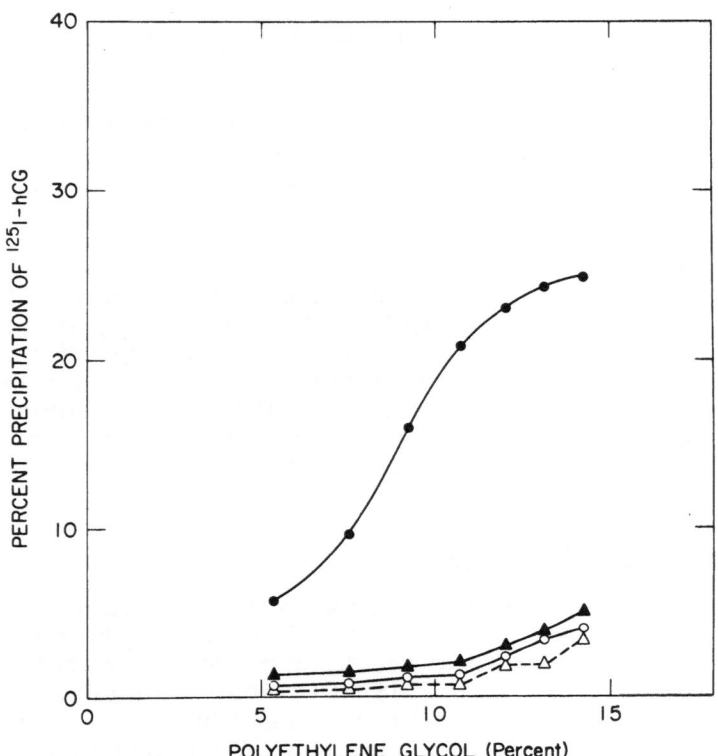

Figure 1. Separation of receptor-bound and free ^{125}I-hCG by
precipitation of the bound complex with increasing concentrations
of polyethylene glycol. In the presence of excess unlabelled hCG,
binding of ^{125}I-labelled hormone is reduced to the level of the
blank value observed in the absence of the soluble receptor.
●——●, soluble receptor, 0——0, soluble receptor + 10^{-7} M hCG,
▲——▲, reagent blank, △– – –△, reagent blank + 10^{-7} M hCG.

The effect of pH on equilibrium binding of hCG by the soluble
gonadotropin receptors was investigated over a wide range of pH
values (pH 5.6 to 9.4), and revealed that maximum binding was
attained at pH 7.4 upon incubation with ^{125}I-hCG for 16 hrs. at

4° C. The rate of binding of ^{125}I-hCG by soluble testis receptors at 4, 24 and 34° C was studied for various times up to 24 hours (Figure 2). The initial rate of association was more rapid at 24° C and 34° C than at 4° C, whereas maximum binding was much higher at 24° C and 4° C due to inhibition of receptor degradation as shown by preincubation studies at three temperatures.

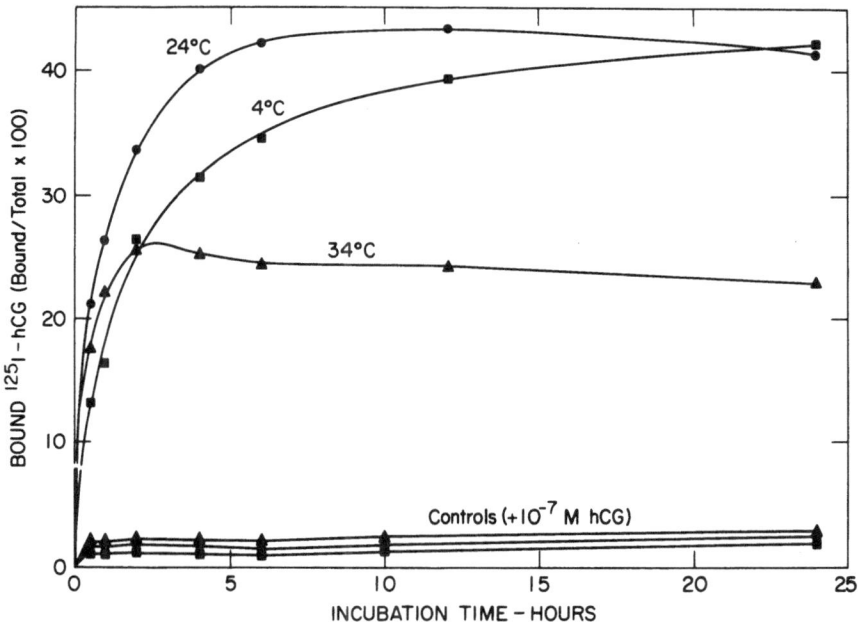

Figure 2. Time course of association of ^{125}I-hCG with soluble gonadotropin receptors during incubation at 4, 24 and 34° C for 24 hours. Nonspecific control levels for each time interval were determined by addition of 100 I.U. (10^{-7} M) of hCG.

The association data were consistent with a second-order reaction, with association rate constant of 6.1×10^5 M^{-1} min^{-1} at 4° C. Dissociation of the hormone receptor complex at pH 7.4 was extremely slow, with first order dissociation rate constant of 0.5×10^{10} min^{-1} at 4° C. The slow dissociation of the complex at low temperature facilitated fractionation and physico-chemical studies of the hormone receptor-complex (5).

Equilibrium binding of ^{125}I-hCG by the soluble testis receptors after incubation for 16 hr. at 4, 24 and 34° C showed progressive binding-inhibition in the presence of increasing

concentrations (1-100 ng) of unlabelled hCG. Other pituitary
hormones (FSH, TSH, GH, and Prolactin) caused no inhibition of
^{125}I-hCG binding. Scatchard plots of such ^{125}I-hCG binding
studies with solubilized testis receptors revealed a single order
of binding sites, with equilibrium association constant of 0.5-1
x 10^{10} M^{-1} at 4°C and 24°C, and 0.4 x 10^{10} M^{-1} at 34°C (Fig. 3).

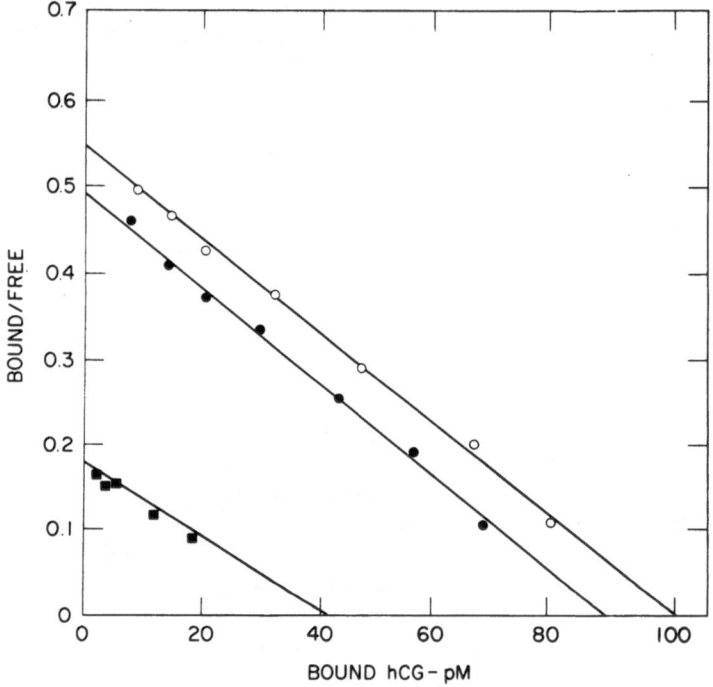

Figure 3. Scatchard plots of receptor-hCG binding studies at
different temperatures. Similar binding affinities were obtained
at the three temperatures, O———O, 4°C Ka = 0.53 x 10^{10} M^{-1} ;
●———● 24°C Ka = 0.56 x 10^{10} M^{-1} ;■———■34°C Ka = 0.4 x 10^{10}
M^{-1} . However, significant reduction in binding capacity of
soluble receptor sites was observed at 34°C.

The binding capacity of the soluble receptor preparation was
significantly reduced when incubations were performed at 34°C.
Scatchard plots of hCG binding studies with solubilized ovarian
receptors at 4°C have shown binding affinity and binding capacity
similar to those observed with the soluble testis receptor (Ka
0.5 x 10^{10} M^{-1}, binding capacity 0.10 to 0.50 x 10^{-12} mol/mg
protein) (3).

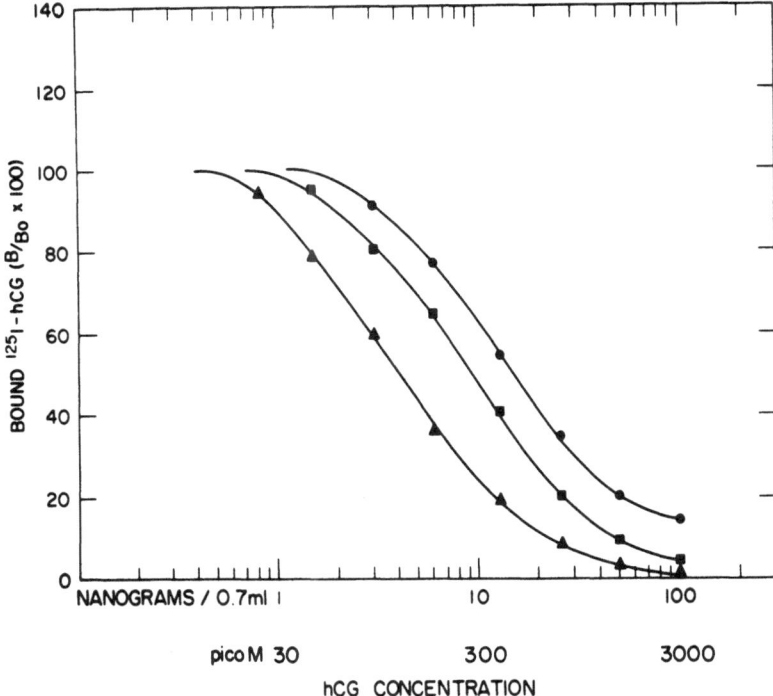

Figure 4. Comparison of ^{125}I-hCG binding-inhibition curves obtained with soluble receptors (●————●), 27,000 g interstitial cell fragments (▲————▲) and 1500 g rat testis homogenate (■————■).

Binding-inhibition curves obtained with the soluble receptor were similar to those observed during incubation of ^{125}I-hCG with rat testicular homogenate, and with the interstitial cell fraction from which the soluble receptor was extracted by treatment with Triton X-100 (Fig. 4). The association constant of the soluble receptor was 3 to 5 times lower than that of the parent particulate preparation, and the binding capacity was also reduced (Table 1).

When the soluble free receptor preparation was allowed to age, either by standing at 4° C for 16 hours or by dialysis against buffer containing 0.1% Triton, subsequent binding studies gave Scatchard plots which showed two sets of binding sites. The major site was of similar affinity to that observed in the freshly-prepared soluble receptors, with $Ka = 0.6 \times 10^{10}$ M^{-1}. However, a marked reduction of total binding sites has occurred at this

Table 1

Association Constant (Ka) and Binding Capacity
of Particulate and Soluble Testis Binding Fractions
for hCG at 24°C

Testis fraction	Ka	Binding Capacity
Testis homogenate (1,500 g sediment)	1.2×10^{10} M^{-1}	3.3×10^{-12} mol g^{-1}
Interstitial cell particles (27,000 g sediment)	1.2×10^{10} M^{-1}	0.4×10^{-12} mol mg^{-1} protein
Soluble receptor	0.56×10^{10} M^{-1}	0.13×10^{-12} mol mg^{-1} protein

time, revealing the presence of a small number of high affinity
receptor sites (Ka 3-4 x 10^{10} M^{-1}) with similar association constant to that found in the original particulate receptor preparation.
If aging of the preparation was extended for a further period of
time, the lower affinity site has completely disappeared, leaving
only a small quantity of the high-affinity sites. This was demonstrated by binding studies on a receptor preparation aged for
48 hrs at 4° C (Ka 3 x 10^{10} M^{-1}). The lability of the solubilized
receptor preparations during storage was much more marked
for the free receptors than for the hormone-receptor complex.
With further purification of the free receptors, these also were
found to be relatively stable when kept at 0-4° C.

Physical Properties of Soluble Gonadotropin Receptors

Gel Filtration and Density Gradient Centrifugation

A. Receptors extracted from testis particles with Triton X-100
and subsequently equilibrated with ^{125}I-hCG particles

The elution profile obtained by gel filtration of the ^{125}I-hCG
receptor complex on Sephadex G-200 in 0.1% Triton showed a
prominent peak of radioactivity coincident with the void volume
indicated by blue Dextran, and also a retarded peak of free hCG
with Kav of 0.33. The elution pattern obtained with gel filtration
on Sepharose 6B also exhibited a major radioavtive component
which was coincident with the front peak of blue Dextran, and a
peak of free hCG with Kav = 0.56 (Fig. 5). These results suggested that the receptor-hormone complex was absorbed to the

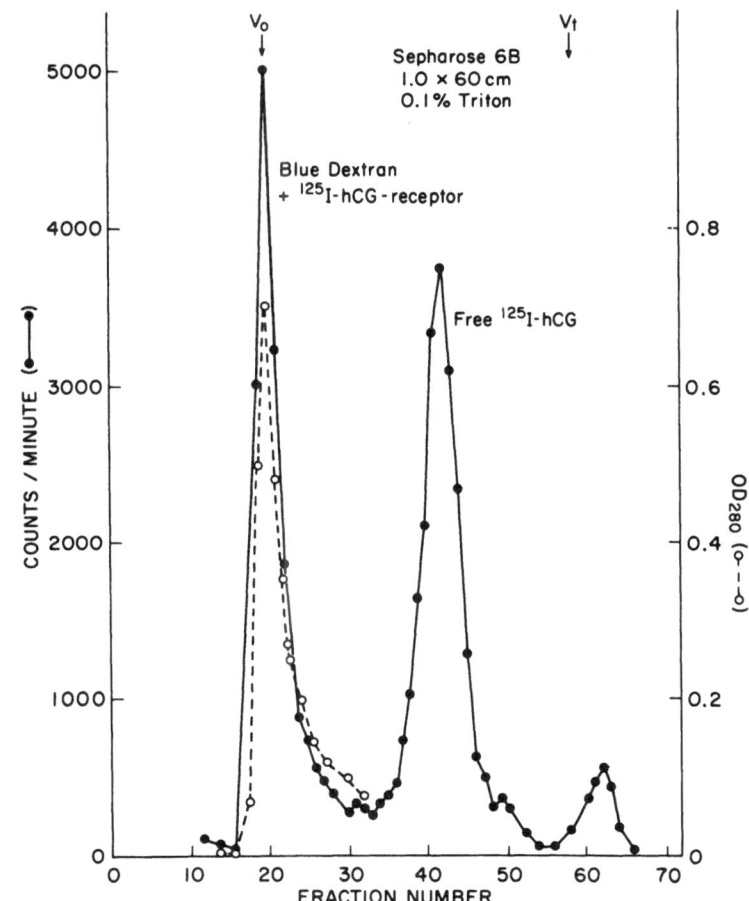

Figure 5. Gel filtration of ^{125}I-hCG-receptor equilibration mixture on Sepharose 6B. A major radioactive peak of hormone-receptor complex was eluted coincident with the void volume shown by the Blue Dextran marker, and the free hormone was eluted with Kav 0.56.

front marker of blue Dextran during gel filtration, and this phenomenon was confirmed by gel filtration performed in the absence of blue Dextran. A similar effect has been observed with certain other proteins, including pyruvate kinase, blood coagulation factors, and erythrocyte glutathione reductase (6, 7).

Dissociation of the hormone-receptor complex and free receptor from blue Dextran could be achieved by passing the blue Dextran-receptor complex through a small column of DEAE-Sephadex A-50 previously equilibrated with 5% ammonium sulfate in 0.1 M phosphate buffer. Elution of the receptor from the column was performed with the same buffer, the blue Dextran remaining adsorbed to the column. The association between protein ligands and blue Dextran is believed to depend upon ionic interaction with the negatively charged chromophore. If such a mechanism is also operative in the association of blue Dextran with testicular and ovarian receptors, it would suggest the presence of a net positive charge on the receptor molecule at pH 7.4.

The elution profile of ^{125}I-hCG receptor complex during gel filtration on Sephadex G-200 in the absence of blue Dextran showed that the hormone-receptor complex was eluted as a broad peak immediately behind the void volume. This peak could be abolished by preceding incubation with excess unlabeled hCG; also, the radioactivity in fractions from the hormone-receptor peak were 80 to 98% precipitable with polyethylene glycol.

Resolution of equilibrium mixtures of the hormone-receptor complex and free ^{125}I-hCG was performed by gel filtration on a calibrated Sepharose 6B column equilibrated with 0.1% Triton in 50 mM Tris-HCl buffer, in the absence of blue Dextran. A small radioactive front peak of aggregated material at the void volume was followed by two closely adjacent peaks of receptor-bound hormone and free hCG. The receptor-hormone complex appeared as a shoulder on the larger peak of free hCG (Fig. 6), above). When fractions corresponding to the hCG-receptor peak were pooled and concentrated, refiltration on Sepharose 6B showed two clearly defined peaks, the hCG-receptor complex with Kav of 0.32, and free hCG with Kav of 0.56 (Fig. 6, below). By comparison of the Kav of the testicular receptor-hormone complex with reference proteins by the method of Laurent and Killander (8), the hydrodynamic radius of the complex was estimated to be 64 A (Fig. 7). By similar methods, the Stokes' radius of the ovarian receptor-hormone complex was found to be 60A, and was not significantly different from that of the testicular complex (3).

When the receptor-hormone mixture was subjected to density gradient centrifugation in 5-20% sucrose for 16 hrs. at 100,000 g, two discrete radioactive components were resolved, one peak at 2.9S corresponding to free hCG, and the hormone-receptor complex at 7.5S (Figures 8 and 9). The 7.5S peak was 98% precipitable by polyethylene glycol and could be completely abolished by preincubation in the presence of excess hCG. A similar sedimentation pattern was obtained with the soluble ovarian hormone-receptor peak, with free hCG (2.9S and a 7.5S

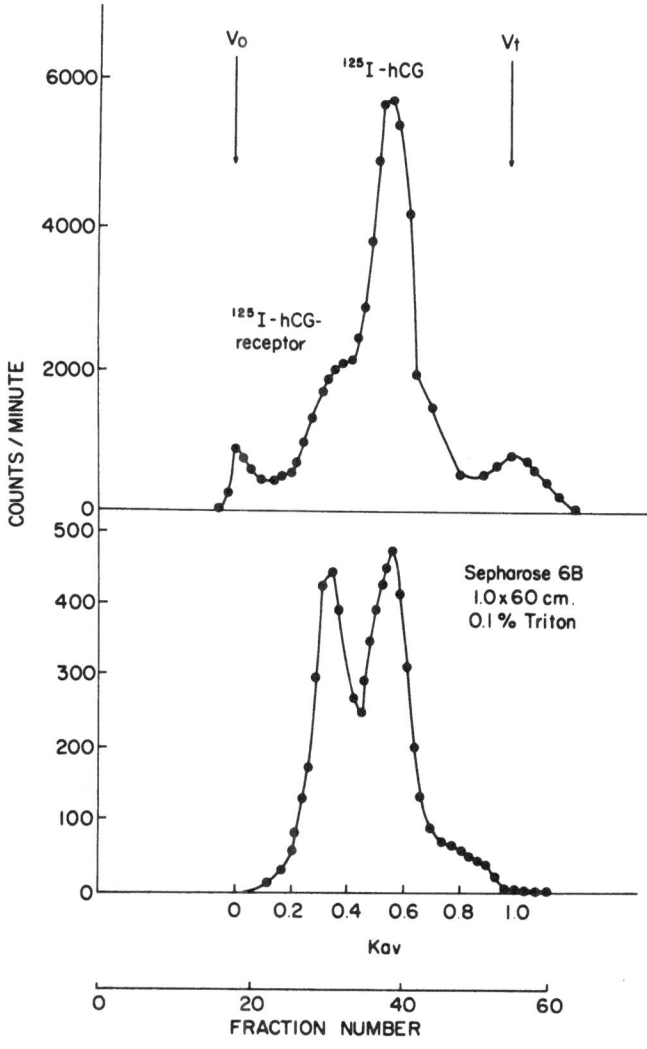

Figure 6. (Above) Elution profile of hCG-receptor complex during gel filtration on Sepharose 6B, in the absence of Blue Dextran. A small peak of radioactivity was present at the void volume, coincident with a minor and a constant peak of aggregated protein. The hCG-receptor complex was eluted as a shoulder preceding the major peak of free hCG. (Below) Fractions corresponding to the hCG-receptor peak were pooled and concentrated five-fold with Sephadex G-25. An aliquot containing 6000 cpm was then subjected to further gel filtration on Sepharose 6B. The elution profile shows two clearly separated radioactive peaks corresponding to free hCG and the hormone-receptor complex.

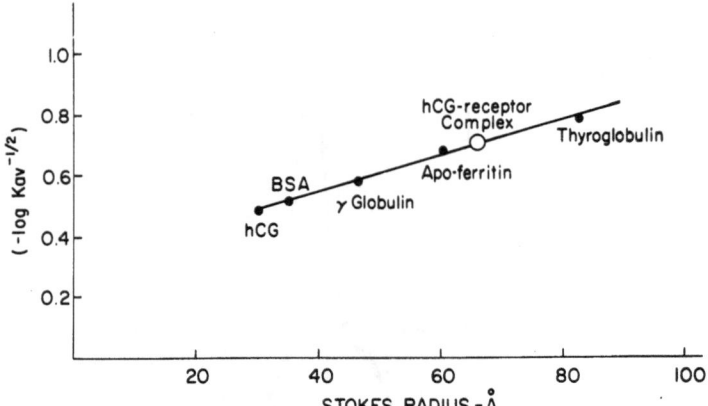

Figure 7. Stokes radius of Triton solubilized ^{125}I-hCG-receptor complex calculated from gel filtration experiments. The ^{14}C and ^{3}H acetylated standard proteins gave linear calibration plots according to the method of Laurent and Killander (8).

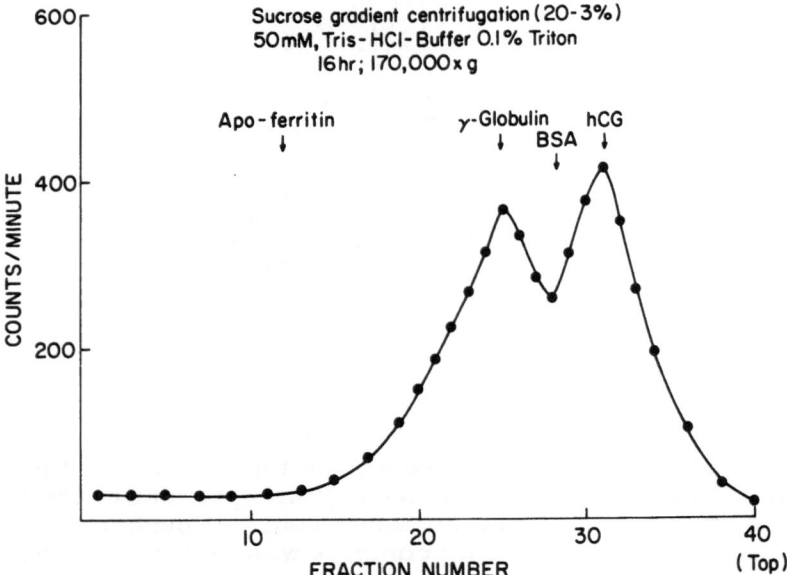

Figure 8. Sucrose density gradient centrifugation of the hormone-receptor complex previously fractionated on Sepharose 6B (Fig. 7, above). Two discrete peaks of radio-activity were resolved, corresponding to free hCG (2.9s) and the hormone receptor complex (7.5S), which was 98% precipitable by polyethylene glycol.

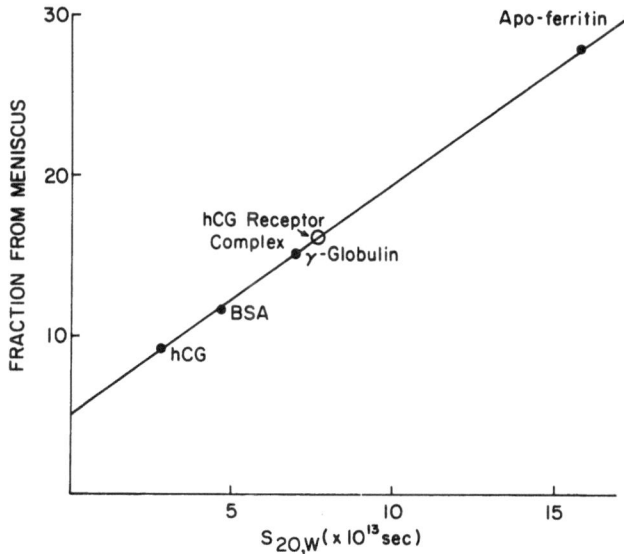

Figure 9. Sedimentation coefficient of gonadotropin receptor extracted from testis particles and subsequently equilibrated with labeled gonadotropin, as determined in 5-20% sucrose gradients. The results are averages of 3-5 experiments.

hormone-receptor complex (3). The density of the receptor-hormone complex obtained by centrifugation studies on 50% CsCl isopycnic gradients was found to be 1.289.

The elution pattern of 'free' or 'uncharged' gonadotropin receptor on Sepharose 6B was also determined. For such experiments, gel filtration was followed by binding assay of the column fractions. Aliquots were equilibrated with ^{125}I-hCG, and bound radioactivity was isolated by polyethylene glycol precipitation. The Kav of the free receptor was the same as that of the receptor-hormone complex, indicating a similar Stoke's radius for the free and combined form of the receptor (Fig. 10).

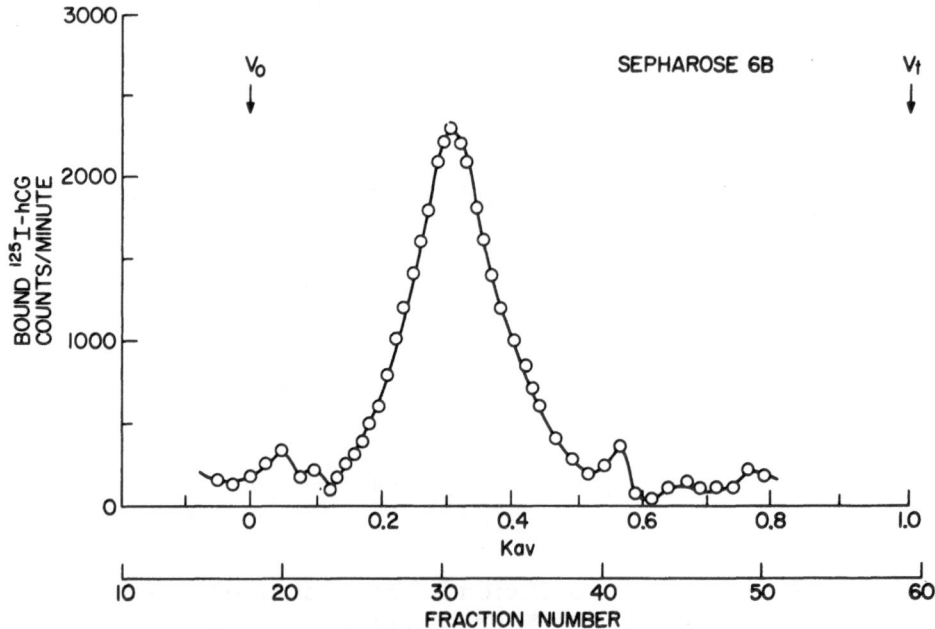

Figure 10. ^{125}I-hCG binding by gonadotropin receptor after gel filtration in 0.1% Triton. Gel filtration of free gonadotropin receptor on Sepharose 6B. After elution, 0.7 ml of each fraction was incubated with 15,000 cpm of ^{125}I-hCG in the presence or absence of 10^{-7} M hCG for 16 hours at 4° C, and the bound radioactivity isolated by polyethylene glycol precipitation. Non-specific values determined in tubes containing excess hCG were subtracted from the total precipitable radioactivity.

Density gradient centrifugation of the free receptor revealed a single peak of binding activity with sedimentation coefficient of 6.5S, which was significantly different (P < 0.02) from the 7.5S hormone-receptor complex (Fig. 11).

Combining the data from gel filtration and sucrose gradient centrifugation, as described by Siegel and Monty (9), the approximate molecular weights calculated for the free receptor and hormone-receptor complex were 194,000 and 224,000, respectively. The molecular weight of free hCG was also calculated by the same manner to be about 38,000. The difference between the free and combined forms of the receptor is consistent with binding of one molecule of gonadotropin by each receptor molecule.

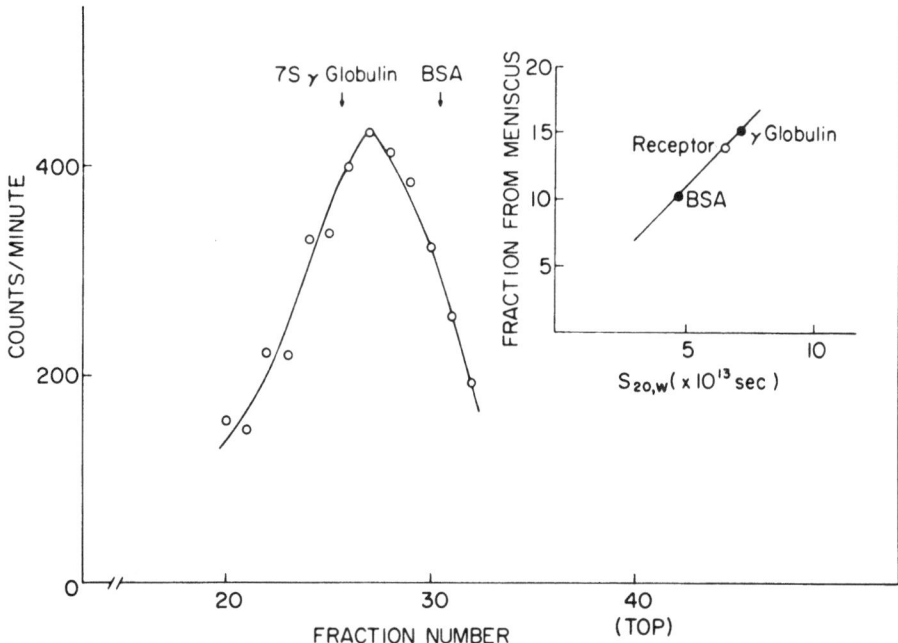

Figure 11. ^{125}I-hCG binding by gonadotropin receptor after sucrose gradient centrifugation (5-20% in 0.1% Triton). Sucrose gradient centrifugation of the soluble free gonadotropin receptors. After fractionation, 100 µl aliquots were incubated with 5000 cpm of ^{125}I-hCG in the presence or absence of 10^{-7} M hCG for 16 hours at 4° C, and the bound radioactivity was determined by precipitation with polyethylene glycol.

The frictional ratios of the receptor and the receptor-hormone complex were calculated to be 1.65 and 1.56, corresponding to the prolate axial ratios of 12.0 and 10.2. These values suggest that the solubilized forms of the gonadotropin receptor exist in solution as highly asymmetric molecules.

When the hormone-receptor complex (7.5S) and the free receptor (6.5S) were dialyzed against detergent-free buffer and subjected to gel filtration on Sepharose 6B, the elution profile of the dialyzed hormone-receptor complex showed three radioactive peaks. An early peak at the void volume was probably due to aggregated complexes. A further peak with Kav = 0.27 represented the hormone-receptor complex. This peak could be abolished by preincubation of the soluble receptor with excess unlabeled hCG, and was significantly different from the Triton forms of the free receptors (6.5S) and the hormone-receptor complex (7.5S). A third peak of free hCG with Kav

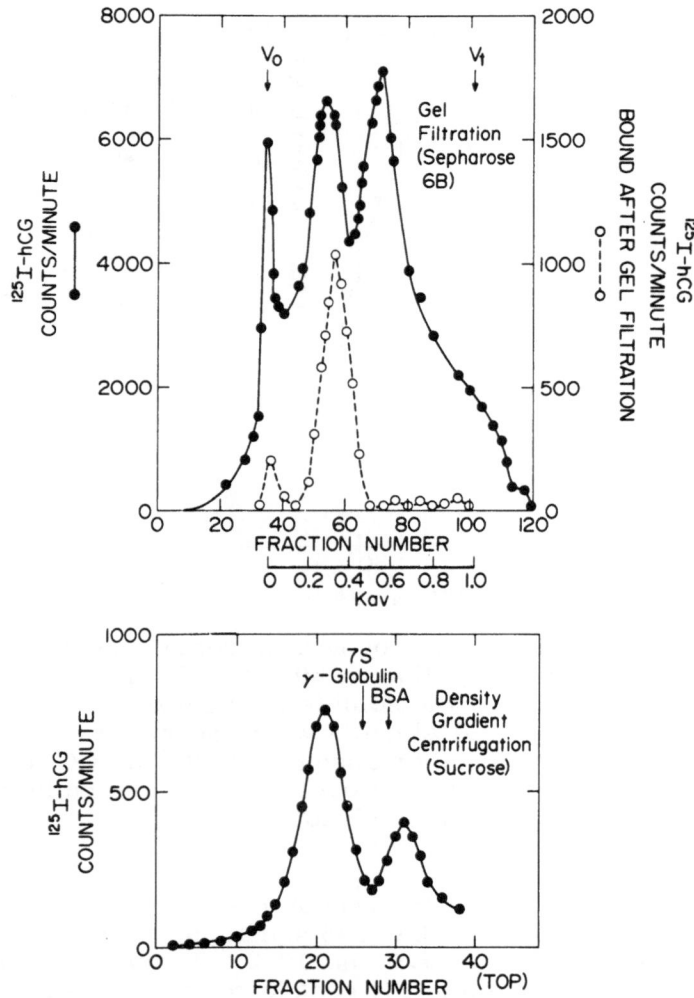

Figure 12. (Above) Elution profile of dialyzed, Triton-extracted free gonadotropin receptors extracted by Triton X-100 (o———o) and hCG-receptor complex (●———●) during gel filtration on Sepharose 6B. After elution of the free receptor, 0.7 ml of each fraction was incubated with 32,000 cpm of ^{125}I-hCG in the presence or absence of 10^{-7} M hCG for 16 hours at 4°, and the bound radioactivity was isolated by polyethylene glycol precipitation. Nonspecific values determined in tubes containing excess hCG were subtracted from the total precipitable radioactivity.

0.56 was also observed. The elution of the free dialyzed receptor was monitored by incubating the eluted fraction with [125]I-
hCG in the presence or absence of 10^{-7} M hCG, and determination
of bound radioactivity by PEG precipitation, giving a value of
0.27 for the Kav of the free receptor as well as for the dialyzed
form of the hormone-receptor complex (Fig. 12, above).

Fractions corresponding to the hCG-receptor peak were
pooled and concentrated, and an aliquot was then subjected to
density gradient centrifugation. Two discrete peaks were
resolved, corresponding to free hCG (2.9S) and the dialyzed
hormone-receptor complex. The latter exhibited a mean sedimentation coefficient coefficient of 8.8S + 0.30 (SD), and was
significantly different from the 7.5S Triton form of the hormone-
receptor complex (Fig. 12, below). The 8.8S form of hormone-
receptor complex obtained after dialysis was converted to the
original 7.5S form after re-equilibration with 0.1% Triton.

The increased sedimentation velocity of the dialyzed 7.5S
complex in sucrose density gradients could be due to removal
of a significant proportion of the bound detergent molecules,
with consequently increased density of the soluble complex.
Also, the markedly hydrophilic properties of the heavily
sialylated glycoprotein hormone molecule may contribute to
the maintenance of the soluble form of the extracted hormone-
receptor complex after dialysis against detergent-free solutions.

B. Extraction of prelabeled testis particles with non-ionic and
ionic detergent

The 200-27,000 g fraction of testis interstitial tissue or
ovarian homogenates was labeled by incubation with ^{125}I-hCG
(2-10 ng) for 16-24 hours at 4° C. The labeled particulate
binding sites remaining after washing to remove free hCG was
then extracted as a preformed complex, rather than as the
uncharged or free receptors described above. Extraction
of prelabeled particles with Triton X-100 gave a soluble hormone-
receptor complex which sedimented as an 8.8S species in sucrose
gradients. However, the elution of this complex during gel

(Below) Fractions corresponding to the hCG-receptor peak
(above) were pooled and concentrated with Sephadex G-25. An
aliquot containing 5000 cpm then was subjected to density gradient
centrifugation. Two discrete peaks of radioactivity were
resolved, corresponding to free hCG and the hormone-receptor
complex, which was 99% precipitable by polyethylene glycol.

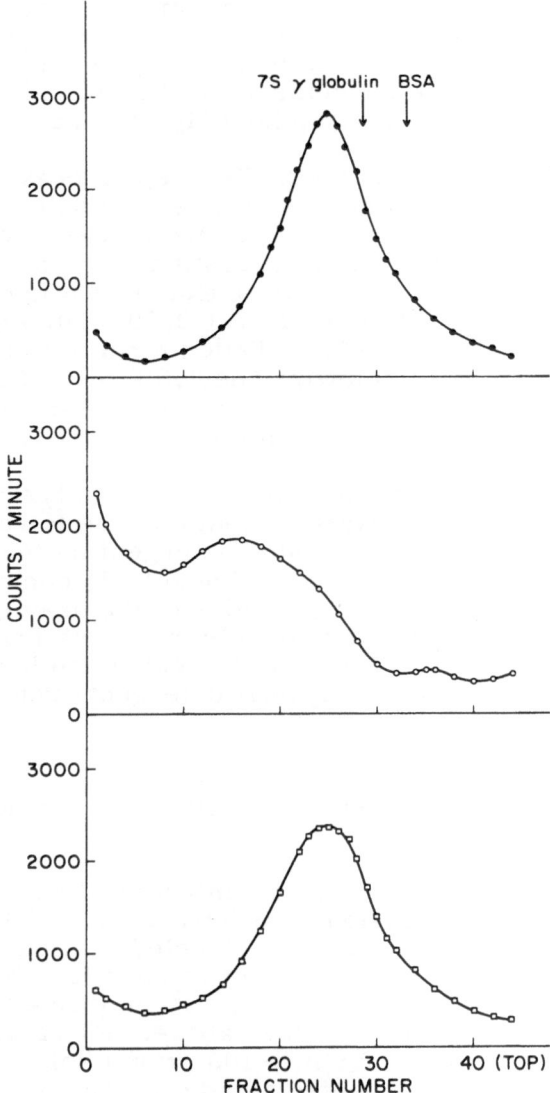

Figure 13. (Above) Sucrose gradient centrifugation of ^{125}I-hCG-receptor solubilized from prelabeled testis particles with Triton X-100, showing a single 8.8S peak of radioactivity. (Middle) Dialysis of the above preparation caused aggregation of the 8.8S complex, to more rapidly sedimenting forms. (Below) Effect of Triton X-100 on the aggregated receptor-hormone complex, with reversion to the 8.8S form.

filtration on Sepharose 6B was identical with that of the 7.5S and 6.5S forms, indicating a Stokes radius of 60-64 A (Fig. 13, top).

When the detergent concentration was reduced by dialysis, the preformed 8.8S hormone-receptor complex was converted to a broad and rapidly sedimenting peak. This pattern was consistent with the formation of aggregates, and such dialyzed preparations were eluted in the void volume on Sepharose 6B (Fig. 13, middle). Such aggregation was reversible upon addition of Triton X-100 to a concentration of 0.1%, which converted the rapidly-sedimenting complexes to the original 8.8S form (Fig. 13, lower). The increased sedimentation properties of the 8.8S receptor-hormone complex extracted from prelabeled testis particles is probably due to solubilization of a larger or less asymmetric species than that extracted from unlabeled particulate receptors.

Dissociation of the hormone-receptor complex was favoured by low pH and denaturing agents. Decreasing the pH to 3.5 for 1-5 minutes by addition of acetic acid immediately dissociated the hormone from the receptor sites. Subsequent reassociation in 0.1% Triton after neutralization to pH 7.4 gave the 7.5S form of the complex (Fig. 14). Exposure to 2M urea or guanidine HCl also caused complete dissociation of the hormone from receptor sites. No effects on dissociation of the receptor-hormone complex were observed after incubation with a variety of steroid hormones from the androsten, androstan, and pregnen series (including estradiol, testosterone, dihydrotestosterone progesterone at concentrations 10^{-7} M). In addition, cyclic AMP (5 mM), ATP (5 mM) and GTP (1 mM) were without effect on hormone binding and dissociation, and variations in medium calcium concentration from 0-3 mM caused no change in binding.

While solubilization of the prelabeled particles with Triton X-100 gave only the 8.8S form of the receptor, extraction with other detergents led to the formation of soluble hormone-receptor complexes other than the 8.8S form. For example, extraction with Lubrol PX (1%) gave a 7S form of the complex. Dialysis of this preparation caused the hormone-receptor complex to aggregate, and addition of Triton to 0.1% concentration reverted the aggregated complex to the 8.8S form. In addition, treatment of prelabeled testis particles with 1% Lubrol WX or 0.2% sodium deoxycholate gave 7S and 8.8-9S forms, respectively, of the hormone-receptor complex.

Gel filtration of the 7S complex extracted by Lubrol WX and Lubrol PX upon Sepharose 6B showed elution profiles with Kav of 0.26 and 0.32 corresponding to Stokes radii of 77A and 64A respectively. The density of the 7S Lubrol WX form determined

Table 2. Comparison of physico-chemical characteristics of Triton X-100 solubilized testicular and ovarian receptors

Parameter	Ovarian Receptors	Testicular Receptors
Association constant (Ka)	$0.66 \times 10^{10} M^{-1}$	$0.60 \times 10^{10} M^{-1}$
Binding capacity of initial extract	0.15×10^{-12} mole/mg protein	0.12×10^{-12} mole/mg protein
Partition coefficient (Kav) Stokes radius (A)		
Free receptor	0.36 (60A)	0.32 (64A)
hCG-receptor complex formed after extraction	0.36 (60A)	0.32 (64A)
hCG-receptor complex extracted from prelabeled particles	0.29 (66A)	0.32 (64A)
Sedimentation constant:		
Free receptor	6.0-6.8S	6.5S
hCG-receptor complex formed after extraction	7.5S	7.5S
hCG-receptor complex extracted from prelabeled particles	8.8S	8.8S

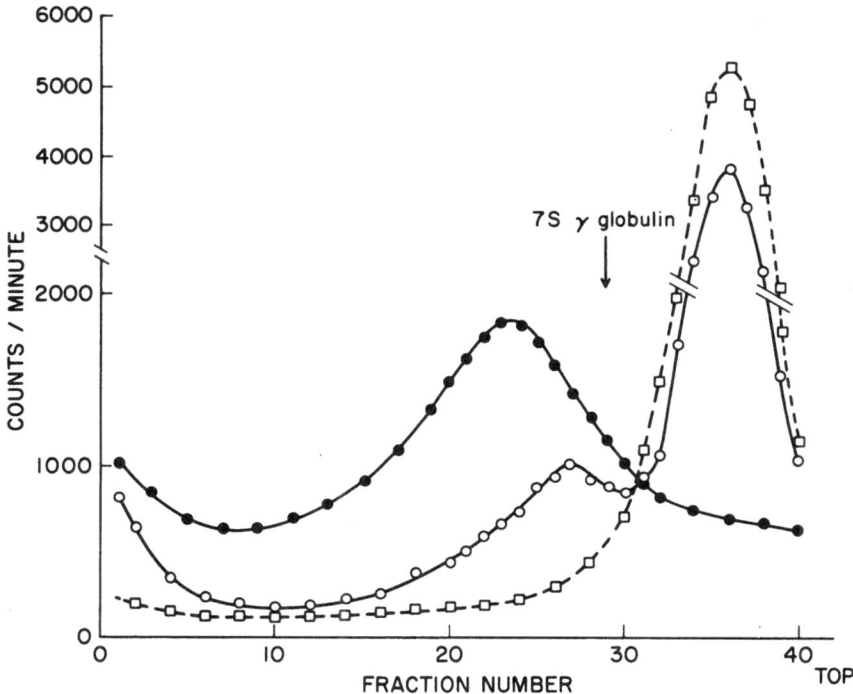

Figure 14. Effect of pH on ^{125}I-hCG-receptor extracted from prelabeled testis particles. Soluble receptor in 0.1% Triton X-100, pH 7.4,•———•. Soluble receptor adjusted to pH 3.5 for 1 min, reincubated at pH 7.4 for 16 hours,o———o. Soluble receptor adjusted to pH 3.5 for 1 min, reincubated with 20 µg of hCG at pH 7.4 for 16 hours,◻– – –◻.

by isopycnic density gradient centrifugation was 1.3150. Since the density of the 7.5S Lubrol WX-extracted form of the receptor complex (1.315) is greater than that of the Triton-solubilized form (1.277) and the apparent frictional ratio is higher (1.6 vs. 1.4 for the 8.8S form), the lower sedimentation velocity of the Lubrol form in sucrose gradients is probably caused by extraction of a more highly asymmetric form of the receptor.

Parallel studies carried out in the ovary have given almost identical results as those obtained with the testis receptors (Table 2). A notable feature of these studies was the reproducibility with which the several forms of the receptor complex could be extracted under defined conditions by various detergents.

Interpretation of the several forms of the gonadotropin receptors extracted from testis particles is complicated by differential actions of detergent binding and molecular conformation upon sedimentation velocity during density gradient centrifugation sucrose solutions. Because the changes in density of the complexes extracted under various conditions are not sufficient to account for the observed sedimentation behavior of the hormone-receptor complexes, it is likely that changes in the symmetry or degree of association of the complexes are responsible for the multiplicity of forms detected under different conditions of detergent extraction. The glycoprotein nature of the ligand, and a degree of assymmetry in the receptor molecule, probably all contribute to the observed disparity between Stokes radius and sedimentation velocity, and combine to accentuate the apparent asymmetry of the receptor-hormone complex as calculated from the hydrodynamic properties.

Enzymic and Chemical Treatment of Soluble
Gonadotropin Receptors

The actions of enzymic and chemical treatment upon hormone binding by particulate and soluble receptors have provided useful information about certain of the structural features of the gonadotropin binding sites. Brief exposure of the free receptors to trypsin (1 mg/ml) destroyed the binding activity of the soluble testis receptor. This effect, which was accompanied by abolition of the 7.5S complex during sucrose density gradient centrifugation (Fig. 15), indicates that protein forms an essential component of the gonadotropin receptor. The action of proteolytic and other enzymes may also be responsible for the degradation of receptors which occurs during storage of solubilized binding fractions, particularly during incubation at 34° C.

When ^{125}I-hCG binding after enzyme treatment of the soluble receptor at 34° C was analyzed by sucrose density gradient centrifugation, the presence of significant receptor degradation was apparent in control tubes pre-incubated at 34° C when compared with 4° C preincubation (Fig. 16). Exposure to phospholipase C and neuraminidase caused an increase in the magnitude of the 7.5S hormone-receptor peak, and was accompanied by the appearance of aggregated material seen in the lower left part of the gradient. By contrast, substantial loss of binding activity was found after exposure to phospholipase A.

The enhanced binding after neuraminidase treatment of the soluble receptor is probably attributable to desialylation of the labeled gonadotropin, since asialo-hCG has been shown to possess higher affinity for gonadotropin receptors. Also, exposure of

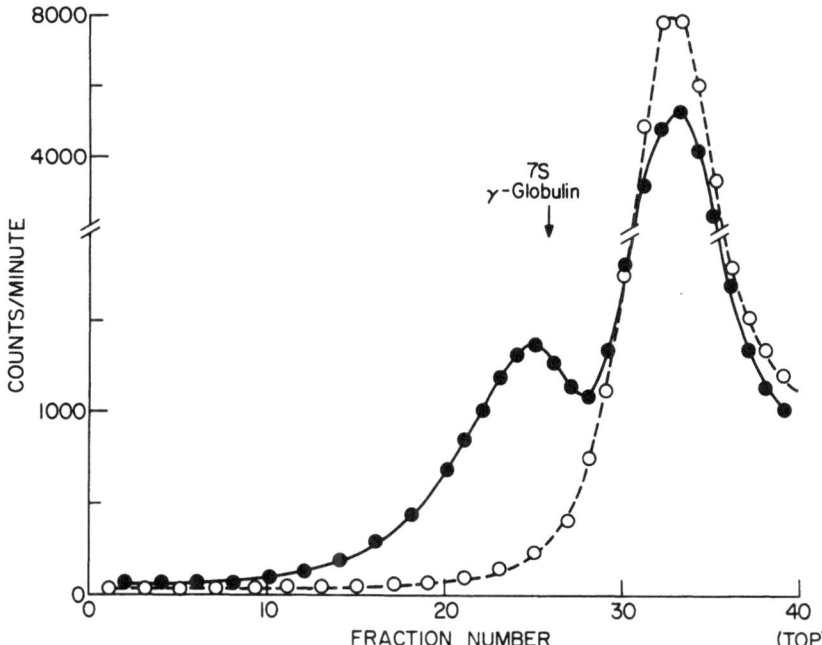

Figure 15. Effect of trypsin on gonadotropin receptor binding activity. Aliquots of soluble gonadotropin binding fraction (400 μg protein) were incubated with 1 mg of trypsin for 10 min at 25°; after addition of 2 mg of soybean trypsin inhibitor the samples were incubated with 50,000 cpm (1.5 ng) of ^{125}I-hCG for 16 hours at 4°. The patterns of sucrose gradient centrifugation show complete abolition of binding activity by trypsin treatment (0– – –0) when compared to the control (●———●).

particulate receptors to neuraminidase did not cause increased binding on subsequent incubation with ^{125}I-hCG. The marked reduction of the gonadotropin-receptor peak after exposure to phospholipase A may reflect an important function of phospholipids in the biological activity of the gonadotropin receptor. The lipid content of the soluble gonadotropin receptor is probably quite small, in view of the high density of the molecules, but appears to play a significant role in hormone binding.

No effect of phospholipase A and C upon the receptor-hormone complex formed after Triton X-100 extraction of testis particles by subsequent equilibration with ^{125}I-hCG (i.e., the 7.5S complex) was observed. Treatment of the dialyzed 7.5S ^{125}I-hCG-receptor complex (8.8S) with phospholipase A did not dissociate

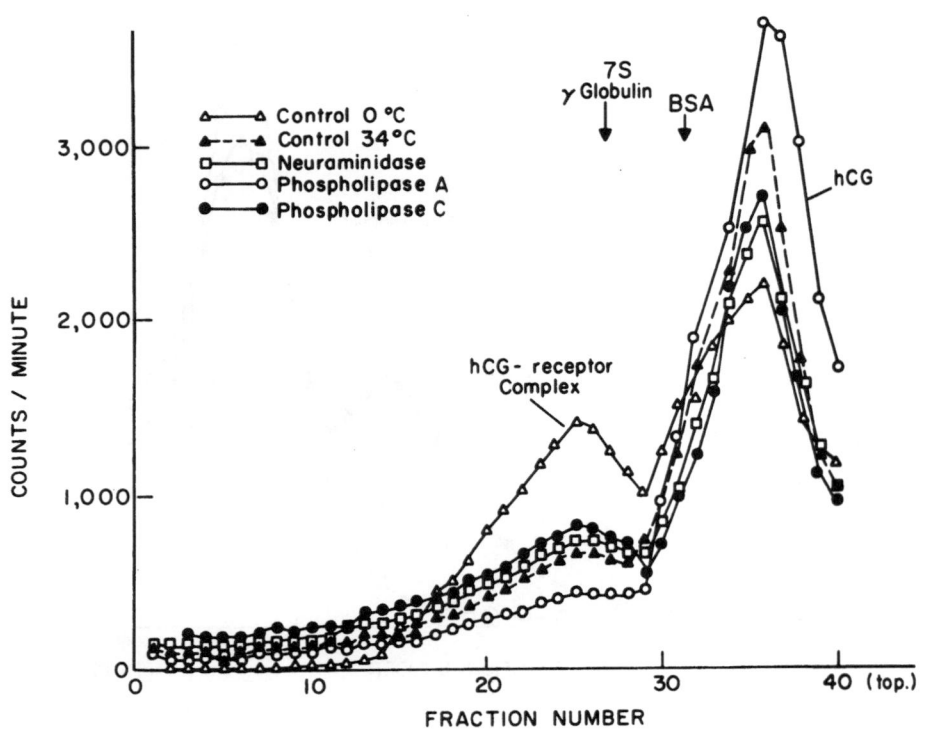

Figure 16. ^{125}I-hCG binding after preincubation and enzyme treatment of soluble gonadotropin receptor.   Effects of neuraminidase and phospholipase on gonadotropin binding activity of solubilized receptors during incubation at 34°.   Sucrose density gradient centrifugation revealed the presence of significant receptor degradation in control tubes incubated at 34°C.   Treatment with neuraminidase and phospholipase C slightly increased the peak of binding activity, and phospholipase A caused a marked decrease in binding.

or otherwise alter the complex, although phospholipase C caused a moderate degree of aggregation (Fig. 17).

Treatment of prelabeled testis particles with phospholipases A and C before extraction with Triton X-100 caused considerable aggregation of the hormone-receptor complexes as shown by sucrose density gradient centrifugation (Fig. 18A).   The 8.8S hormone-receptor complex extracted from prelabeled particulate fractions with Triton X-100 was also aggregated by exposure to phospholipase C, while phopholipase A had virtually no effect

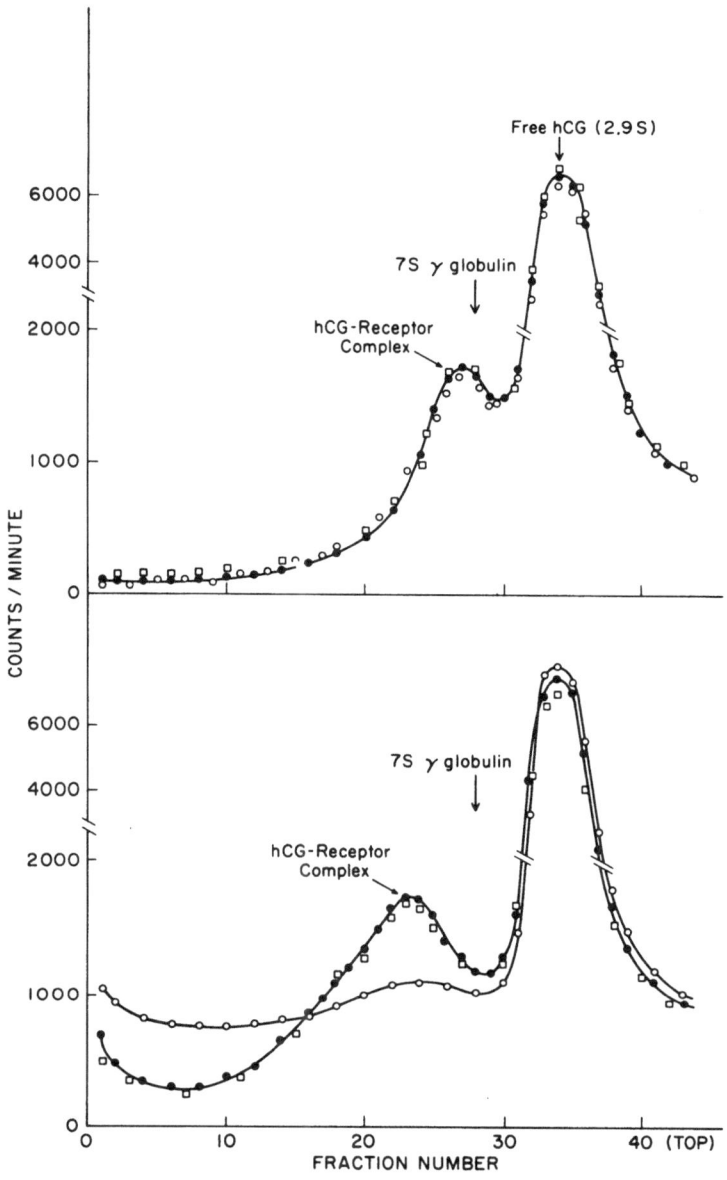

Figure 17. Effects of phospholipase A and C upon the sucrose density gradient centrifugation pattern of the 7.5S ^{125}I-hCG-receptor complex prepared by Triton X-100 extraction of testis particles and subsequent equilibration with ^{125}I-hCG (top). Effects of phospholipase A and C on 8.8S complex formed by dialysis of the 7.5S ^{125}I-hCG-receptor complex. Control, ●——●; phospholipase A, 0.05 unit,□——□; phospholipase C, 1.0 unit, ○——○.

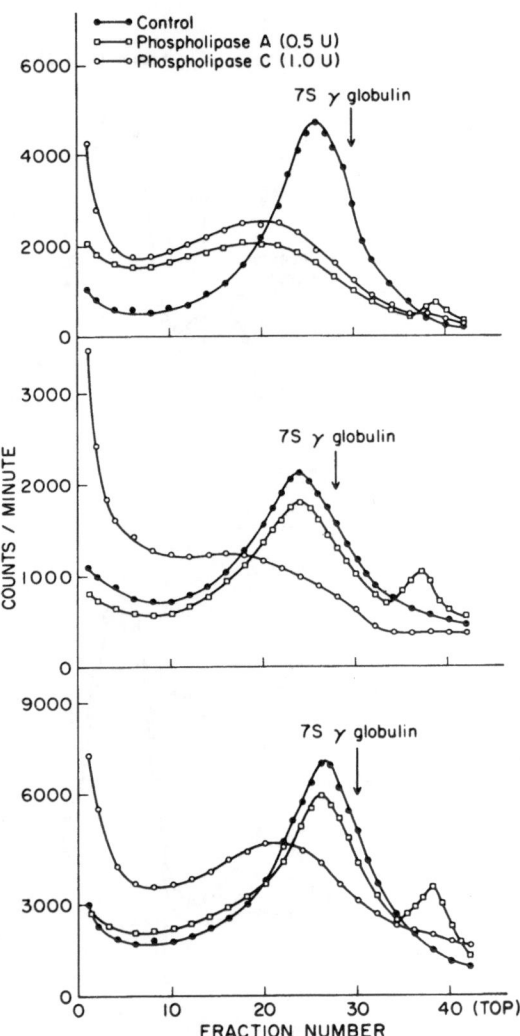

Figure 18. Effects of phospholipase A and C upon the sucrose density gradient centrifugation pattern of the 8.8S ^{125}I-hCG-receptor complex extracted from prelabeled testis particles with Triton X-100. A, enzyme treatment of particles; B, enzyme treatment after solubilization; C, enzyme treatment of soluble receptor fractionated by precipitation with 25 to 50% $(NH_4)_2 SO_2$.

upon this species (Fig. 18 B). Identical results were observed with the 8.8S receptor-hormone complex subjected to ammonium sulphate fractionation at 25-50% saturation. Phospholipase C caused aggregation of the receptor-hormone complex while phospholipase A did not change the sedimentation behaviour of the 8.8S hormone-receptor complex (Fig. 18 C). The presence of a small but definite peak of free hCG (2.9S) suggested that some dissociation of the hormone from the receptor (8.8S) occurred during treatment with phospholipase A (Fig. 18, B, C). Other enzymes tested, including neuraminidase, RNase and DNase, did not reduce the uptake of ^{125}I-hCG by the soluble receptor preparation.

Although these various results are not simple to interpret, it is clear that phospholipase A has a more pronounced effect upon the unoccupied binding sites of the soluble and particulate receptor than on the soluble and particulate preformed receptor complexes. By contrast, phospholipase C was never observed to destroy binding activity, though it frequently caused aggregation of the extracted complexes. Therefore, it appears likely that phospholipids form an important component of the receptors and that binding activity in particular is strongly influenced by a phospholipid moiety which is susceptible to hydrolysis by phospholipase A.

The importance of membrane lipids in peptide hormone binding and activation of adenylate cyclase has been noted in several other systems. Binding of labeled glucagon by liver membranes, and of labeled thyrotropin-releasing hormone by pituitary membranes, are markedly reduced by treatment with phospholipase A (10,11). In general, the effects of phospholipases C and D upon binding of peptide hormones to all membrane receptors are less destructive than that of phospholipase A. The more marked effects of phospholipase A have been attributed to two mechanisms, disruption of membrane structure by ß-ester bond cleavage (12), and the detergent effect of the lyso-phospholipid end products of phospholipase A digestion (11).

The role of protein sulphydryl and disulphide groups for gonadotropin binding has been investigated by determination of ^{125}I-hCG binding activity after reduction and/or alkylation of soluble and particulate receptors, receptor-hormone complexes and gonadotropins (13). After such treatment, the alkylating or reducing agent was washed or dialyzed out from particulate or soluble fractions before binding studies were performed.

Soluble gonadotropin receptors extracted from testis particles with Triton X-100 were treated with reducing agents for 30 minutes at 37° C, and subsequently equilibrated with ^{125}I-hCG for 16 hours at 4° C. Subsequent analysis by sucrose gradient cen-

trifugation showed a significant decrease in the magnitude of the
7.5S hormone-peak after treatment with 2 mM DTT, and complete
abolition occurred after treatment with 10 mM dithiotreitol or 42
mM cysteine.

Studies on reduction and/or alkylation of free receptors on
the binding of ^{125}I-hCG by particulate or soluble receptors have
demonstrated that binding of labeled hormone after treatment of
particulate receptor with 20 mM NEM alone was similar to that
of the control experiments, indicating that the accessible SH
groups of the receptor molecule are not involved in the binding
process. The slight but significant increase of ^{125}I-hCG binding by soluble receptors treated with NEM could be due to reduced
receptor degradation, caused by the blocking of thiol groups in
degradative enzymes.

Significant impairment of ^{125}I-hCG binding by particulate
and soluble receptor was apparent after exposure to 4 mM DTT,
and complete abolition of binding occurred after treatment of
the reduced soluble receptors with 20 mM NEM. In particulate
receptors, complete loss of hormone binding was observed when
particles were treated with 10 mM DTT followed by 50 mM NEM
(Fig. 19, top).

Reduction and alkylation of the preformed soluble or particulate hormone-receptor complexes (i.e. previously equilibrated
with ^{125}I-hCG) have shown that treatment with reducing agents
and NEM does not cause dissociation of the preexisting hormone-
receptor complex (Fig. 19, below). This lack of effect upon the
hormone-receptor complex suggests that the relevant S-S groups
may be adjacent to the receptor site, and play an essential role
in the binding mechanisms. Exposure of DTT-reduced particles
to mild oxidative conditions, including 5 mM methylene blue,
mixing under oxygen for a period of two hours, and up to 20 mM
DTNB for 4 hours, caused no restoration of gonadotropin binding
activity.

In addition, the binding of reduced ^{125}I-hCG by untreated
receptors was also examined. Treatment with DTT and or NEM
considerably diminished the binding of ^{125}I-labeled hCG by both
particulate and soluble receptors, while treatment with NEM
alone did not significantly alter binding of the hormone (Fig. 20).
The α and ß subunits of hCG contain 5 and 6 disulphide bridges
respectively, and it is not surprising that reduction of at least
some of these bonds causes a major loss of binding activity of the
molecule.

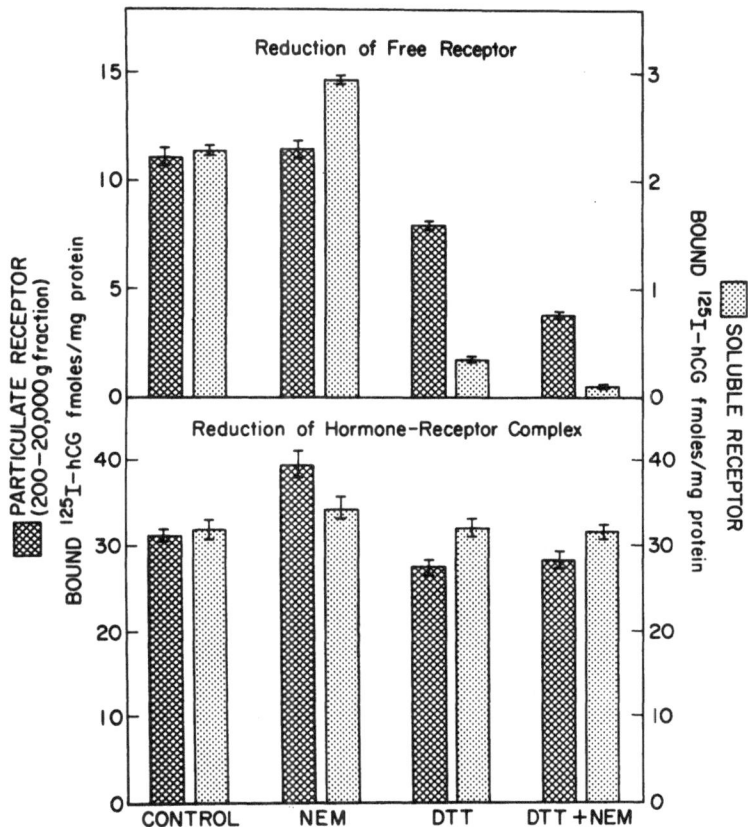

Figure 19. (Above) Reduction and alkylation of free receptors: binding of ^{125}I-hCG by particulate and soluble gonadotropin receptors previously treated with dithiothreitol (DTT) (4 mM for 60 min at 22° C) and/or N-ethylmaleimide (NEM) (20 mM, for 120 min at 22° C). Specific gonadotropin binding is expressed as fmoles/mg protein, each value being the mean ± SD of four determinations.

(Below) Reduction and alkylation of preformed hormone-receptor complex: retention of bound ^{125}I-hCG by particulate and soluble testis receptors, following treatment of the hormone-receptor complex with DTT and/or NEM.

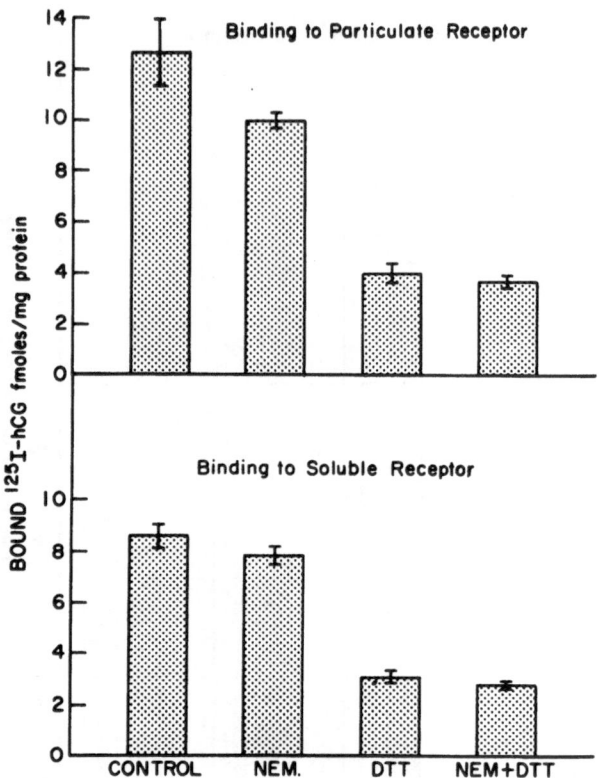

Figure 20. Reduction and alkylation of ^{125}I-hCG binding of intact, reduced and reduced alkylated gonadotropin by particulate and soluble gonadotropin receptors. Specific gonadotropin binding is expressed as fmoles/mg protein, each value being the mean $\pm$ SD of four determinations.

The lack of effect of alkylation alone is also not unexpected, since hCG has been reported to contain no free sulfhydryl groups (14). In these experiments, the use of denaturing conditions in conjunction with the reducing agents was omitted because we have previously found that treatment with urea or guanidine significantly impairs the binding properties of the receptor. Therefore, the present treatment with reducing agents was probably selective for accessible disulfide bonds, without necessarily affecting buried intrachain disulfide bridges. Such treatment is likely to produce relatively less disruption of tertiary structure than would occur after reduction in the presence of denaturants. The dependence of ^{125}I-hCG binding upon the integrity of accessible disulfide bonds indicates that these groups are essential for the specificity of the molecular conformation of the hormone receptor site. The lack of effect of reduction upon preformed hormone-receptor complexes suggests that S-S bonds may be directly involved in the binding process, and are possibly protected from reduction when the receptor site is occupied by gonadotropin. Alternatively, the participating disulphide bonds of the receptor may not be essential for maintenance of gonadotropin binding once the hormone-receptor complex has formed. Whichever of these two possibilities is correct, the present findings provide direct evidence for the importance of disulphide bonds in the structural organization of the specific testicular receptors for gonadotropins.

Studies on the Purification of Gonadotropin Receptors

For affinity chromatography of the LH/hCG receptors, partially purified hCG (Pregnyl, Organon) was coupled to agarose beads by a number of procedures. When hCG was coupled directly to cyanogen bromide-activated sepharose, or to sepharose-concanavalin A by glutaraldehyde conjugation, the uptake of receptors from solution by such preparations was almost complete. However, subsequent recovery of gonadotropin receptors from the affinity gel could not be achieved in adequate yield by a variety of eluting agents. The most satisfactory medium for affinity chromatography was prepared by conjugation of hCG to agarose beads bearing a 10 Å side arm terminating in N-hydroxy succinimide ester (Affigel 10, Biorad). The complex was prepared by shaking the Affigel 10 beads with hCG at 4° C for 16 hours, followed by extensive washing of the gel with phosphate-buffered saline pH 7.4 (5 L), 0.025 M acetic acid pH 3.2 (2 L) and again with the initial buffer (2 L). The uptake of hCG by the gel particles was equivalent to 1500 μg of pure hCG per gm of gel. No dissociation of the hormone from the gel particles was observed at any time. For purification studies, uptake of the Triton X-100 solubilized LH-hCG receptor of testis and ovary was performed by shaking with the gel-hCG for 16 hr at 4° C. The gel-hCG-receptor complex was then washed with phosphate buffer pH 7.4 at 22° C, to remove non-receptor proteins of the solubilized gonadal particles. Elution of the receptor was accomplished with high efficiency by shaking the gel-hCG-receptor with 0.025 M acetic acid for 1 hr at 4° C, followed by column elution with the acetic acid solution. This elution step was repeated 4 to 5 times, to obtain the most satisfactory recovery.

The eluted fractions were immediately neutralized and the binding activity was determined by incubation at 4° C with ^{125}I-hCG for 16 hrs. followed by polyethylene glycol precipita-

Table 3

LH-hCG Receptor Purification.

Receptor Preparation	Specific Activity (cpm/mg)	Binding Capacity (pmole/mg)
Triton-solubilized particles	2.07×10^3	0.15
From affinity column	3.13×10^6	225*
Pure receptor		5000**

* Purification Factor:	1500
** For complete purity:	30,000

tion.   The percent of binding capacity recovered was 68% of the capacity of the original samples measured at zero time, i.e., the moment the gel was mixed with the receptor.   The capacity of the original solution measured at the time of acid elution was somewhat lower, and the calculated recovery of the eluted receptor was then 168%.   This difference is due to the relatively rapid degradation of the non-purified receptor.   By contrast, the purified receptor is very stable and no loss of binding activity was observed during several days at 4° C, while the non-purified receptor decayed rapidly after a few hours.   The sedimentation constant of the complex formed after binding of ^{125}I-hCG by the purified receptor was determined by sucrose gradient centrifugation to be 7.5S, a form identical to that observed in the original soluble receptor preparation.   The association constant of the purified receptor determined by equilibrium binding studies was 1.0×10^{10} M^{-1}.   The hCG binding capacity of the original Triton-solubilized material was 0.15 pmole/mg protein, while the capacity of the purified receptor was 225 pmoles/mg protein, representing a 1,500 fold purification factor.   The expected binding capacity for the completely pure receptor, based on the molecular weight of 200,000, is about 5000 pmole/mg.   Based upon this value, an overall purification factor of 30,000 will be needed to achieve complete homogenity of the receptor (Table 3).   The purification obtained by this single step in affinity chromatography is quite substantial, and is of comparable magnitude to those reported for other receptors using similar techniques.   It appears very likely that a combination of the affinity chromatography procedure with other purification methods will be necessary to achieve complete homogeneity of the receptor molecule.

References

1. Dufau, M. L. and Catt, K. J., Nature New Biol. 242: 246, 1973.

2. Dufau, M. L., Charreau, E. H. and Catt, K J., J. Biol. Chem. 248: 6973, 1973.

3. Dufau, M. L., Charreau, E. H., Ryan, D. and Catt, K. J., FEBS Letters 39: 149, 1974.

4. Dufau, M. L., Tsuruhara, T. and Catt, K. J., Biochim. Biophys. Acta 278: 281, 1972.

5. Charreau, E. H., Dufau, M. L. and Catt, K. J., Biol. Chem. 294: 4189, 1974.

6. Swart, A.C.W. and Hemker, H. C., Biochim. Biophys. Acta 222: 692, 1970.

7. Staal, G.E.J., Koster, J. F., Kamp, H., Millingen Boersma, L. and Veerger, C., Biochim. Biophys. Acta 227: 86, 1971.

8. Laurent, T. C. and Killander, J., J. Chromatogr. 14: 317, 1964.

9. Siegel, L. M. and Monty, K. J., Biochim. Biophys. Acta 112: 346, 1966.

10. Rodbell, M., Krans, H.M.J., Pohl, S. L. and Birnbaumer, L., J. Biol. Chem. 246: 1861, 1971.

11. Barden, N., and Labrie, F., J. Biol. Chem. 248: 7601, 1973.

12. Simpkins, H., Tay, S., and Panko, E., Biochemistry 10:3579 (1971).

13. Dufau, M. L., Ryan, D. and Catt, K. J., Biochim. Biophys. Acta 343: 417, 1974.

14. Belisario, R., Carlsen, O. P., Swaminathan, N., Bahl, O. P., J. Biol. Chem. 248: 6180, 1973.

APPARENT POSITIVE COOPERATIVITY IN THE MECHANISM OF

ACTION OF LUTEINIZNG HORMONE

David Rodbard

Reproduction Research Branch, National Institute of Child Health
and Human Development, National Institutes of Health
Bethesda, Maryland 20014

W. Moyle* and J. Ramanchandran

Hormone Research Laboratory, University of California
San Francisco, California 94143

Dose response curves for cyclic AMP accumulation and testosterone prodduction were analyzed with respect to the apparent K_m (ED_{50}), apparent "Hill coefficient", and basal and maximal production rates using a new computer program for a "four parameter" logistic function, employing weighted nonlinear least-squares regression. Results indicate the presence of apparent positive cooperativity for cyclic AMP production, with a Hill coefficient between 1.76 and 2.60, which is highly statistically significantly different from 1.0. For testosterone production, the calculated Hill coefficients were 1.44, 1.71 and 2.95. However, due to the large standard errors, these Hill coefficients were not significantly different from unity. These results are suggestive of the presence of positive cooperativity, or the presence of "quantal" mechanism at a level intermediate between binding and cyclic AMP production, or some other type of "threshhold" phenomenon. The methods employed should be generally useful for analysis of dose response curves from hormone-receptor binding systems.

---

* Present Address: Laboratory of Human Reproduction and Reproductive Biology, Harvard Medial School, Boston, Massachusetts.

CHAPTER 4

INTRODUCTION

Moyle and Ramachandran have previously reported techniques for measurement of testosterone production and cyclic AMP accumulation in rat Leydig cell preparations and mouse tumor Leydig cells (1). The dose response curves had a fairly usual sigmoidal appearance when the nanograms of testosterone synthesized or picomoles of cyclic AMP accumulated per flask are plotted versus the logarithm of the dose of exogenous luteinizing hormone (LH). In a previous report, attention was called to the marked dissociation between the apparent "ED_{50}" for cyclic AMP production and for steroid production. These findings are similar to those of Catt and Dufau (2). In these and most other previous studies, no attempt was made to describe the dose response curve by a computerized least-squares method using a specific model.

In related studies, one of us has developed a computer program permitting weighted nonlinear least-squares regression specifically for the four parameter logistic function. This approach makes it possible to estimate the response for zero dose (blank, control, "basal", nonspecific) and also the maximal response (V_{max}, B_{max}, etc.), simultaneously with estimation of the ED_{50} or the apparent Michaelis-Menten constant (K_m) and the apparent Hill coefficient. Details of this statistical approach are presented elsewhere (3).

The Model

The equation is

$$Y = \frac{a - d}{1 + (X/c)^b} + d \qquad (1)$$

where a, b, c and d are constants.

The weighting function is based on the relationship:

$$w_i = \frac{1}{\sigma_y^2} \quad ; \quad \sigma_y^2 = a_0 + a_1 Y + a_2 Y^2 \qquad (2)$$

The coefficients for the weighting function (a_0, a_1, a_2) were estimated as described previously (3,4) (Fig. 1A, 1B). These results indicated that for analysis of the testosterone production data, it was reasonable to assume uniformity of variance. Thus, unweighted regression could be used by setting $a_0 = 1$; $a_1 = a_2 = 0$ in equation 2. For cyclic AMP production it appeared that there was nonuniformity of variance following the form $a_0 = a_1 = 0$, $a_2 = 0.01$. This corresponds to a constant percentage error (coefficient of variation) for the response variable. Only the relative magnitudes of a_0, a_1,

Table 1

Expt.	cAMP				Testosterone			
	a pmoles	b –	c µg/ml	d pmoles	a ng	b –	c ng/ml	d ng
7/24/72	*14.42 .42	2.60 .29	.60 .05	182 7	138.2 13.2	2.95 1.90	3.54 .60	327 11
	14.35 1.99	2.70 .23	.58 .03	181 3				
6/13/72	*22.49 .85	1.76 .10	.55 .04	277 8				
	23.55 3.50	1.98 .13	.52 .02	272 4				
8/10/72	*19.77 .76	2.53 .16	.40 .02	405 13	.467 .057	1.44 .37	7.68 1.61	1.305 .037
	18.58 5.46	2.29 .22	.41 .02	408 7				
5/5/72					.058 .031	1.71 .46	64. 13.	.711 .046

Values for a, b, c and d given with their approximate (asymptotic) standard errors. Values for Testosterone were obtained using unweighted regression. Values for cAMP were obtained using weighted *(a_0 = a_1 = 0, a_2 = 1) and unweighted regression. Values of a and d cannot be compared between experiments because the number of cells per flask varies.

and a_2 are important, since the sum of the weights of all observations was normalized to be equal to the number of observations.

RESULTS

Results are shown in Table 1 and Figures 1 and 2. The parameters of equation 1 are summarized in Table 1. The results
indicate that the cyclic AMP dose response curve has a b value (Hill
coefficient) which is significantly different from unity. This was
true irrespective of the nature of the weighting function: With unweighted regression in Experiment 1 b was equal to 2.70 whereas
with weighted regression ($a_o = a_1 = 0$, $a_2 = 0.01$) b was equal to
2.60.

This difference in the Hill coefficient is very much smaller than
the approximate standard errors obtained by either method (0.225
and 0.285, respectively). Both weighted and unweighted regression
provide approximately the same values for a, b, c and d. However,

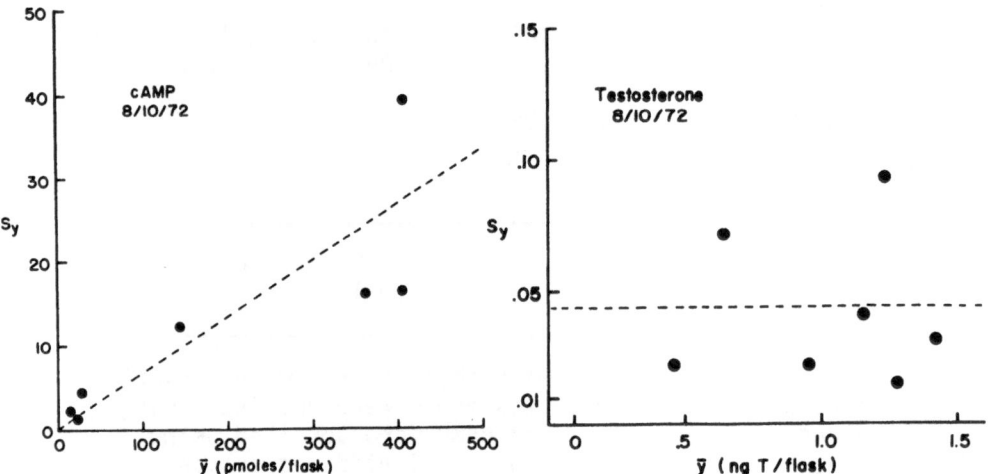

Figure 1. Relationship between standard deviation of replicate
responses versus mean response. (A) cAMP. Note σ_y is proportional to Y. (B). Testosterone. Here the relationship (if any)
between σ_y and Y is less obvious, so unweighted regression may be
used.

In both cases A and B, the estimates of σ_y^2 are subject to considerable sampling error, due to the small number of replicates and low
degrees of freedom. Analyses such as this must be performed for
several experiments and the results combined.

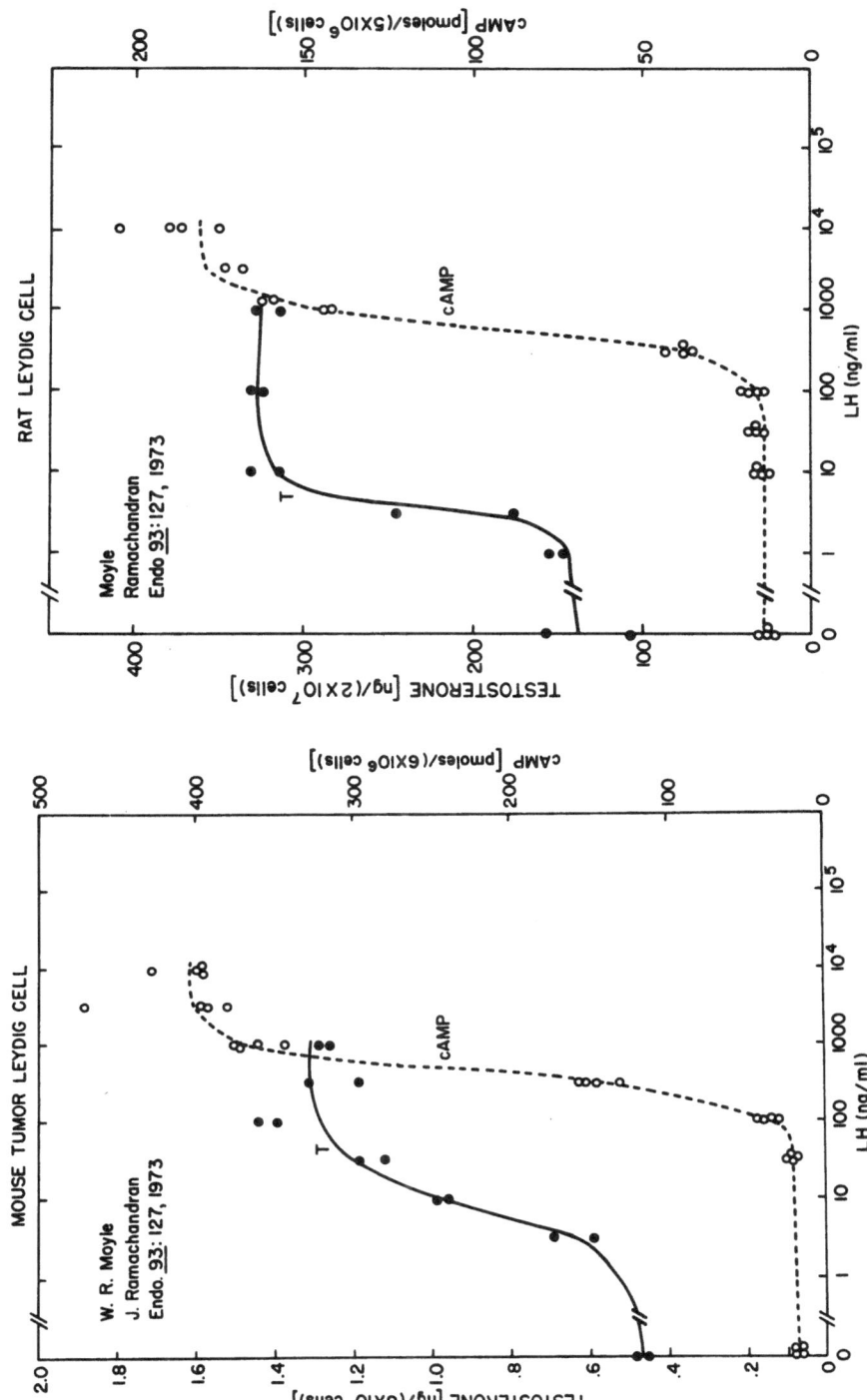

Figure 2. Dose response curves for cAMP and testosterone in the mouse tumor Leydig cell (A) and rat Leydig cell (B). The dose response curves shown are the computer generated least squares "fit" to equation 1, with parameters as shown in Table 1.

the standard errors assigned to these values differ considerably. When weighted regression was used, the standard error for a was reduced from 1.99 to 0.42, whereas the standard error for d was increased from 2.93 to 7.10. In Experiment 2, the standard error for a was reduced from 5.46 to 0.75, whereas the error for d increased from 6.55 to 13.02. The standard errors obtained by the weighted regression appear to be more reasonable, in view of the decreased precision of the response at higher values.

Testosterone. The b values which were obtained for testosterone were $2.95 + 1.90$, $1.44 + .37$ and $1.71 + .46$. These are suggestive of the presence of positive "cooperativity" although the b values are not statistically significantly different from 1.0 when considered individually. Using an unpaired t test, the mean b value ($2.03 + .46$ sem) was not significantly different from unity, due to the low degrees of freedom. Additional studies will be necessary in order to permit more refined estimation of these Hill coefficients.

DISCUSSION

These findings indicate that a newly developed computational method for radioimmunoassays, immunoradiometric (labeled antibody) assays, binding curves, and dose response curves can be applied to the analysis of testosterone and cyclic AMP production by the testis in response to luteinizing hormone. This approach provides a method for computerized curve fittings for this type of dose response curves. The apparent Hill coefficients for cyclic AMP production are significantly greater than unity, which is highly suggestive of the presence of a cooperative interaction, such as an allosteric enzymatic step intermediate between binding and cyclic AMP production. However, several alternative hypotheses must be considered:

1) One must consider the possibility that the b value is elevated due to the presence of phosphodiesterase. It is possible, that at low concentrations of LH, the cyclic AMP is produced in such small quantity that it is virtually immediately destroyed by the phosphodiesterase. However, as the LH concentration is increased, cyclic AMP production might exceed the ability of phosphodiesterase to degrade it, and as a result a type of "threshhold" is introduced. From the data of the type analyzed here, it is impossible to distinguish between these two mechanisms. By recalculation of data from a closely analogous study of the action of ACTH on the adrenal by Richardson, Schulster and Mackey (5), it appears that the introduction of theophylline into the system resulted in a dramatic change in the parameter b for corticosterone production from 1.5 to 1.0. In other words, the introduction of theophylline appeared to abolish the "cooperative" effect with respect to the production of corticosterone by the adrenal in response to ACTH.

2) A spuriously elevated "b" value or Hill coefficient will arise, if one uses <u>total</u> ligand (LH) concentrations in lieu of <u>free</u> ligand concentration <u>for the</u> abscissa, and if <u>binding exceeds 25%</u> (Fig. 3). In the present studies, "total" <u>ligand concentration was</u> used for the abscissa, but the percent of ligand bound (B/T ratio) was almost certainly less than 10% under the conditions employed.

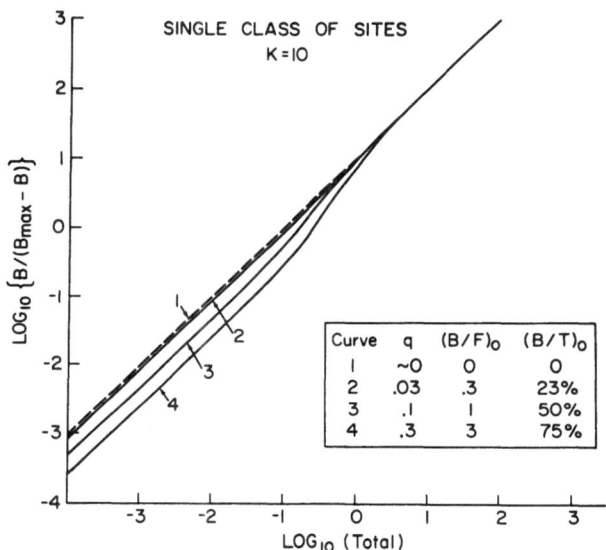

Figure 3. Hypothetical "Hill plots" (never actually used by Hill) of log $B/B(B_{max}$ -B) vs. log(hormone concentration). A "correct" Hill plot uses log(Free) on the abscissa. If log(Total) is used instead, one may have an apparent positive cooperativity (slope > 1), if "Free" and "Total" differ seriously. In practice, if the % bound (B/T) for ligand is less than 25%, then log(Total) may be used without serious error.

The results with respect to b for testosterone are not statistically significant within any one experiment. However, once again there is a suggestion of a positive cooperative effect, when the data from three experiments are considered simultaneously.

Reanalysis of the data of Catt and Dufau (2) in view of the present findings are also highly suggestive of the presence of positive cooperativity (b > 1) for testosterone production and possibly cAMP production. This indicates that the present findings are not restricted to one experimental system, procedure or laboratory. Also, similar results are seen for the ACTH → adrenal → cAMP→corticosterone system (4, 5).

Presently available data regarding the binding of hCG to Leydig cells (2), with the presence of a linear Scatchard plot, suggests that there is no positive cooperativity at the level of hormone-receptor binding. Thus, the apparent "cooperativity" must arise at a step intermediate between binding and cyclic AMP production.

3) Studies such as these are complicated by the fact, that the testis preparations are likely to be contaminated with some endogenous LH. This could result in a spurious elevation of the parameter a, and may have an appreciable effect on the apparent value for b and the shape of the entire dose-response curve.

4) Presence of an elevated "b" value for testosterone would be compatible with the "quantal" model (6). However, it by no means establishes this model. Further, the presence of an elevated "b" value for cyclic AMP, would be in contrast to the assumption (6) that cyclic AMP production would be directly proportional to binding of hormone. However, the elevated b value would be compatible with the presence of a "quantal" mechanism at a level intermediate between binding and cyclic AMP, although it would not exclude the possibility of a second "quantal" mechanism intermediate between cyclic AMP and corticosterone production.

These findings suggest a number of lines for further experimentation. Kinetic studies will be necessary to examine the possibility of cooperativity. The effect of theophylline on the parameter b should be studied. Further, studies of the type utilized by DeMeyts (7) would be useful in indicating whether cooperative phenomenon occur at the level of hormone-receptor binding.

Summary

In vitro accumulation of cyclic AMP by rat Leydig cell preparation and mouse tumor Leydig cells in response to exogenous LH appears to display an apparent Hill coefficient of 2.5. This is suggestive of positive cooperativity at a level intermediate between binding and cyclic AMP production, although several alternative hypothesis cannot be excluded on the basis of these data alone. The Hill coefficient for testosterone is higher than unity, although it has not been established with adequate precision in these experiments.

Acknowledgements

Dr. P. Schulster kindly provided access to his original data. Dr. P. DeMeyts provided many stimulating discussions of cooperativity.

References

1. Moyle, W. R., and Ramachandran, J., J. Endocrinology 93, 127, 1973.

2. Catt, K. J., and Dufau, M. L., Adv. Expt. Med. Biol. 36, 379, 1973.

3. Rodbard, D., and Hutt, D. M., Proc. Symposium on RIA and Related Procedures in Clin. Med. and Research, Int. Atomic Energy Agency, Vienna, Austria, in press.

4. Rodbard, D., Endocrinology, in press.

5. Mackie, D., and Schulster, D., Biochem. Biophys. Res. Comm. 53, 1973.

6. Rodbard, D., Adv. Expt. Med. Biol. 36, 342, 1973.

7. DeMeyts, P., Roth, J., Neville, D. M., Gavin, J. R., and Lesniak, M. A., Biochem. Biophys. Res. Comm. 55, 154, 1973.

FUNCTIONAL GROUPS IN OVINE LUTEINIZING HORMONE AND THEIR RECEPTOR SITE INTERACTIONS - A Chemical Study

Wan-Kyng Liu, Kuo-Pao Yang, Bruce D. Burleigh and
Darrell N. Ward

Department of Biochemistry, The University of Texas System
Cancer Center, M. D. Anderson Hospital and Tumor Institute
6723 Bertner Avenue, Houston, Texas 77025

Introduction

Selective chemical reactions have long been used in the field of hormone research for the study of functional group relationships to biological activity. An early example of such a study applied to ovine LH is that of Li, Simpson and Evans (1) who employed ketene to acetylate LH (ICSH) and found that acetylation under very mild conditions inactivated the hormone. Geschwind and Li (2) found periodate oxidation inactivated ovine LH. Although in that study periodate was selected for its attack on vicinal hydroxyl groups in the carbohydrate moiety, these authors appreciated that other reactions might be taking place. In a later study from that same laboratory Gan et al. (3) demonstrated that periodate oxidation of ovine LH not only attacked the carbohydrate moiety but also the disulfide bonds in the molecule. Thus, although periodate oxidation inactivates ovine LH it is not known whether this inactivation results from destruction of the carbohydrate moieties, destruction of the disulfide bonds, or both. Our own laboratory made an extensive study of the effect of several reagents and various conditions upon the activity of ovine LH (4). Included in those studies were some on the effects of oxidation by performic acid which attacks the disulfide bonds and the thioether group of methionine. This reagent completely inactivated ovine LH. We also studied the effect of reduction with sodium and liquid ammonia on the biological activity of the hormone. Although the hormone was virtually inactivated by this treatment, it is difficult to be certain in such an experiment that there was not some reoxidation to the native hormone to account for the small residual activity observed. There are also other technical difficulties in dealing with a

TABLE 1

SUMMARY OF THE LH-NITRATION STUDIES OF CHENG AND PIERCE (22) AND SAIRAM, PAPKOFF, AND LI (21)

MATERIALS STUDIED	NITRATION CONDITIONS					NO. Tyr NITRATED*	BIOLOGICAL ACTIVITY**
	Temp.	pH	TNM/Tyr$^+$	Time	Protein Conc.		
Sairam et al. (21)							
oLH (Control)							2.06 (100)
oLH††	23°	8.0	8.6	2 hr	10mg/ml	6.1 (7)	0.15 (7)
"	0°	8.0	8.6	2 hr	10mg/ml	3.1 (7)	0.04 (2)
oLH	23°	8.0	8.6	2 hr	10mg/ml	4.6 (7)	0.68 (33)
"	0°	8.0	0.58	1 hr	10mg/ml	1.0 (7)	
oLHα‡	23°	8.0	8.6	1 hr	6mg/ml	4.2 (5)	
oLHβ‡	23°	8.0	8.6	1 hr	10mg/ml	2.0 (2)	
Recombinations							
oLHα + oLHβ							1.2 (58)
[5 NO$_2$]LHα + oLHβ							0.07 (3)
oLHα + [2 NO$_2$]LH							0.22 (11)
Cheng & Pierce (22)							
bLH (Control)							1.74 (100)
bLH	23°	8.0	1.4	1 hr	1mg/ml	1.5 (7)	
bLHα	23°	8.0	2.0	1 hr	0.5mg/ml	1.3 (5)	
bLHβ	23°	9.0	5.0	1 hr	0.5mg/ml	0.8‡‡ (2)	
Recombinations							
bLHα + bLHα							2.16 (120)
bLHα + [2 NO$_2$]LHβ							1.02 (60) or 1.6 (95)
[2 NO$_2$]bLHα + bLHβ							0.25 (14)

hormone in the reduced form at the very dilute concentrations which must be used for bioassay.

In our early studies (4) we also observed that simple dissociating conditions, e.g. urea, guanidine hydrochloride, led to inactivation of ovine LH. We also observed that low pH led to inactivation. These studies preceded or were probably even contemporary with the memorable demonstration by Li and Starman (5) that low pH in itself is a dissociating condition for ovine LH. This very important finding on the physical properties of ovine LH we were quick to confirm (6) using different methodology. Although initially this dissociation was regarded as a simple monomer-dimer type dissociation (7,8), by 1965, it became obvious that a dissimilar subunit model of the LH molecule was more appropriate, as we then proposed (9). Procedures for the separation of the subunits were devised; the first to be reported was that of Papkoff and Samy (10), although several alternatives have been provided for the subunit separation of LH and the other glycoprotein hormone subunits (11-16).

The availability of the isolated subunits eventually led to the establishment of the complete amino acid sequence for ovine luteinizing hormone from studies in two laboratories (17,18 and 19,20). These sequences are in essential agreement, except for two or three points of difference.

With our growing knowledge of the structure of ovine luteinizing hormone it is possible to design more selective chemical studies that have bearing on the biological activity of LH. Two studies dealing with the selective nitration of LH have been reported. One study utilized ovine LH (21) while the other utilized bovine LH (22). It is known, however, that the amino acid sequence of this hormone from the two species is identical (23).

Legend to Table 1.

* Measured on monomeric form which ranged from 10-15% of the original weight of hormone.

** Determined by OAAD assay, potency relative to NIH-LH-S1. Values in parentheses are % of native hormone potency.

† Molar ratio of tetranitro methane per mole of tyrosine residues in the protein.

†† Reacted in 5 M-guanidine hydrochloride.

‡ Reacted in 1 M-NaCl.

‡‡ No free tyrosine detected.

There are some apparent discrepancies in the two nitration studies, but we hope to lend some clarification to this in the present report.

In the studies we now report we take advantage of the dissimilar subunit nature of LH to provide an additional tool to study the functional groups in the LH molecule. We have studied both acylation and selective nitration as they affect biological activity as measured by two bioassays, the ovarian ascorbic acid depletion assay (24) and the testicular homogenate radioligand assay (25-27).

Nitration Studies on LH and LH Subunits

Before presenting our studies on the nitration of ovine LH it will be well to summarize the results of the two laboratories reporting nitration studies on ovine or bovine LH (21,22). In Table 1 are summarized the reports of Cheng and Pierce (22) and of Sairam, Papkoff and Li (21). For brevity Table 1 has only selected data. For example Cheng and Pierce (22) also studied the effect of varying the tetranitromethane concentration from 0.5 to 14.0 x the molar ratio to tyrosine. We have simply selected those products they characterized most extensively. In general, Cheng and Pierce (21) observed lower degrees of nitration than Sairam et al. (21). Perhaps the most singular difference in the conditions employed by the two groups of investigators lies in the more dilute protein concentrations employed by Cheng and Pierce (22).

For the nitration studies we are reporting herein we have utilized protein concentrations of 2 mg per ml. The nitration reaction was conducted at pH 8.0 in 0.05 M Tris buffer. Tetranitromethane (TNM) was dissolved in 95% ethanol and added dropwise to the reaction mixture; the reaction was carried out at 4° C to minimize polymerization which is an important side reaction for this reagent. Rather than carry the reaction for a fixed time we also followed the reaction spectrophotometrically at 428 nm until the reaction reached a plateau indicating completion. At that point the solution was frozen and lyophilized, then chromatographed on Sephadex G-100 with 0.126 M NH_4HCO_3 as eluent. In Figure 1a is shown the extent of reaction of ovine LH as a function of time and with three different molar ratios of tetranitromethane to tyrosine residues in the molecule. In curve C the TNM/Tyr ratio was 1 to 1, in curve B the ratio was 5 or 10 to 1 (in either case a similar curve was obtained) and in curve A the ratio was 25 or 50 to 1. For the product in curve C, one tyrosine was nitrated of the 7 total; the product in curve B, two tyrosines were nitrated; and for the product shown in curve A three to four tyrosines were nitrated.

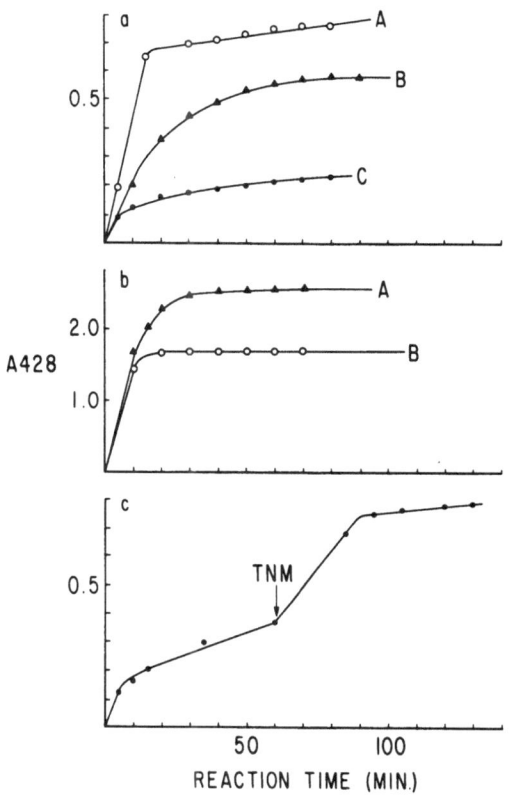

Figure 1 (a). Nitration of tyrosine in oLH as followed by increase in A_{428}. Curve A, protein 2 mg/ml, 0.05 M-Tris buffer pH 8, tetranitromethane (TNM) 50 to 1 molar ratio to tyrosine residues (the curve at 25 to 1 ratio was equivalent). Curve B obtained with molar ratios of TNM/Tyr of 10 to 1 (5 to 1 ratios gave a similar curve). Curve C, obtained with TNM/Tyr molar ratio of 1 to 1. (b). Nitration of oLHα. Curve B, nitration of TNM/Tyr molar ratio of 25 to 1 stops with 4 residues nitrated, but in the presence of 8 M-urea (Curve A) all five tyrosines are nitrated. (c). Nitration of oLHß, molar ratio TNM/Tyr (initially), 25 to 1. After 1 hr (arrow) an additional charge of TNM was added to bring the total ratio to 50 to 1.

Nitration of the subunits followed a somewhat different pattern. At TNM/Tyr ratios demonstrated in the three curves in Figure 1a, the oLHα subunit showed a pattern similar to Figure 1b,

TABLE 2

SUMMARY OF TYROSINE ANALYSES FOR VARIOUS NITRATION PROCEDURES

Sample*	Spectrophotometric Method[a] 3-nitrotyrosine	Amino Acid Analysis[a] Tyrosine	3-nitrotyrosine
Native oLH	0	6.45	0.0
[1 nitro] oLH	1.12	5.50	0.73
[2 nitro] oLH	1.98	4.70	1.54
[3 to 4 nitro] oLH**	2.70 to 3.2	2.7 to 3.3	2.3 to 3.5
[2 nitro] oLHß	1.82	0	1.61
[4 nitro] LHα	3.59	0.61	3.70
[5 nitro] LHα	4.5	0	4.20

---

*Prepared as indicated in Fig. 1 and 2. The numbers in brackets refer to number of nitro groups per molecule and should not be confused with the position of the $-NO_2$ group on the phenolic ring.

[a]Values are residues per mole of protein.

**These analyses are from the pooled data of six different preparations using TNM/Tyr ratios ranging from 25-fold (in molar ratio to tyrosine) to 50-fold. Values given are the extreme ranges on the analyses.

curve B. On analysis, four of the five tyrosine residues had been nitrated. However, if the nitration were done in the presence of 8 M urea (Fig. 1b, curve A) all five residues were nitrated.

In the case of oLHß subunit, nitration proceeded in a much more sluggish fashion. In Figure 1c, although the TNM/Tyr ratio was 20 to 1, after 1 hour a plateau had not yet been reached. At that point an additional charge of reagent was added and the nitration proceeded to completion within approximately 2 hours total reaction time.

In spite of slow addition of reagent and conducting the reaction at low temperature, polymerization was a very significant side reaction during nitration. This can be shown in Figure 2a for intact ovine LH -- only 25 to 30% was isolated as the monomeric form (solid bar) following reaction as in Figure 1a, curve A. As shown in Figure 2b, only 5 to 10% of the ovine LH was isolated in a monomeric form following reaction under conditions shown in Figure 1b, curve A. The oLHß subunit, although it nitrates more sluggishly and requires higher reagent concentration, exhibits less polymerization (Fig. 2c). In this experiment 60% of the subunit was recovered as a monomeric form. In this figure Ve/Vo ratios indicated are those characteristic of the intact LH or its subunits when chromatographed on Sephadex G-100. The solid bars indicate the fractions collected for further study.

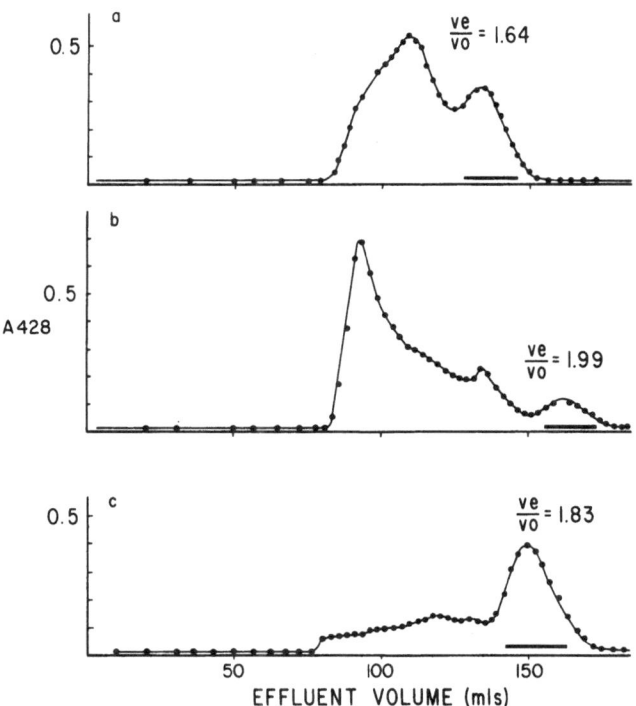

Figure 2 (a). Sephadex G-100 pattern for nitrated oLH (Curve A, Fig. 1a). Columns, 1.6 x 140 cm; eluant, 0.126 M-ammonium bicarbonate; flow rate, 25 ml/hr. Solid bar, material collected for study of composition and bioassay, Ve/Vo approximates that of native oLH. (b). Chromatography of oLHα nitration reaction product (Curve A, Fig. 1b); conditions as in 2a. (c). Chromatography of oLHß nitration reaction product (Fig. 1b). Conditions as per 2a.

The extent of nitration in the nitrated LH or nitrated LH subunits as isolated in Figure 2 was measured in two ways. First, the quantity of 3-nitrotyrosine detected by amino acid analysis following acid hydrolysis and its ratio to tyrosine (and

TABLE 3

YIELD AND POTENCY OF VARIOUS NITRATED LH DERIVATIVES

			Potency**	
Sample		Yield*	OAAD Assay	RLA Assay
Native oLH		-	2.54 (1.4-4.7)	1.00 (16.5 ng)
[1 nitro] oLH		30%	1.05 (0.5-2.4)	0.60 (27.5)
[2 nitro] oLH		25%	0.27 (0.2-0.5)	0.23 (80.0)
[3 to 4 nitro] oLH		25%	0.20 (0.09-0.4)	0.10 (160.0)

Recombination Products

oLHα +	oLHβ	85%	1.47 (0.7-3.1)	0.47 (35.0)
oLHα + [2 Nitro]	oLHβ	75%	0.65 (0.5-0.9)	0.54 (31.5)
[4 Nitro] oLHα +	oLHβ	40%	0.12 (0.07-0.2)	0.06 (280.0)
[5 Nitro] oLHα +	oLHβ	25%	0.03 (0.006-0.12)	<0.01

* Yield: Weight recovery as the designated fraction relative to
the nitration reaction starting material or, for recombinations,
the fraction of the theoretically possible yield with 100% efficiency.

**Potency: In the OAAD assay relative to NIH-LH-S18, values in
parentheses are 95% C.L.; in the RLA, relative to the native oLH
as estimated by ID_{50} (see text), values in parenthesis are ng at
50% Inhibition Dose.

phenylalanine as an internal standard) was measured. The spectro-
photometric determination of 3-nitrotyrosine at 428 nm was estimated on the isolated product using the molar extinction coefficient
reported by Riordan et al. (28). These analyses are summarized
in Table 2. The sum of the tyrosine and 3-nitrotyrosine residues
accounts for all of the tyrosine in the original molecules except in
the case of the higher degree of nitration in the intact LH. In this
case only six of the seven residues could be accounted for. The
results shown for the sample identified as [3 to 4] nitro LH represents the data range obtained with six different preparations and
separate analyses. In this respect our results more closely follow
the values presented by Cheng and Pierce (22), since Sairam et al.
were able to account for all seven of the tyrosine residues in their
most highly nitrated preparations. Whether the difference here
represents a labile nature for a certain portion of the nitrotyrosine
residues or further nitration products which are undetected under
our conditions of reaction and analysis cannot be stated.

We next studied the efficiency of recombination of the native
subunits and the native subunit plus nitrated subunit counterpart.

The results are summarized in Table 3. In this table the yield represents that portion of the sample on a weight basis which was recovered from a Sephadex chromatogram in the area representing the molecular weight of native LH (Fig. 3). For these studies only the monomeric form of the nitrated subunit has been employed for recombination. Recombination was done in 0.01M phosphate

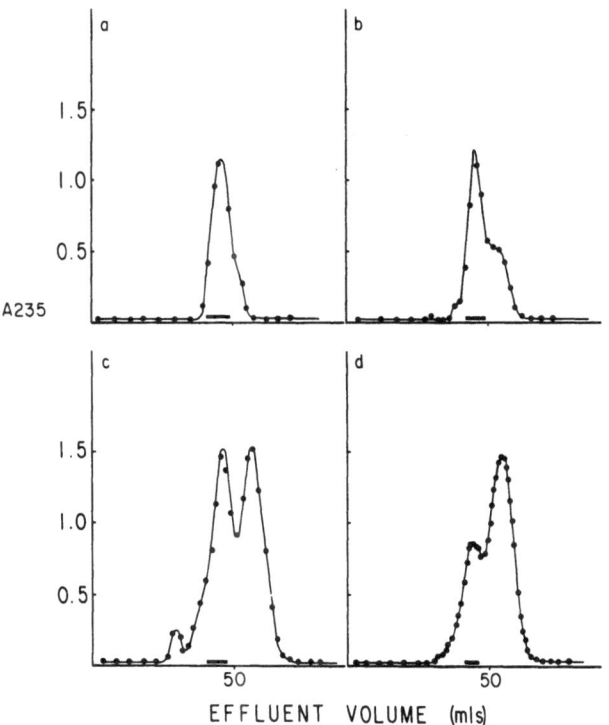

Figure 3. Sephadex G-100 chromatography of: a.) Recombined oLHα + oLHß. b.) oLHα + nitrated oLHß. c.) 4-nitro oLH + oLHß. d.) 5-nitro oLHα + oLHß. Solid bar designates fractions with Ve/Vo similar to native oLH, tubes pooled for further study.

buffer at pH 7, 37° for 24 hours with a total protein concentration of 2 mg/ml. Under these conditions the native oLHα recombined with the nitrated oLHß almost as well as did the two native subunits. The [4 nitro-] oLHα, plus the native beta subunit recombined about one-half as well as the native subunits. When the [5 nitro-]α alpha subunit was recombined with the beta subunit only one-third of the expected material was obtained with the molecular weight equivalent to that of LH.

From these results one may conclude that nitration of the
tyrosine residues in the beta subunit does not materially interfere
with the binding of the two subunits. On the other hand, it should
be recalled that nitration of the two tyrosines on the beta subunit
does not occur in the nitration of the intact LH (21, 22). This observation has also been confirmed in our studies. Separation of
the subunits from the nitrated LH preparations shown in Table 1
showed all the nitro-tyrosine was in the α-subunit. Yang and
Ward found a similar situation with regard to the iodination of the
tyrosines in intact LH (29).

In Table 3 are summarized our bioassay data for the nitrated
LH products as a function of the degree of nitration. Concerning
the nitration of the native LH, the biological potency of OAAD
assay or testicular radioligand assay of the one-nitro derivative
showed a potency of approximately 40% in the OAAD assay; the
two nitro derivative approximately 10% of the native LH; and
the three-to-four-nitro derivative of LH was not appreciably
reduced from the latter potency. The potency estimates in the
ovarian ascorbic acid depletion assay were based on assays
which had good parallelism in response. However, in the radioligand assay using the testicular homogenates the response of
various LH-derivatives was less likely to be parallel. For this
this reason we have adopted the practice of expressing potency
as that dose at which a 50% inhibition of binding of labeled LH
was obtained. This point will be further clarified by reference
to Figure 4. The radioligand assay showed good correlation

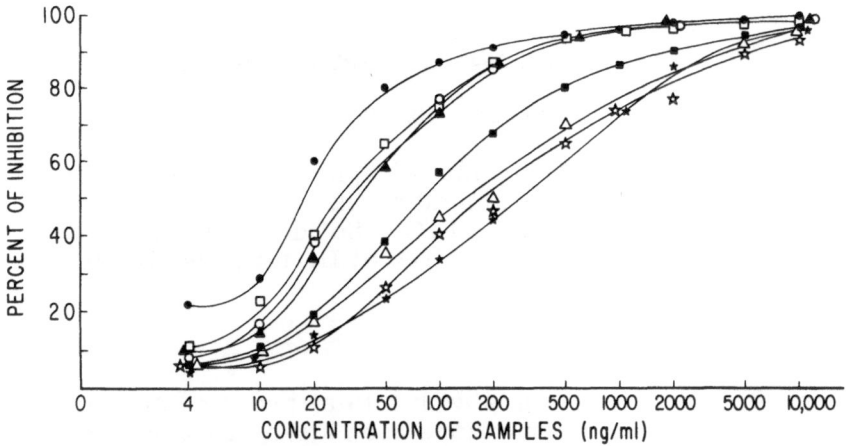

Figure 4. Competetive inhibition studies, radioligand assay.
Native oLH, •—•; [1-Nitro] oLH,□—□; oLH + oLHß,▲—▲; oLHα
+ nitrated -oLHß, o—o ; [2-Nitro]-oLH, ■—■; [3 to 4 nitro]-oLH
(2 separate preparations), △—△ or ☆—☆; and [4-nitro]oLHα +
oLHß, ★—★.

with the OAAD assay up through the [two-nitro] derivative. However, the difference between the [three-to-four-nitro] LH and
the [two-nitro] LH derivatives was much more apparent with
the radioligand assay than with the OAAD assay. The potency
of the recombined native subunit was about 65% that of the native
LH when measured by the OAAD assay. When native oLH*was
combined with the nitrated oLHß the potency was about 25%
that of the native LH in the OAAD assay. However, this derivative
showed a slightly, although not significantly, better ability
to compete with native LH for the receptor sites in the radioligand
assay than did the native subunit recombination product. The
[four-nitro] oLH*a* recombined with oLHß gave a potency only
5% that of the native LH and its slope in the competitive
binding assay was of a much different character than the native LH (Fig. 4). The recombination product from the five-nitro
oLH*a* plus native oLHß, gave a very slight response in the OAAD
assay and showed a detectable competition with labeled oLH in the
radioligand assay, comparable to the [4 nitro] oLH*a* plus oLHß
(curve for [5-nitro] oLH*a* + oLHß not shown).

From these results we conclude that the nitration of the tyrosine residues in the beta subunit does not sigificantly affect the
ability of the two subunits to recombine nor does it materially
affect the biological potency of the molecule as measured by its
ability to combine with the receptor site in the radioligand assay;
nevertheless, the activity as measured in the OAAD assay is significantly lower in this instance. When one nitrates more than one
residue of tyrosine on the alpha subunit the potency of the molecule
drops rapidly as studied by either the OAAD assay or the radioligand assay.

Our potency estimates by the OAAD method for the nitrated derivatives seem to agree quite closely, for comparable preparations, with the values reported by Sairam et al. (21). The estimates of potency reported by Cheng and Pierce (22), in general,
are considerably higher than ours or those of Sairam et al. (21)
wherever the direct comparisons may be applied.

We are unaware of comparable data for radioligand assays
versus in vivo bioassays with derivatives of a hormone. Others
have reported good correlation of radioligand data with data from
in vivo bioassays where similar materials are being compared
(30). In this sense the discontinuity in the relative potency
measurements between the two assays as one goes from the [3-
nitro]-derivatives to the [4-nitro]-derivative is noteworthy (Figure
4 and Table 5).

Amino Group Acylation Studies

In this portion of our studies we investigated the effect of

Table 4

Degree of Acylation of LH and its Subunits Expressed
as Epsilon - Amino Groups of Lysine Reacting

Material	Reaction*	
	Maleylation	Carbamylation
oLH	10 (12)	10 (12)
oLHα	9 (10)	9 (10)
oLH β	2 (2)	2 (2)

---

*Values are lysine residues reacting as determined by the method
of Habeeb (32) or the dinitrophenylation reaction (33). Values
in parentheses are total groups available in the molecule. The
NH_2-terminal amino acids were completely acylated in each reaction
(values not tabulated).

changing the charge on the amino groups in ovine LH and its subunits. For our present considerations we will refer to charge as
the anticipated charge on the fuctional group in consideration at
physiological pH range. Under these conditions the amino group
has a positive charge which we may convert to a neutral group,
in this study by carbamylation, or to a negative charge by maleylation. Using these treatments we have produced a series of derivatives which allow us to evaluate the charge effect on subunit-subunit interaction and hormone or hormone derivative interaction
with the hormone receptor site.

From the amino acid sequence studies (17-20) it is known that
there are 10 residues of lysine in oLHα and 2 in oLHß. There are
also free amino groups in the NH_2-terminal position of each subunit, although it has not been settled to our satisfaction that there
is not a portion of the molecules in the oLHß subunit which may
also be acylated to the extent of 50 to 60% on the NH_2-terminus.
The maleylation and carbamylation reactions employed in the present studies will be detailed elsewhere (31). It is sufficient to
state for our present purposes that these reactions were carried
out by conventional procedures, the carbamylation with cyanate
at pH 8 and the maleylation with maleic anhydride at pH 8. To
estimate the number of amino groups reacting we employed the
method of Habeeb (31) or the Sanger reaction as detailed by
Fraenkel-Conrat et al. (32), coupled with amino acid analysis.

These acylation reactions were carried out on the intact oLH,
or the isolated alpha and beta subunits. The final products were

The final products were purified by chromatography on Sephadex G-100. In Figure 5 are presented typical chromatograms obtained in the purification and isolation of the respective derivatives for the maleylation series. A similar set of chromatograms was obtained for the carbamylation studies.

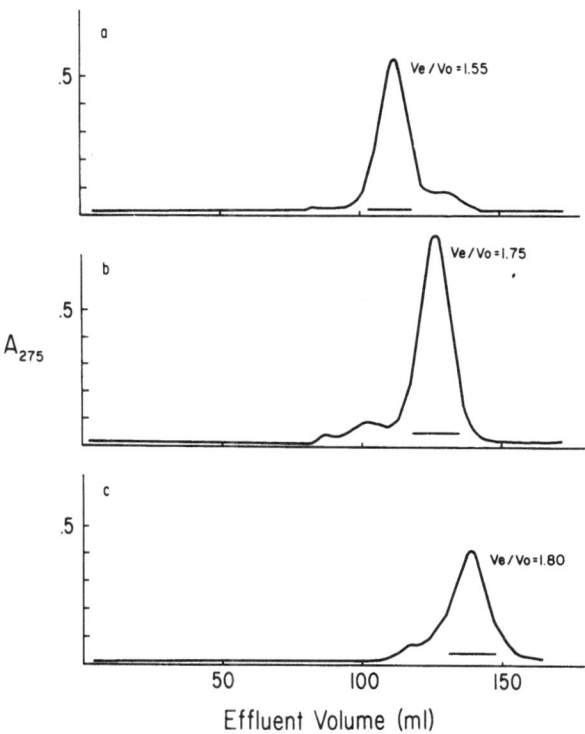

Figure 5. The elution pattern of maleylated oLH and its modified subunits on Sephadex gel G-100 column, 1.6 x 140 cm; eluant, 0.126 M NH_4HCO_3; flowrate: 30 mls/hr; solid bar: fractions pooled for study. a) maleylated oLH; b) maleylated oLHα ; c) maleylated oLHß.

It was clear that not all of the amino groups were available for reaction with either the maleylation or carbamylation reagents. In Table 4 is summarized the number of epsilon amino lysine groups reacting in the preparation of each derivative. The data are tabulated in terms of epsilon lysine amino groups reacting, but it should be noted that in no instance was there evidence that the amino terminal group did not react, e.g. all the amino termini were blocked at the end of the acylation reactions.

TABLE 5

YIELD AND POTENCY OF VARIOUS ACYLATED LH DERIVATIVES

		Potency*	
Sample	Yield*	OAAD Assay	RLA Assay
Native oLH		2.54 (1.4-4.7)	1.00 (16.5 ng)
maleylated oLHα + oLHβ	60%	0.04 (0.03-0.07)	0.02 (1100.)
oLHα + maleylated oLHβ	80%	0.07 (0.02-0.1)	0.03 (510.)
maleylated oLHα + maleylated oLHβ	30%	0.07 (0.01-0.15)	< 0.001
Native oLHα + oLHβ	85%	1.47 (0.7-3.1)	0.47 (35.0)
Carbamylated oLHα + oLHβ	75%	0.04 (0.02-0.07)	0.01 (2350.)
oLHα + carbamylated oLHβ	80%	1.46 (0.7-2.9)	0.71 (23.0)
carbamylated oLHα + carbamylated oLHβ	75%	0.04 (0.02-0.07)	< 0.001

*See Footnotes to Table 3 for description.

    With the availability of the foregoing LH and LH-subunit deri-
vatives we next studied the efficiency of recombination of the subunit derivatives as a measure of the effect of the substituent group
on this ability, and the biological activity of the resulting product
with a molecular weight approximating that of the native LH. (As
a course measure of the substituent's effect on the ability of the
subunits to recombine we have taken the percent yield of an LH-
like molecular weight product as defined by chromatography on
Sephadex G-100.) The respective chromatograms have been summarized in Figures 6 and 7 for the maleyl and carbamyl derivatives. The material with a molecular weight similar to that of
native LH thus defined was obtained after a "standard" recombination period (24 hours at pH 7.0 with 0.01 M phosphate buffer at
37° C). From the material pooled as indicated by the heavy bar
in Figures 6 and 7, the numerical estimate of the recombination
product shown in Table 5 was obtained. In this Table is also
summarized the biological activity for the various fractions and
combination products. As in the previous section, biological
activity has been estimated by both the ovarian ascorbic acid depletion assay (24) and by the radioligand assay (26). Again, with

Figure 7. The elution patterns of the various recombined products of carbamylated subunits on Sephadex gel G-100 column.
Condition same as Fig. 3. a) oLHα + oLHß; b) carbamylated oLHα
+ oLHß; c) oLHα + carbamylated oLHß; d) carbamylated oLHα +
carbamylated oLHß.

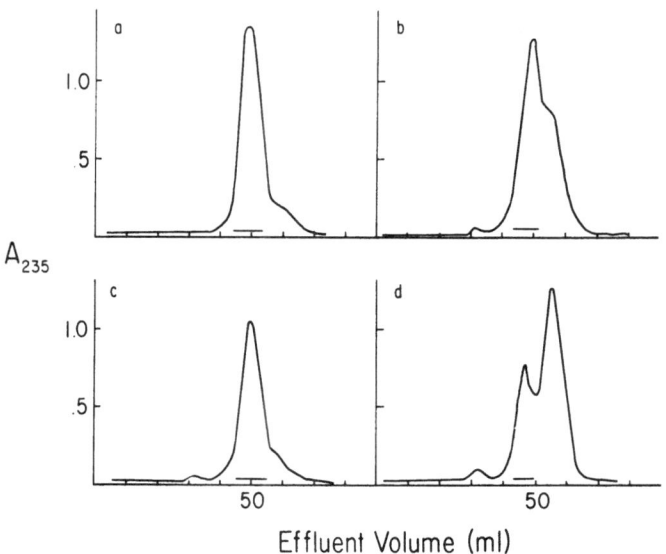

Figure 6. The elution patterns of the various recombined products of maleylated subunits on Sephadex gel G-100 column. Column size: 0.9 x 150 cm; eluant: 0.126 M NH$_4$HCO$_3$; flow rate: 5 ml/hr; solid bar: pooled fraction; a) native oLH α + oLHß; b) maleylated oLH α + oLHß; c) oLH α + maleylated oLHß; d) maleylated oLH α + maleylated oLHß.

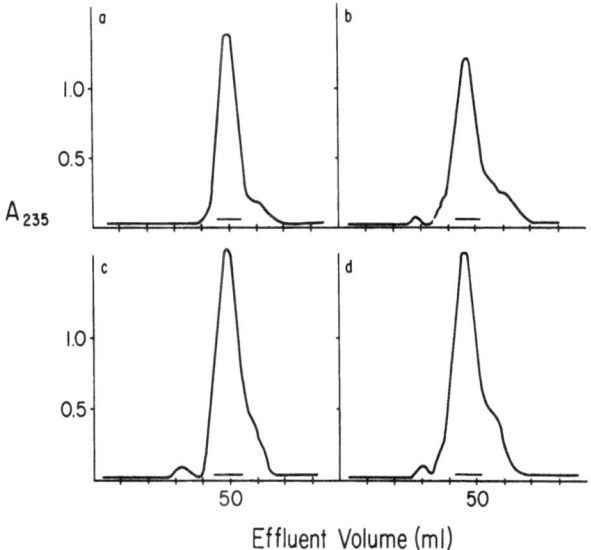

the latter assay it was expedient to use a 50% inhibition point as
a measure of potency rather than comparative dose responses in
parallel line assays.

Directing our attention to the maleyl derivatives we may draw
the following conclusions: The maleylated oLHß combined with its
native counterpart as well as the native subunits recombine, however, the maleylated oLHα did not combine with native oLHß as
well as the native subunits. When combination of the two
maleylated subunits was attempted the recombination was very
poor, giving rise to only 30% weight recovery of a product
approximating the size of native oLH. Concerning the biological
activity of the maleylated derivatives, it is clear that maleylation
of intact LH inactivated the hormone. As one might expect from
this finding the recombinant of the two maleylated subunits also
gave a product which was virtually devoid of activity. The combined products of oLHα + maleylated oLHß and maleylated oLH α +
oLHß also gave very little activity.

From the fact that two amino groups do not react when intact
LH is maleylated we may conclude that two epislon amino lysine
groups are "buried" or "masked" by the subunit interaction. We
may then presume that there are two such groups which are not
available for interaction with the hormone receptor site. It may
also be concluded that the remaining amino groups, either all or
part of them, are essential for hormone receptor site interaction
in that blockage with a maleyl (i.e. negative) group prevents this
expression of biological activity.

If we turn now to the carbamylation studies we may draw still
further conclusions. There were two residues "buried" or
"masked" in the subunit interaction and therefore not carbamylated in the intact ovine LH. This is similar to what was shown in
the maleylated LH series. Again the carbamylated oLH, the carbamylated oLH α + native oLHß and the carbamylated oLHα + carbamylated oLHß showed very little activity by either assay. On
the other hand, native oLH α combined with carbamylated oLHß
showed an activity equivalent to that of the recombined native subunits. From this we conclude that the amino groups on the beta
subunit may be either positively charged (e.g. the native subunit
series) or neutral (the carbamylated derivative of the beta subunit)
without significantly impairing either the ability of the subunits to
combine with each other or the hormone receptor site. We favor
the interpretation that this is a charge effect rather than a steric
effect of the acylating reagent, since the difference between the
neutral carbamylated derivative and the negatively charged maleylated derivative is so great. Nonetheless, the experiments provide no absolute distinction between charge effects and steric
effects for the acylating reagents.

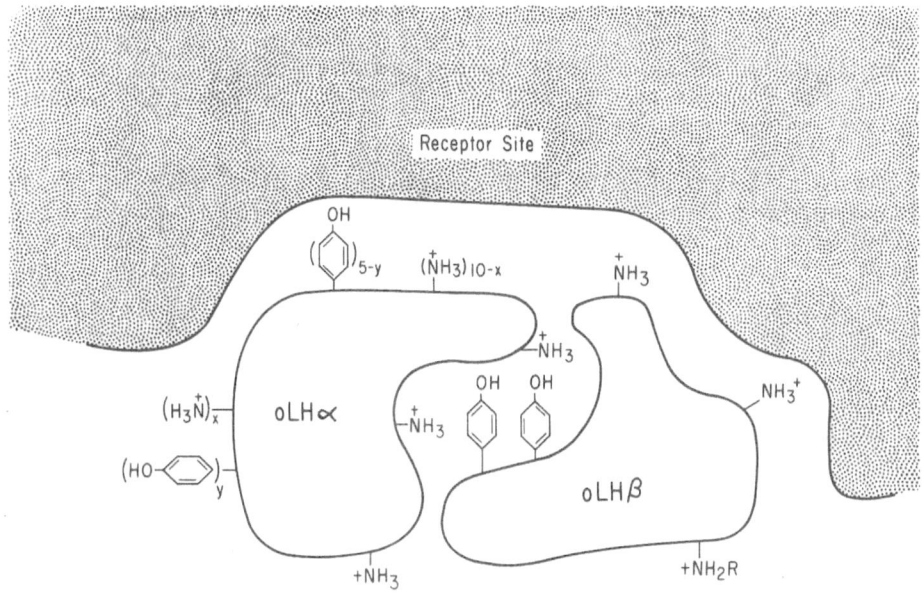

Figure 8. (This figure was added at the conference in response to a request for a summarizing diagram and has been refined from the extemporaneous diagram presented then.) This figure is intended to convey the following ideas which derive from the presentation: a) The receptor site requires a conformational fit generated by the alpha and beta subunit working ensemble and not individually. b) Two tyrosine residues on the ß-subunit are buried in the interaction between the two subunits. Although non-reactive (nitration or iodination) in native LH they may undergo nitration in the isolated subunit without deleterious effect. c) The remaining 5 tyrosines are on the α-subunit; y of these tyrosines are not affected by nitration and/or do not participate in the receptor site interaction, while 5-y of these tyrosines are essential to biological activity or receptor site interaction. The data suggest y may be any integer from 1 to 4. d) The amino termini (drawn at the bottom of the figure) appear from present and previous data not to be involved in subunit association or receptor site interaction. For the ß-subunit R may be either H or an unidentified acyl group. e) Two amino groups on the ß-subunit are involved in the receptor site interaction and must be either neutral or positively charge. f) Two amino groups on the α-subunit appear involved in subunit-subunit interaction and are masked to acylation reactions. g) There are x epislon lysine amino-groups on the α-subunit which are not involved in the receptor site interaction or the subunit-subunit interaction and 10-x epsilon lysine amino groups involved in receptor site interaction. The data suggest x may be any integer from 2 to 8.

Studies are in progress which will identify the individual reacting (or not reacting) lysine or tyrosine residue under the various conditions employed in the studies presented in this paper.
However, the number of preparations to be examined is large and
these data are not yet available.

In summary, the results of the nitration studies indicated that
the two tyrosines in oLHß are buried in native oLH and do not react. If they are nitrated in isolated oLHß they do not materially
interfere with subunit recombination nor biological activity.

For the remaining five tyrosine residues in oLHα they show
different degrees of reactivity toward nitration. Depending on the
conditions of nitration a derivative with one, two or three to five
nitro groups may be obtained. If only one group is nitrated biological activity is decreased by approximately 50%, but if more than
one group reacts the activity drops rapidly to less than 10% that
of the native hormone.

The acylation studies showed that the NH_2-termini and ten of
twelve lysine- ε-amino groups are on the periphery of the molecule
(i. e. readily reactive) but two of the latter are buried and do not
react. One of ten lysine residues in the isolated alpha subunit is
also buried to acylation. The two lysine residues on the beta subunit readily acylated. It did not matter what charge was on these
beta subunit residues for good subunit recombination but a requirement for a positive or neutral charge was shown for good biological activity. Acylation of the alpha subunit showed all or part
of the amino groups on this subunit with a positive charge are
essential for biological activity. The method would not distinguish if only a portion of these amino groups were essential. Substitution of a neutral or negative charge on the alpha subunit amino
groups was less crucial to subunit-subunit recombination, a negative charge substitution being the most deleterious.

Acknowledgements

This investigation was supported in part by Contract NIH-69-
2221, Center for Population Research, National Institute of Child
Health and Human Development; Research Grant AM-09801,
Institute for Arthritis, Metabolism and Digestive Diseases; The
Robert A. Welch Foundation (G-147); and the Population Research
Institute of the Southwest Foundation for Research and Education,
San Antonio, Texas.

References

1. Li, C. H., Simpson, M. E., and Evans, H. M., J. Biol.
Chem. 131: 259, 1939.

2. Geschwind, I. I., and Li, C. H., Endocrinology 63: 449, 1958.

3. Gan, J., Papkoff, H., and Li, C. H., Biochim. Biophys. Acta 170: 189, 1968.

4. Adams-Mayne, M., and Ward, D. N., Endocrinology 75: 401, 1964.

5. Li, C. H., and Starman, B., Nature 202: 291, 1964.

6. Ward, D. N., and Arnott, M. S., Anal. Biochem. 12: 296, 1965.

7. Papkoff, H., Gospodarawicz, D., Candiotti, A., and Li, C. H., Arch. Biochem. Biophys. 111; 431, 1965.

8. Papkoff, H., Proceedings of the VIth Pan-American Congress of Endocrinology (Mexico City), Exerpta Medica International Cong. Series, No. 112, 1965, p. 334.

9. Ward, D. N., Fujino, M., and Lamkin, W. M., Fed. Proc. 25: 348, 1966.

10. Papkoff, H., and Samy, T.S.A., Biochim, Biophys. Acta 147: 175, 1967.

11. Ward, D. N., Sweeney, C. M., Holcomb, G. N., Lamkin, W. M., and Fujino, M., in Progress in Endocrinololgy, Gual, C. (ed.), Excerpta Medica, Amsterdam, 1969, p. 385.

12. Swaminathan, N., and Bahl, O. P., Biochem. Biophys. Res. Commun. 40: 422, 1970.

13. Lamkin, W. M., Fujino, M., Mayfield, J. D., Holcomb, G. N., and Ward, D. N., Biochim. Biophys. Acta 214: 290, 1970.

14. Pierce, J. G., Liao, T-H., and Carlsen, R. B., Hormonal Prot. Peptides 1, 17, 1973, Academic Press, New York and London.

15. Morgan, F. J., and Canfield, R. B., Endocrinology 88: 1045, 1971.

16. Ward, D. N., Reichert, L. E., Jr., Liu, W-K., Nahm, H. S., Hsia, J., Lamkin, W. M., and Jones, N. S., Recent Prog. Hormone Res. 29: 533, 1973.

17. Liu, W-K., Nahm, H. S., Sweeney, C. M., Lamkin, W. M., Baker, H. N., and Ward, D. N., J. Biol. Chem. 247: 4351, 1972.

18. Liu, W-K., Nahm, H. S., Sweeney, C. M., Holcomb, G. N., and Ward, D. N., J. Biol. Chem. 247: 4365, 1972.

19. Sairam, M. R., Papkoff, H., and Li, C. H., Arch Biochem. Biophys. 153: 554, 1972.

20. Sairam, M. R., Samy, T.S.A., Papkoff, H., and Li, C. H. Arch. Biochem. Biophys. 153: 572, 1972.

21. Sairam, M. R., Papkoff, H., and Li, C-H., Biochim. Biophys. Acta 278: 421, 1972.

22. Cheng, K-W., and Pierce, J. G., J. Biol. Chem. 247: 7163, 1972.

23. Ward, D. N., and Liu, W-K. Proceed. Sec. Intnl. Symp. Liege, Sept. 28-Oct. 1, 1971, Excerpta Medica, Margoulies, M. and Greenwood, F. C., (eds.), 1972, pp. 80-90.

24. Parlow, A. F., in Human Pituitary Gonadotropins, Albert, A., (ed.), C. C. Thomas Co., Springfield, Ill., 1961, pp. 300.

25. Catt, K. J., Dufau, M. L., and Tsuruhara, T., J. Clin. Endocr. 34: 123, 1972.

26. Leidenberger, F. L., and Reichert, L. E., Jr., Endocrinology 91, 901, 1972.

27. Lee, C-Y., and Ryan, R. J., Proc. Nat. Acad. Sci. USA 69: 3520, 1972.

28. Riordan, J. F., Sokolovsky, M., and Vallee, B. L., Biochemistry 6: 3609, 1967.

29. Yang, K. P., and Ward, D. N., Endocrinology 91: 317, 1972.

30. Reichert, L. E., Jr., Leidenberger, F., and Trowbridge, C. G., Recent Prog. Hormone Res. 29: 497, 1973.

31. Habeeb, A.F.S.A., Anal. Biochem. 14: 328, 1966.

32. Fraenkel-Conrat, H., Harris, J. I., and Levy, A. L., in Methods of Biochemical Analysis 2: 359, 1955.

CONFORMATIONAL AND METABOLIC ASPECTS OF GONADOTROPINS

David Puett, Mario Ascoli, and Leslie A. Holladay

Department of Biochemistry, Vanderbilt University

Nashville, Tennessee 372 32

Introduction

The gonadotropins represent an interesting class of glycoprotein hormones that are comprised of two non-identical subunits, termed α and ß, each with a molecular weight of approximately 15,000. The α-subunit appears common to the gonadotropins and to TSH[1] and it is the ß-subunit that confers hormonal specificity.

Recent studies by a number of investigators have established the primary structure of LH from several species, hCG, and TSH. These hormones are characterized by a high content of prolyl residues and disulfides, and, with but one or two exceptions, the absence of tryptophan. However, little is known regarding the conformation of the gonadotropins. Of particular interest is a comparison of the subunit conformations with that of the intact, biologically active gonadotropins in order to elucidate the conformational changes that may occur upon subunit association.

The molecular mechanisms that are involved in gonadotropin catabolism and clearance are also poorly understood. It is well established that sialic acid is important in the circulatory properties of hCG and human FSH (1), but LH from some species contain little or no sialic acid, e.g. oLH and bLH, and it is of interest to compare their circulatory properties with those of sialic acid containing glycoprotein hormones.

Materials and Methods

oLH was extracted from sheep pituitaries using essentially the method of Koenig and King (2) to obtain the gonadotropin fraction. Purification was achieved by using ion-exchange chromatography, DEAE-Sephadex (3) and CM-Sephadex (4) and gel filtrattion (Sephadex G-100). Small amounts of oLH and bLH were purified from the NIH preparations using the aforementioned anion and cation exchangers and gel filtration. (Identical biological and physico-chemical results were obtained with the two preparations of oLH.) hLH was a highly purified product kindly provided by Dr. Aida Nureddin (5). hCG was purified from the Organon preparation using anion-exchange (DEAE-Sephadex) chromatography essentially as described by Bahl (6). oLH subunits were prepared by counter-current distribution (7) and hCG subunits were prepared using a slight modification of the ion-exchange method following incubation with urea (8).

Ovarian ascorbic acid depletion bioassays were performed according to Parlow (9). The in vitro assays were based on the stimulation of steroidogenesis by rat testis in vitro (10). The CD[1] spectra were obtained using a Cary 60 spectropolarimeter equipped with a CD attachment.

Results and Discussion

Conformation of Gonadotropins

CD spectroscopy has been extremely useful in evaluating certain conformational aspects of proteins (11). The far uv region of the spectrum is due primarily to the peptide group and can yield both qualitative and quantitative information on secondary structure, e. g. α -helicity and ß-structure. For several years, poly-L-lysine has been used as a standard for assessing protein CD spectra. Recently, Chen et al (12)

---

[1]The abbreviations are: CD, circular dichroic; GuHCl, guanidine hydrochloride; NAG, N-acetylglucosamine; NAL, N-acetylgalactosamine; NANA, N-acetylneuraminic acid; R, rotational strength of circular dichroic bands; SDS, sodium dodecyl sulfate; T, testosterone.

Table I

Rotational Strengths of the Major Resolved Gaussian Bands of
Standard Protein Conformations (190-230 nm) and of the Gonadotropins
(200-230 nm) [a]

Conformation	λo, nm	$Rx10^{40}$	Gonadotropin	λo, nm	$Rx10^{40}$
α-helix	222	-21.0[b]	o LH	209	-0.9[d]
α-helix	208	- 6.3[c]	o LH	215	-2.0[b]
α-helix	193	+34.3[c]	b LH	208	-0.7[d]
β-structure	227	+ 3.4	b LH	215	-2.6[b]
β-structure	215	- 7.8[b]	h LH	205	-2.0[d]
β-structure	196	+ 1.4[c]	h LH	214	-2.9[b]
non-helix	226	- 1.7	h CG	207	-1.9[d]
non-helix	197	- 7.3[c]	h CG	215	-2.1[b]

a. The rotational strength, R, in cgs units was determined from
    Gaussian parameters as described elsewhere (13); λo represents
    the wavelength corresponding to the extremum of the resolved
    band.

b. Assigned to the peptide n-π*transition.

c. Assigned to the peptide π-π*transition.

d. Assigned to the N-acetylated amino sugars of the carbohydrate
    moiety.

have determined average CD spectra for α-helical regions, ß-
structure, and non-helix by analyzing the CD spectra of five
proteins whose conformation is known from x-ray crystallographic studies. We have resolved these spectra and the results,
which will be used for comparing gonadotropin CD spectra, are
given in Figure 1 and Table I.

The far uv CD spectrum of LH from three species and of
hCG is shown in Figure 2. and the rotational strengths of the
major resolved bands (13) are given in Table I. The gonadotropin far uv CD spectra are characterized by a negative
extremum in the vicinity of 207-212 nm with a shoulder at about
214 nm. Similar spectra showing the 210-212 nm negative extremum have been reported for oLH (14-16) and bLH (17). Between

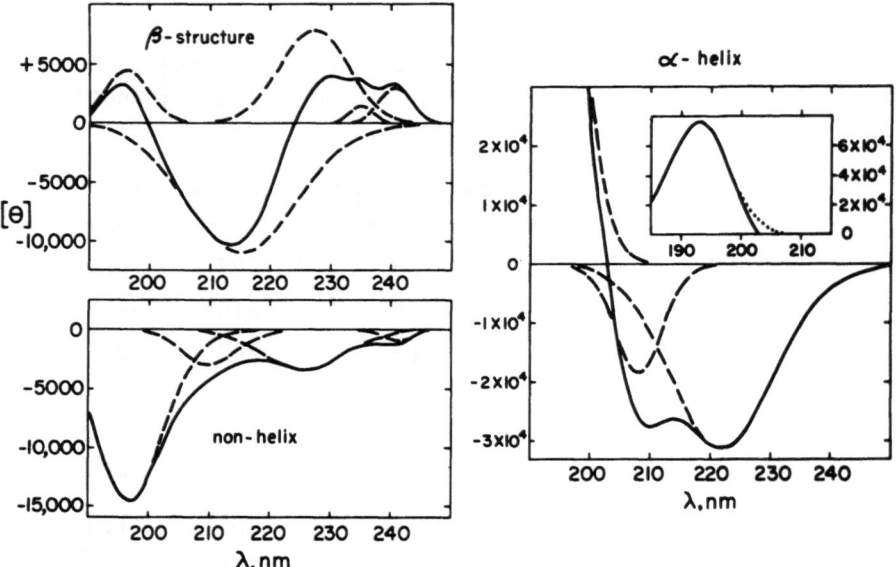

Figure 1. The solid lines denote the average far uv CD spectrum (i.e., reduced mean residue ellipticity vs. wavelength) of the α-helical, ß-structrue, and non-helical conformation in several globular proteins of known crystallographic structures reported by Chen et al. (12). These spectra, arising mainly from the peptide chromophore, have been resolved and the constituent Gaussian bands are indicted by dashed lines.

200-230 nm the major resolved bands occur at about 205-209 nm and 215-216 nm, and it is these Gaussian bands that produce the gonadotropin 207-212 nm negative extremum. The 215-216 nm resolved band probably arises from the peptide n-π* transition associated with ß-structure (Fig. 1). A comparison of the rotational strength of this resolved gonadotropin band with that found from Figure 1, and an analysis of the overall spectrum, indicates the presence of about 20-30% ß-structure in the gonadotropins. In Figure 2 there is no evidence of the peptide n-π* transition at 222 nm that is associated with α-helicity, thus showing the absence of this form of secondary structure in gonadotropins.

The conventional conformations of proteins (Fig. 1) do not exhibit major bands in the region corresponding to the gonadotropin 207-212 extremum, or even to the resolved 205-209 nm band. (The 206-209 nm π-π* component parallel to the helix axis can be ruled out in the case of gonadotropins since this particular band will always be accompanied by the 222 nm n-π* band.) Although

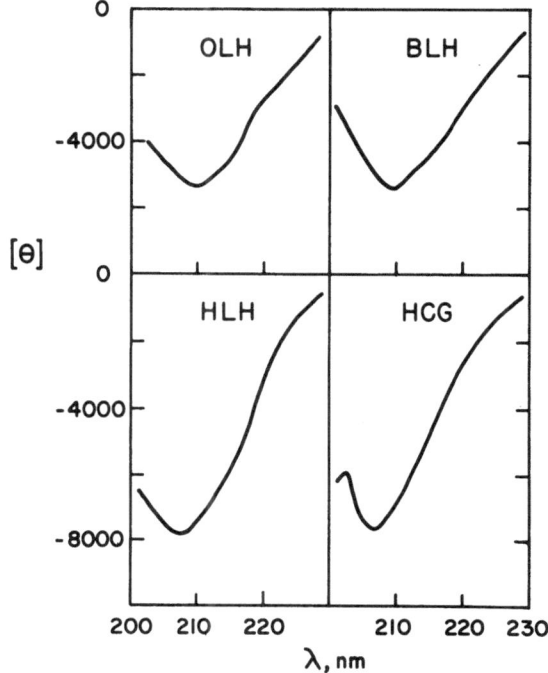

Figure 2. The far ultraviolet CD spectrum of several gonadotropins in 50 mM KCl, 10mM Na$^+$ -phosphate (pH 7). The mean α
residue ellipticity is based on the protein moiety. The spectrum
for hLH is from Puett, D., and Neureddin, A.

many amino-acid side-chains exhibit optically active CD bands
in the far ultraviolet (11), based on the wavelengths of the extrema
it appears doubtful that any of these could be responsible for the
207-212 nm extremum. Bewley and Li (16) concluded that the
carbohydrate component of oLH could not contribute significantly
to the ellipticity in this region. In contrast, we have evidence
which indicates that the carbohydrate moiety of the gonadotropins
makes a major contribution to the CD spectrum in the region of
207-212 nm.

Figure 3 shows the CD spectrum of hCG glycopeptides. These
were prepared by digesting reduced, S-carboxymethylated hCG
with pronase, followed by purification using gel filtration. Chemical analysis indicates that most of the hCG oligosaccharides are
attached (via asn and ser linkages) to very short peptides, e.g.,
2-4 residues, although one of the glycopeptides contains a longer

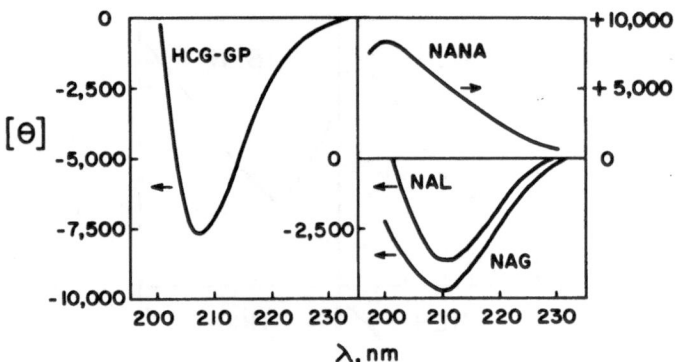

Figure 3. The left panel shows the CD spectrum of the hCG glycopeptides with the ellipticity representing the decimolar ellipticity based on the sum of NAG, NAL, and NANA. The right panels
show the CD spectra of NAG, NAL, and NANA.

stretch of amino-acid residues presumably arising from the C-
terminal region of the ß-subunit. The spectrum is characterized
by a negative band at 207 nm, analogous to the 207 nm extremum
in native hCG. We have also obtained the CD spectra of glycopeptides prepared from ovalbumin, thyroglobulin, and α_1 -acid glycoprotein, and these all exhibit negative CD extrema between 207-
212 nm.[2] The right panels of Figure 3 show the CD spectra of
NAG, NAL, and NANA. The former two N-acetylated amino
sugars exhibit negative CD bands in the vicinity of 211-212
nm, while the ellipticity of NANA is positive and of lower magnitude than the others in this region.

The rotational strength of the resolved 207 nm band in the
hCG glycopeptides is considerably greater than that expected
from the NAG, NAL, and NANA content. This suggests that the
asymmetry of the entire oligosaccharide moiety is considerably
enchanced over that of the component N-acetylated amino sugars.
The rotational strength of 207 nm resolved band in hCG (based on
NAG, NAL, and NANA) is greater than that found for the glycopeptides. This is not surprising since the asymmetric protein
moiety probably restricts the flexibility of the oligosaccharies
and enhances the rotational strength.

Thus, the 207-212 nm negative CD extremum in gonadotropins

[2]Puett, D., Wasserman, B. K., Ford, J. D., and Cunningham,
L. W., unpublished observations.

is believed to represent the net of two negative CD bands. The at 215-216 nm is assigned to the n-π* transition associated with ß-structure in the protein moiety and the band at 205-209 nm is assigned to the N-acetylated amino sugars in the carbohydrate moiety. Within the latter, NAG probably makes the greatest contribution since it is present in the greatest amount, and also has the greatest magnitude of ellipticity (Fig. 3). We have found that the neutral sugars present in the gonadotropins (i.e., mannose, galactose, and fucose) exhibit negligible ellipticity above 200 nm. This represents the first assignment of carbohydrate in CD spectroscopy of glycoproteins.

The near uv CD spectra of proteins can yield valuable information on the localized environment due to tertiary structure of aromatic chromophores and disulfides (11,13). This is shown for hCG in Figure 4 where the near uv CD spectrum is given for native hCG and reduced, S-carboxymethylated hCG in 6 M GuCHl (i.e., an equimolar mixture of unfolded α and ß subunits). The enhanced optical activity of native hCG arises primarily from the tertiary and quaternary structure.

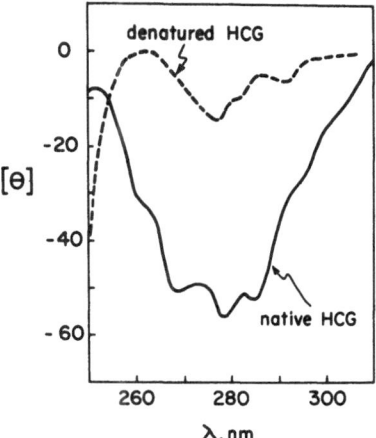

Figure 4. The near uv CD spectrum of native hCG (—) at pH 7 (50 mM KCl, 10 mM Na⁺ -phosphate) and of reduced, S-carboxymethylated hCG in 6 M GuHCl (---), i.e., a mixture of nonstructured α and ß subunits.

The complete CD spectra of hCG, oLH, and their subunits are given in Figures 5 and 6. These spectra have been resolved

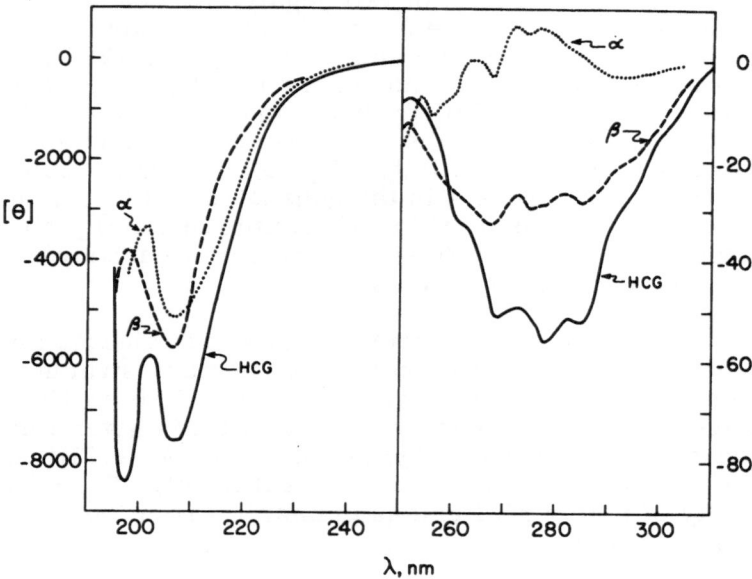

Figure 5. The near (right) and far (left) uv CD spectrum (—) of hCG, hCG-α , and hCG-ß. The ordinate for the near uv CD spectrum represents the mean residue ellipticity based on the protein moiety. The buffer consisted of 50mM KCl and 10 mM Na$^+$ -phosphate (pH 7).

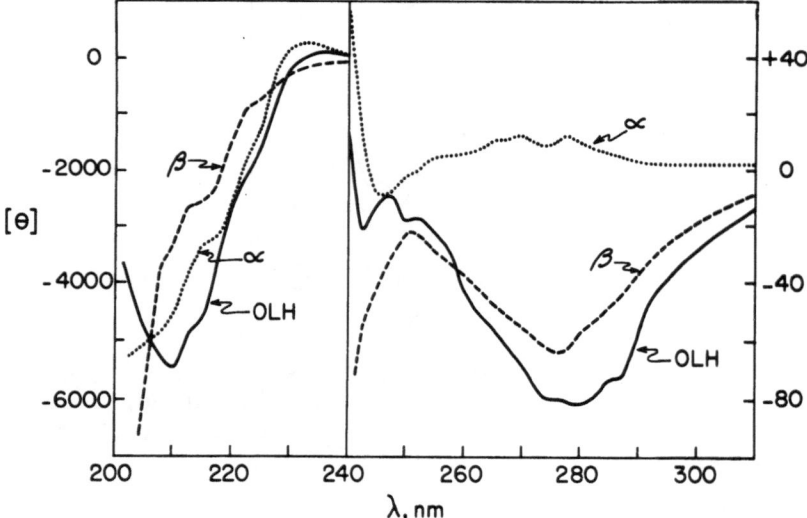

Figure 6. CD spectra similar to Fig. 5 for oLH. To enhance solubility (of the ß-subunit in particular) all buffers contained 6% (v/v) dioxane. The spectrum of oLH either with or without dioxane was essentially the same.

and assignments to the resolved bands will be discussed elsewhere. It can be seen that most of the near uv optical activity of
the intact gonadotropins arises from the ß-subunit. A comparison
of the near uv CD spectra of unfolded hCG in 6 M GuHCl with that
of hCG-ß shows the retention of a considerable amount of tertiary
structure in the ß-subunit. A detailed analysis of the far uv CD
spectra indicates that the subunits probably contain somewhat less
ß-structure than the intact gonadotropin.

Figure 7 shows the near uv CD difference spectrum for hCG
and oLH. The major negative extremum corresponds to tyrosyl
CD bands as does the positive band in oLH. This indicates that
the localized environment of one or more tyrosines is altered.
Such changes could result from the presence of tyrosine(s) at the
subunit interface or from small conformation changes in the subunits upon dissociation.

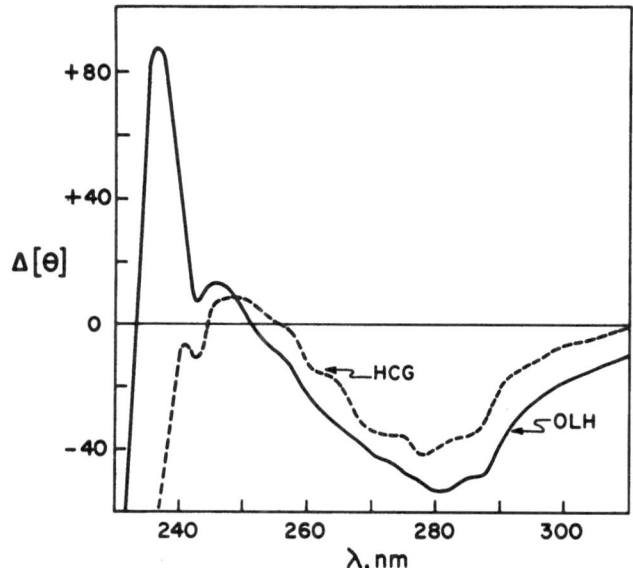

Figure 7. The near uv CD difference spectrum (i.e., the molecular ellipticity for intact hormone minus the sum of the molecular
ellipticities of the subunits) for hCG and oLH. In order to make
the ordinate comparable with Figs. 5 and 6 the difference spectrum has been divided by the number of amino-acid residues in
the intact gonadotropins.

Metabolism of Gonadotropins

Little is known regarding the molecular events responsible for the catabolism and clearance of proteins and hormones. Recent studies by Ashwell and co-workers (1) have shown that sialic acid is an important determinant in the circulatory behavior of many glycoproteins and glycoprotein hormones, e.g., hCG and human FSH. Desialylation results in rapid removal from circulation by the parenchymal cells of the liver.

Some of our data on the glycoprotein fetuin in mature male rats are shown in Figure 8 where the percent of the injectd radio-actively labeled glycoprotein and asialoglycoprotein remaining in plasma is shown as a function of time after injection. The intact glycoprotein circulates with an apparent half-life of about 2 hours, whereas that of the asialo-derivative is only several minutes. These particular data were obtained by using both reductive methylated (18) ^{14}C-fetuin and fetuin labeled with tritium at the carbohydrate moiety (19).

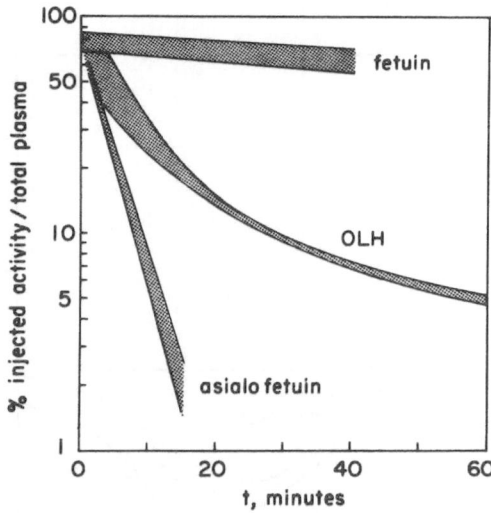

Figure 8. The plasma disappearance profile of radioactivity labeled fetuin, asialo-fetuin, and oLH as a function of time following a single intravenous injection at time zero into mature male rats. The data for fetuin and asialo-fetuin were obtained using both protein and carbohydrate labeled glycoprotein. The results of oLH were obtained on tritiated material; we found that the injection of either 1.6 or 32 μg of ^{3}H-oLH resulted in identical plasma disappearance profiles.

Using reductive methylation (borotritide), we have prepared
^{3}H-oLH with high specific activity (650 μCi/mg) and no loss of
biological activity. For example, the ovarian ascorbic acid
depletion bioassay gave a potency (95% confidence limits) of
1.94 U/mg (1.24-3.60) compared to the value of 1.97 U/mg
(1.27-3.53) before labeling. Analysis of ^{3}H-oLH showed high
specificity in that greater than 95% of the tritium was in the lysyl
groups. Dimethyllysine was the major derivative (82.5%), mono-
methyllysine accounted for 2.6%, and 14.9% of the ϵ-amino groups
unmodified.

Also shown in Figure 8 is the circulatory disappearance profile
of ^{3}H-oLH in mature male rats. On the semi-logarithmic plot
there are at least two distinct phases with apparent half-lives of
about 5-10 minutes and 180 minutes. Thus, the terminal fucose
in oLH does not mimic sialic acid in prolonging the circulatory
half-life of the majority of oLH. We have obtained similar data
on hLH which, despite the fact that it contains sialic acid, behaves
like oLH. This is in contrast to the circulatory behavior of hCG
and human FSH, both of which contain greater amounts of sialic
acid than hLH. We are presently investigating the relative importance of the protein and carbohydrate components of LH in determining its circulatory properties.

The time course of tissue uptake of ^{3}H-oLH is given in
Figure 9 for intact mature male rats. (Similar data were obtained
in hypophysectomized animals). It can be seen that urine and kidney contain the greatest amount of radioactivity. Within the first
60 minutes we estimate that about 0.77 ng of ^{3}H-oLH (per gm of
tissue) are located in the testes; at greater times this approximately doubles. SDS-polyacrylamide gel electrophoresis of urine
samples of rats that had been injected with ^{3}H-oLH failed to
demonstrate the presence of material of smaller size than the
control, i.e., ^{3}H-oLH subunits. This was shown in urine samples obtained up to 60 minutes after injection. These results
suggest that there is little, if any, degradation into low molecular
weight components during renal excretion. Likewise, the plasma
^{3}H-oLH seems to be undegraded as monitored by gel filtration.

Preliminary data have been obtained on the renal catabolism
of ^{3}H-oLH. The results were obtained by injecting rats with
^{3}H-oLH; after various times the animals were sacrificed and the
kidneys were quickly removed and homogenized. The four major
subcellular fractions (i.e., nuclei, mitochondria, lysozomes,
microsomes and cytosol) were obtained by differential

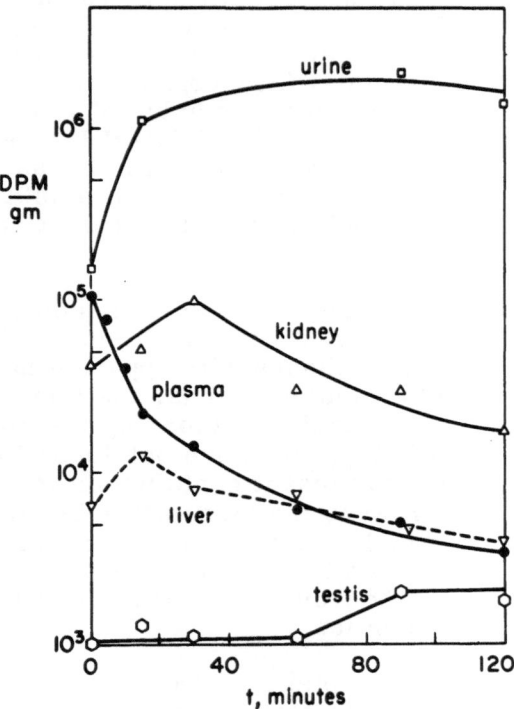

Figure 9. Plasma disappearance and tissue uptake of ^{3}H-oLH following a single intravenous injection of 1.6 μg into mature (intact) male rats at time zero. The ordinate represents dpm/gm of tissue for liver, kidney, and testis and dpm/ml for plasma and urine. The recovered radioactivity in the tissues and fluids was always near 100%.

centrifugation and some of our data are shown in Figure 10. These results show that cytosol contains the greatest percentage of both total and TCA soluble radioactivity. Moreover, the percentage of TCA soluble radioactivity increases with time, at least up to four hours. Liver was also found to promote degradation.

These data demonstrate the importance of renal catabolism and excretion in clearing LH from circulation. We know from the work of Dufau et al. (20) that hCG is neither degraded nor inactivated by the gonadotropin receptors of rat testis. Therefore, it appears that renal excretion of apparently intact LH is important in regulating the level of circulating LH. As yet we do not know if the urinary LH is biologically active.

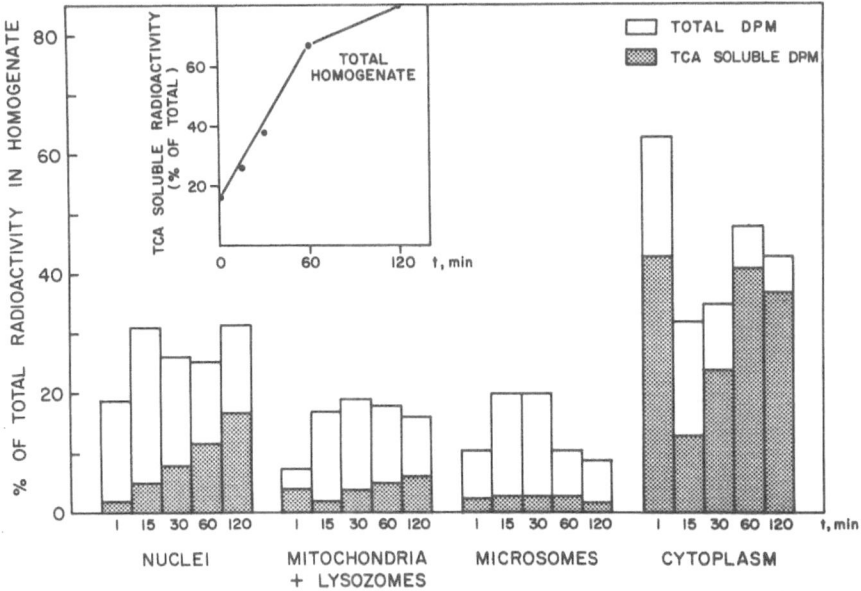

Figure 10. The distribution of radioactivity in various subcellular fractions of rat kidney following an intravenous injection at time zero. Results are given for total dpm and TCA soluble dpm's. The inset shows the variation of the TCA soluble dpm's in the homogenate as a function of time after injection.

Mechanism of Action

A lengthy discussion of the mechanism of gonadotropin action in the testes is outside the scope of this paper. Figure 11 summarizes some of our recent studies involving H-oLH binding and the stimulation of steroidogenesis and of cAMP production by oLH in rat testis. These results show that the level of tissue cAMP is maximal at 30 minutes; in contrast, the stimulation of steroidogenesis continues to increase for several hours (10). The extent of binding is near the maximal value after about 30 minutes. These results on the stimulation of steroidogenesis and cAMP production agree well with those of Rommerts et al. (21) using hCG. Dufau et al. (22), however, found that the tissue levels of cAMP reached a maximum at about 2 hours after hCG stimulation.

Clearly, much remains to be done to elucidate the structural and metabolic relationships of gonadotropins, and to clarify the complex intracellular events involved in gonadotropin action.

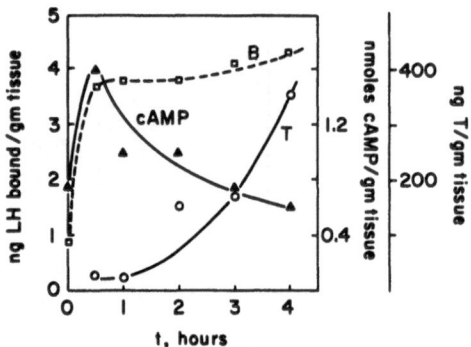

Figure 11. The time dependence of steroidogenesis (T), binding (B), and tissue cAMP levels following the addition of 20 ng of ^{3}H-oLH to rat testis in vitro.

Summary

Circular dichroic spectra are presented for luteinizing hormone from several species and for human chorionic gonadotropin. The far ultraviolet spectrum is interpreted in terms of ß-structure (ca. 20-30%) in the protein moiety and the N-acetylated amino sugars in the carbohydrate moiety. A comparison of the near ultraviolet circular dichroic spectrum of the subunits with that of the intact gonadotropin indicates that the localized environment of one or more tyrosyl residues is altered when the subunits associate to form a biologically active hormone. Also, the subunits appear to have less ß-structure than the intact gonadotropin. Metabolic studies demonstrate the importance of the kidney in the removal of luteinizing hormone from circulation. Following the kinetics of ovine luteinizing hormone binding to rat testis (in vitro), we found that the extent of binding is maximal after about 30 minutes. Testicular cAMP levels reach a maximum in 30 minutes, whereas steroidogenesis increases with time (at least up to four hours).

Acknowledgements

This work was supported by the National Institutes of Health (Research Grant AM-15838, Training Grant HD-00334, and the Center for Population Research and Studies in Reproductive Biology, HD-05797) and in part by the Camille and Henry Dreyfus Foundation. It is a pleasure to thank Betty Kay Wasserman, Gudrun Moustafa, John D. Ford and Rodger Liddle for expert technical assistance.

References

1. Morell, A. G., Gregoriadis, G., Scheinberg, I. H., Hickman, J., and Ashwell, G., J. Biol. Chem. 246: 1461, 1971.

2. Koenig, V. L., and King, E., Arch. Biochem. Biophys. 26: 219, 1950.

3. Pierce, J. G., Liao, T. H., Howard, S. M., Shome, B., and Cornell, J. S., Recent Progr. Hormone Res. 27: 165, 1971.

4. Ward, D. N., McGregor, R. F., and Griffin, A. C., Biochim. Biophys. Acta 32: 305, 1959.

5. Neureddin, A., Hartree, A. S., and Johnson, P., in Saxena, B. B., and Gandy, H. M. (eds.) Gonadotropins, Wiley-Interscience, New York, pp. 167, 1972.

6. Bahl, O. P., J. Biol. Chem. 244: 567, 1969.

7. Papkoff, H., and Samy, T. S., Biochim. Biophys. Acta 147: 175, 1967; Reichert, L. E., Jr., Rasco, M. A., Ward, D. N., Niswender, G. D., and Midgley, A. R., Jr., J. Biol. Chem. 244: 5110, 1969.

8. Swaminathan, N., and Bahl, O. P., Biochem. Biophys. Res. Comm. 40: 422, 1970.

9. Parlow, A. F., in Albert, A. (ed.) Human Pituitary Gonadotropins, C. C. Thomas, Springfield, pp. 300, 1961.

10. Dufau, M. L., Catt, K. J., and Tsuruhara, T., Endocrinology 90: 1032, 1972.

11. Adler, A. J., Greenfield, N J., and Fasman, G. D., Met. Enzymol. 27D: 675, 1973.

12. Chen, Y., Yang, J. T., and Martinez, H. M., Biochemistry 11: 4120, 1972.

13. Puett, D., Biochemistry 11, 1980, 1972; Zahler, W. L., Puett, D., and Fleischer, S., Biochim. Biophys. Acta 255: 365, 1972.

14. Jirgenson, B., and Ward, D. N., Texas Rep. Biol. Med. 28: 553, 1970.

15.   Pernollet, J. C., and Garnier, J., FEBS Letters 18: 189, 1971.

16.   Bewley, T. A., Sairam, M. R., and Li, C. H., Biochemistry 11: 932, 1972.

17.   Cheng, K. W., Glazer, A. N., and Pierce, J. G., J. Biol. Chem. 248: 7930, 1973.

18.   Means, G. E., and Feeney, R. E., Biochemistry 7: 2192, 1968; Rice, R. H., and Means, G. E., J. Biol. Chem. 246: 831, 1971.

19.   Morell, A. G., and Ashwell, G., Met. Enzymol. 28B: 205, 1972, Van Lenten, L. and Ashwell, G., ibid., 209, 1972.

20.   Dufau, M. L., Catt, K. J., and Tsuruhara, T., Proc. Natl. Acad. Sci. 69: 2414, 1972.

21.   Rommerts, F.F.G., Cooke, B. A., Van Der Kemp, J.W.C.M., and Van Der Molen, H. J., FEBS Letters 24: 251-1972.

22.   Dufau, M. L., Watanabe, K., and Catt, K. J., Endocrinology 92: 6, 1973.

THE ROLE OF CARBOHYDRATE IN THE BIOLOGICAL
FUNCTION OF HUMAN CHORIONIC GONADOTROPIN

Om P. Bahl, Leopold März and William R. Moyle
Department of Biochemistry
State University of New York at Buffalo
Buffalo, N. Y. 14214

and

Laboratory of Human Reproduction
and Reproductive Biology
Harvard Medical School
Boston, Mass. 02115

The binding sites or the so-called receptors for polypeptide and glycoprotein hormones such as insulin (1), glucagon (2), adrenocorticotropin (3), human chorionic gonadotropin (4-6), luteinizing hormone (7-9), and follicle stimulating hormone (10, 11) are located on the plasma membranes of the target cells. The binding is characterized by the high degree of affinity and hormonal specificity, which suggests that the binding sites must have highly specific chemical structures. It is not clearly understood whether all of the sites are equivalent. Moyle and Ramachandran have suggested the presence of more than one type of receptor on Leydig cells for LH with different affinities for the hormone; the sites which induce steroidogenesis have higher affinity than those which stimulate the accumulation of cyclic AMP (12). That the receptors are protein in nature is indicated by their properties after solubilization from the corpora lutea or interstitial tissue from testes with nonionic detergents (13). It is not known, however, whether the receptors are composed of one or several proteins or if any prosthetic groups such as lipids or polysaccharides are also present. The precise chemical elucidation of the receptors must await until all of its components are identified and purified.

The bulk of the evidence, derived from several lines of

125

experiments, strongly suggests that these hormones including gonadotropins exert all of their biological effects by interaction with the plasma-membrane sites without entrance in the cells. It is not understood, however, how the signal from the exterior of the cell is transmitted into the cell, triggering various molecular events. Consequently, the first step in the understanding of the molecular mechanism of hormone action is to elucidate the nature of the binding of the hormone to the receptors and the precise chemical nature of the receptors.

The glycoproteins and glycolipids are essential components of cell surfaces and play an important role in diverse cell surface phenomena such as interaction with macromolecules, cell recognition, cell adhesion, and contact inhibition. It is, therefore, conceivable that the carbohydrate may be involved in the interaction of hCG with its receptors and as a result may effect the various metabolic functions including the stimulation of accumulation of cyclic AMP by hCG, protein synthesis and steroidogenesis. The present work is an attempt to evaluate the role of carbohydrate in the hormone-receptors interactions and in the various biological properties of the hormone. hCG is a glycoprotein which binds to the plasma membranes with an association constant of the order of 10^{10} M^{-1} (4, 6). In fact, gonadotropins provide good model compounds for the evaluation of the function of carbohydrate in glycoproteins at the target site level (14) in addition to their previously postulated role in the secretion (15), and metabolic clearance of proteins (16, 17).

Carbohydrate moiety of hCG. hCG contains approximately 30% carbohydrate (18) which is distributed in seven carbohydrate units, four of them being linked N-glycosidically to the asparaginyl residues and the remaining three O-glycosidically to the seryl residues (19-21). The asparagine-linked carbohydrate units are bulky, complex and multiple-branched (19), and are located at positions 52 and 78 (Fig. 1) in the a subunit (20), and at positions 13 and 30 (Fig. 2) in the ß subunit (21). The serine-linked carbohydrate units are short linear oligosaccharide chains and are present only in the ß subunit at positions 118, 129, and 131. The average monosaccharide sequence (Fig. 3) in a single branch of the complex carbohydrate unit, determined by sequential removal of the monosaccharides with specific glycosidases, is NANA(Fuc)-Gal-GluNAc-Man- (22). The monosaccharide sequence (Fig. 3, structure III) in a serine-linked carbohydrate unit is reported to be NANA-Gal-GalNAc-. Evidently, hCG has two types of carbohydrate-protein linkages in the same molecule. Only a few other examples of glycoproteins of this type have been reported thus far (20).

Experimental approach. hCG and plasma membranes were sequentially hydrolyzed with purified specific glycosidases (22).

H-Ala-Pro-Asx-Val-Glx-Asx-Cys-Pro-Glx-Cys-Thr-Leu-Glx-Glx-Asx-Pro-Phe-Phe-Ser-Glx- (10) (20)

Pro-Gly-Ala-Pro-Ile-Leu-Gln-Cys-Met-Gly-Cys-Cys-Phe-Ser-Arg-Ala-Tyr-Pro-Thr-Pro- (30) (40)

Leu-Arg-Ser-Lys-Lys-Thr-Met-Leu-Val-Gln-Lys-[Asn(CHO)]-Val-Thr-Ser-Glx-Ser-Thr-Cys-Cys- (50) (60)

Val-Ala-Lys-Ser-Tyr-Asn-Arg-Val-Thr-Val-Met-Gly-Gly-Phe-Lys-Val-Glx-[Asn(CHO)]-His-Thr- (70) (80)

Ala-Cys-His-Cys-Ser-Thr-Cys-Tyr-Tyr-His-Lys-Ser-OH (90)

Figure 1. Linear amino acid sequence of hCG-α.

H-Ser-Lys-Gln-Pro-Leu-Arg-Pro-Arg-Cys-Arg-Pro-Ile-[Asn(CHO)]-Ala-Thr-Leu-Ala-Val-Glu-Lys- (10) (20)

Glu-Gly-Cys-Pro-Val-Cys-Ile-Thr-Val-[Asn(CHO)]-Thr-Thr-Ile-Cys-Ala-Gly-Tyr-Cys-Pro-Thr- (30) (40)

Met-Thr-Arg-Val-Leu-Gln-Gly-Val-Leu-Pro-Ala-Leu-Pro-Glx-Leu-Val-Cys-Asn-Tyr-Arg- (50) (60)

Asp-Val-Arg-Phe-Glu-Ser-Ile-Arg-Leu-Pro-Gly-Cys-Pro-Arg-Gly-Val-Asn-Pro-Val-Val- (70) (80)

Ser-Tyr-Ala-Val-Ala-Leu-Ser-Cys-Gln-Cys-Ala-Leu-Cys-Arg-(Arg)-Ser-Thr-Thr-Asp-Cys- (90) (100)

Gly-Gly-Pro-Lys-Asp-His-Pro-Leu-Thr-Cys-Asp-Asp-Pro-Arg-Phe-Gln-Asp-[Ser(CHO)]-Ser-Ser- (110) (120)

Lys-Ala-Pro-Pro-Pro-Ser-Leu-Pro-[Ser(CHO)]-Pro-[Ser(CHO)]-Arg-Leu-Pro-Gly-Pro-Pro-Asx-Thr-Pro- (130) (140)

Ile-Leu-Pro-Gln-Ser-Leu-Pro-OH

Figure 2. Linear amino acid sequence of hCG-ß.

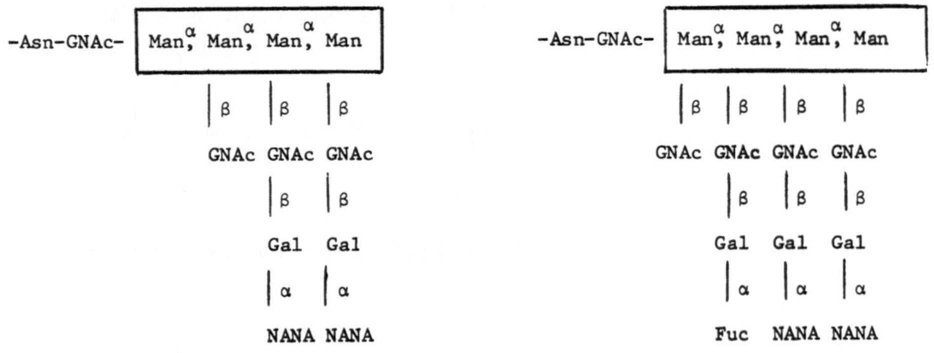

-Asn-GNAc- | Man $\overset{\alpha}{,}$ Man $\overset{\alpha}{,}$ Man $\overset{\alpha}{,}$ Man |

|β |β |β

GNAc GNAc GNAc

|β |β

Gal Gal

|α |α

NANA NANA

Structure I

-Asn-GNAc- | Man $\overset{\alpha}{,}$ Man $\overset{\alpha}{,}$ Man $\overset{\alpha}{,}$ Man |

|β |β |β |β

GNAc GNAc GNAc GNAc

|β |β |β

Gal Gal Gal

|α |α |α

Fuc NANA NANA

Structure II

-Ser-GalNAc-Gal-NANA

Structure III

Figure 3. Structure I, sequence of the monosaccharides in the carbohydrate of the α subunit; Structure II, sequence of the monosaccharides in the asparagine-linked carbohydrate of the ß subunit; Structure III, sequence of the monosaccharides in the serine-linked carbohydrate of the ß subunit.

The resulting modified forms of hCG were examined for their ability to compete for binding to the membrane receptors using ^{125}I-labeled hCG, prepared by the method of Greenwood and Hunter (23). The 2000 g fraction of the rat testes homogenate (4) or partially purified membrane preparations (24) were used in these studies. In order to further ascertain the role of the carbohydrate in the binding, monosaccharides, oligosaccharides, and glycoproteins were tested for their inhibitory properties. Such an approach is analogous to the inhibition of agglutination of red cells by phytoagglutinins by specific haptenes, monosaccharides or oligosaccharides (25). Also, the possible involvement of the cell surface glycosyltransferases in the binding, by carrying out the binding experiments in the presence of appropriate nucleotides as inhibitors, has been considered. The effect of the inhibitors of glycosidases on the binding has been investigated.

The effect of glycosidase-treated hCG derivatives on the

Table I

Preparation of hCG derivatives by glycosidases

Sample	% hydrolysis
hCG	
N-hCG[a]	99.
NG-hCG	60.0
NGA-hCG	52.5
NGAM-hCG-1	19.0
NGAM-hCG-2	b

[a]hCG treated sequentially with V. cholerae neuraminidase (N-hCG), then with A. niger β-D-galactosidase (NG-hCG), then with A. niger β-N-acetylglucosaminidase (NGA-hCG), and finally with A. niger α-D-mannosidase (NGAM-hCG-1).

[b]NGAM-hCG-2 was obtained by treating hCG with all of the glycosidases simultaneously. The percent of each sugar hydrolyzed is as follows: NANA, 99; Gal, 45; GluNAc, 39; Man, 14.

accumulation of cyclic AMP by hCG and steroidogenesis was measured by using a suspension of Leydig cells (26). The cyclic AMP was determined by protein binding method with or without the presence of theophylline (26) as described earlier (12) and testosterone by radioimmunoassay (27).

Digestions of hCG and plasma membranes with glycosidases. The following glycosidases vibrio cholerae neuraminidase (22), Aspergillus niger ß-D-galactosidase, ß-N-acetylglucosaminidase (28), and α-D-mannosidase (29), free of cross contamination and proteases, were employed. The hormone was treated sequentially with the glycosidases at 37° under nitrogen for an extended period of time. After each enzyme treatment, the sugar released was separated from the enzymatic digest by dialysis and was estimated by gas chromatography (22). Each modified form of the hormone was freed of the enzyme by chromatography (Fig. 4) on DEAE-cellulose (DE-52, Whatman). Table I gives the percentage of each monosaccharide removed from the hormone by the various enzymes. The neuraminidase hydrolyzed almost all of the sialic acid. The ß-D-galactosidase, ß-N-acetyl-glucosaminidase, and α-Dmannosidase liberated approximately 60, 55 and 20% of the total galactose, N-acetylglucosomine, and mannose residues

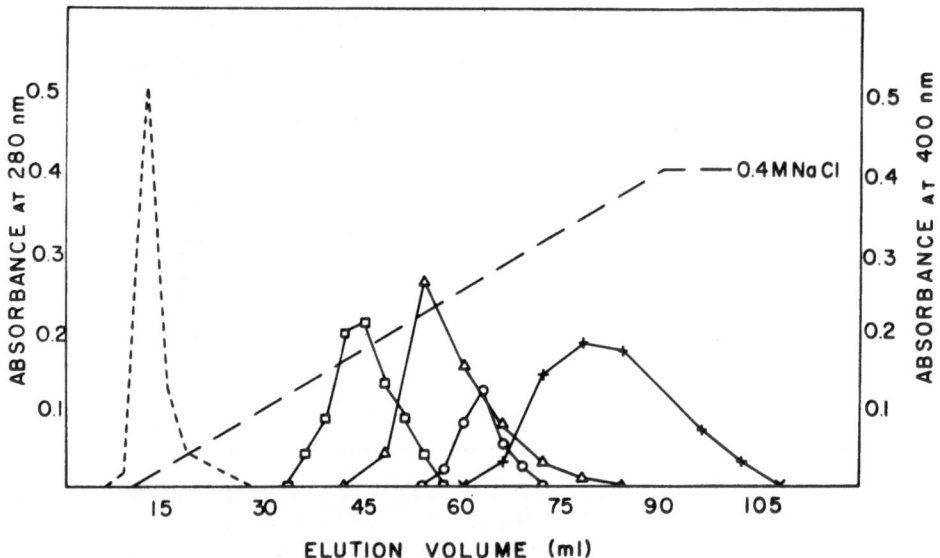

Figure 4. Separation of the hCG derivatives from glycosidases on a DEAE-cellulose column (0.7 x 18 cm), previously equilibrated with 0.05 M sodium acetate. After elution with 10 ml of the starting solution a linear salt gradient was set up between 0 and 0.4 M NaCl in 0.05 M sodium acetate (40 ml each). 3 ml fractions were collected. ------, hCG derivatives, □—□—□—□ , neuraminidase; —Δ—Δ—Δ . ß-galactosidase x-x-x-x , ß-N-acetylglucosaminidase; o—o—o , α-mannosidase.

present in hCG, respectively. The hormone was also degraded using all of the above enzymes simultaneously (NGAM-hCG-2).

The resulting modified forms of hCG, neuraminidase-(N-hCG), neuraminidase-ß-galactosidase-(NG-hCG), neuraminidase-ß-galactosidase-ß-N-acetylglucosaminidase (NGA-hCG), and neuraminidase-ß-galactosidase-ß-N-acetylglucosaminidase-α-mannosidase treated hCG (NGAM-hCG-1) were characterized chemically by analyzing for amino acids, hexosamines, and neutral sugars. The results summarized in Table II indicate that there was no apparent degradation of the polypetpide chain during the modification of the carbohydrate. Also, an examination of the various derivatives of hCG on Sephadex G-100 ensured that the dissociation of the hormone had not occurred during the hydrolysis of the carbohydrate. This was further supported by their high immunological activities as determined by radioimmunoassay.

Table II

Amino acid[a] and hexosamine compositions of hCG
and glycosidase-treated hCG derivatives

Amino Acid	N-hCG[b]	NG-hCG	NGA-hCG	NGAM-hCG-1	hCG
Lysine	10.4	11.8	12.1	11.1	12.1
Histidine	4.1	4.1	4.3	3.1	4.1
Arginine	15.2	15.6	18.7	19.5	18.8
Aspartic acid	17.7	18.0	18.0	17.2	15.5
Threonine	16.9	17.3	17.7	14.9	16.3
Serine	19.0	19.5	21.0	22.4	16.5
Glutamic acid	19.1	18.4	18.3	18.2	17.1
Proline	29.9	30.2	29.1	32.0	33.5
Glycine	13.2	14.7	14.3	18.9	13.8
Alanine	13.5	14.4	12.9	14.4	12.6
Half-cysteine	21.8	19.7	18.0	16.0	20.4
Valine	18.6	18.1	18.6	18.8	18.7
Methionine	3.9	3.4	2.9	1.3	3.2
Isoleucine	6.8	5.7	6.1	6.5	6.2
Leucine	15.3	15.2	15.1	14.7	16.6
Tyrosine	6.9	6.0	5.7	4.8	7.3
Phenylalanine	6.3	6.1	5.6	4.8	6.3
N-acetyl-glucosamine	9.6		5.2		
N-acetyl-galactosamine	1.7		2.0		

[a]Represents the number of residues.

[b]hCG treated sequentially with V. cholerae neuraminidase (N-hCG), then with A. niger β-galactosidase (NG-hCG), then with A. niger β-N-acetylglucosaminidase (NGA-hCG), and finally with A. niger α-D-mannosidase (NGAM-hCG-1).

The plasma membranes were also treated with glycosidases
in a similar manner. However, one of the problems encountered
during their digestion was that the membrane receptors were
partially inactivated at the pH optima of the enzymes (pH 4 to
5.5). Therefore the duration of the hydrolysis was kept at a
minimum for 5 hours, and a large excess of the enzymes was
used. Under these restricted conditions, only neuraminidase
and ß-D-galactosidase caused considerable hydrolysis as measured by the liberation of neuraminic acid and galactose.

Immunological activities of the glycosidase-treated hCG
derivatives. The removal of almost all of the sialic acid did not
cause any significant loss in the immunological activity of hCG
as determined by radioimmunoassay. Subsequent cleavage of 60%
galactose residues, however, resulted in a slight drop in the
immunological activity. This is contrary to the report by
Tsuruhara et al. (14) in which the authors did not find any change
in the activity on the removal of galactose. In fact, we observe
a slight decrease in the activity with the cleavage of each of the
monosaccarides (Table III, Fig. 5). This may be due to the
element of instability or the conformational change introduced in

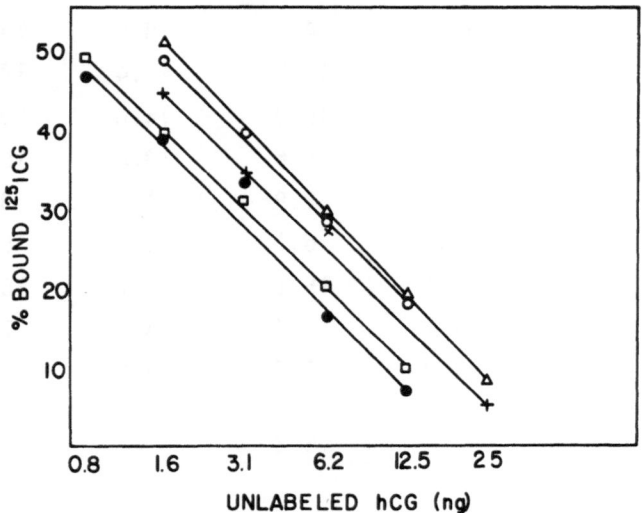

Figure 5. Radioimmunoassay of hCG derivatives: ●—●—● ,
native hCG;   □ —□—□ , N-hCG; △—△—△ , NG-hCG,
x—x—x , NGA-hCG; o—o—o , NGAM, hCG.

the molecule as a result of the degradation of the carbohydrate
since a sample of NGAM-hCG-1, stored at -10° for several weeks,
resulted in a considerable loss in the immunological activity

Table III

Immunological and binding properties of hCG
and glycosidase-treated hCG derivatives

Sample	Immunological[a] activity (%)	Binding activity[b] ng
hCG	100	17.5
N-hCG[d]	93 ± 10	7.5
NG-hCG	78 ± 10	11.0
NGA-hCG	68 ± 10	21.0
NGAM-hCG-1	71 ± 10	c

[a] Determined by radioimmunoassay; values are averages of four assays.

[b] Amount of protein required to decrease the binding of ^{125}I-hCG by 50%.

[c] 10 ng decreased the binding of ^{125}I-hCG by 16%, 20 ng by 19%, and 40 ng by 25%.

[d] hCG treated sequentially with V. cholerae neuraminidase (N-hCG), then with A. niger β-D-galactosidase (NG-hCG), then with β-N-acetyl-glucosaminidase (NGA-hCG), and finally with A. niger α-D-mannosidase (NGAM-hCG-1).

whereas the freshly prepared derivatives, NGAM-hCG-1 and NGAM-hCG-2, invariably were found to be active. It is, therefore, believed that the antigenic determinants are probably not located in the carbohydrate part of the molecule particularly in the sialic acid, galactose, N-acetylglucosamine, and mannose residues. The role of the fucose residues in the antigenicity has not been evaluated so far.

Effect of carbohydrate on the binding. The removal of sialic acid resulted in a twofold increase in the binding activity as evidenced by the decreased amount of asialo-hCG required to

Table IV

Effect of mono- and oligosaccharides, glycoproteins,
lactones, and nucleotides on the binding
to the homogenate[a] and to the membranes

Sample	% Binding homogenate[a]	Membranes
Fetuin (400 µg)	100	99
Desialyzed fetuin (400 µg)	81	62
α_1-Acid glycoprotein (400 µg)	99	100
Desialyzed α_1-acid glycoprotein (400 µg)	71	38
Thyroglobulin (500 µg)	100	100
hCG-α (0.5 µg)	-	25
hCG-β (0.5 µg)	-	30
Monosaccharides (galactose, mannose, fucose (NANA)	104	
Methyl-α-D-mannopyranoside	101	
Methyl-β-D-galactopyranoside	100	
Methyl-α-D-fucopyranoside	109	
Man $1 \overset{\rightarrow}{\alpha} 4$ GluNAc	110	
Man $1 \overset{\rightarrow}{\alpha} 6$ GluNAc	99	
Man $1 \overset{\rightarrow}{\alpha} 3$ GluNAc	102	
Lactofucopentaose I	106	
Lactofucopentaose II	100	
Lactofucopentaose III	98	
2-O-α-fucosyl galactose	102	
3-Fucosyl lactose	98	
Sugar lactones	101	
Nucleotides (CMP, UDP, GDP)	100	

[a] 2000 g fraction.

displace 50% of the ^{125}I-labeled hCG from the membranes (Table III, Fig. 6). Furthermore, the removal of sialic acid from hCG

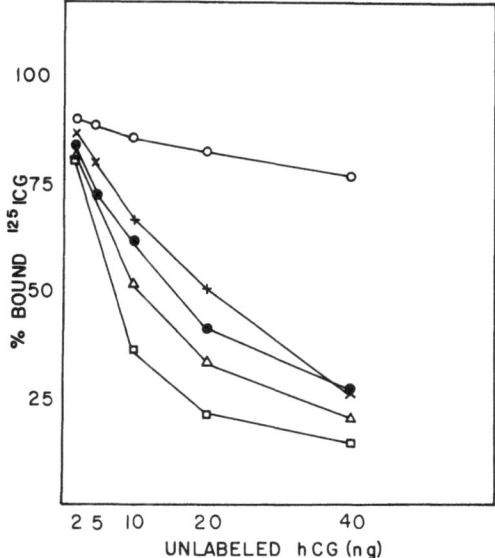

Figure 6. Competitive binding of hCG derivatives to membrane receptors using rat testes homogenate. The assay was carried out for 4 hours at 25° C; ● — ● — ● , native hCG; □—□ —□ , N-hCG; △− △—△ , NG-hCG, x— x—x , NGA-hCG; o— o—o , NGAM-hCG.

increased the uptake of asialo ^{125}I-hCG by about 50% (Fig. 7). This enhancement in binding was most likely due to the charge effect. Only a small portion of it might be attributed to the non-specific binding of asialo ^{125}I-hCG, possibly to sialyl transfer-ases, since about 10% of the radioactivity remained bound to a 2000 g pellet in the presence of an excess of hCG (Fig. 8). This was further supported by the fact that hCG was able to compete for asialo ^{125}I-hCG or vice versa indicating that hCG and asialo hCG were binding to the same sites (Fig. 8). The native and asialo glycoproteins such as α_1-acid glycoprotein and fetuin which possess carbohydrate structures similar to those present in hCG, failed to compete for binding with native or asialo ^{125}I-hCG unless used in several thousand fold excess (Fig. 8). If, however, the 2000 g pellet of rat testes homogenate or partially purified plasma membranes were preincubated with the above asialo glycoproteins for 1 hour at 30° , the binding of ^{125}I-hCG was reduced by 40 to 60% (Table IV). Under similar conditions the native glycoproteins did not cause any change in the binding. It appears that either the asialo glycoproteins have

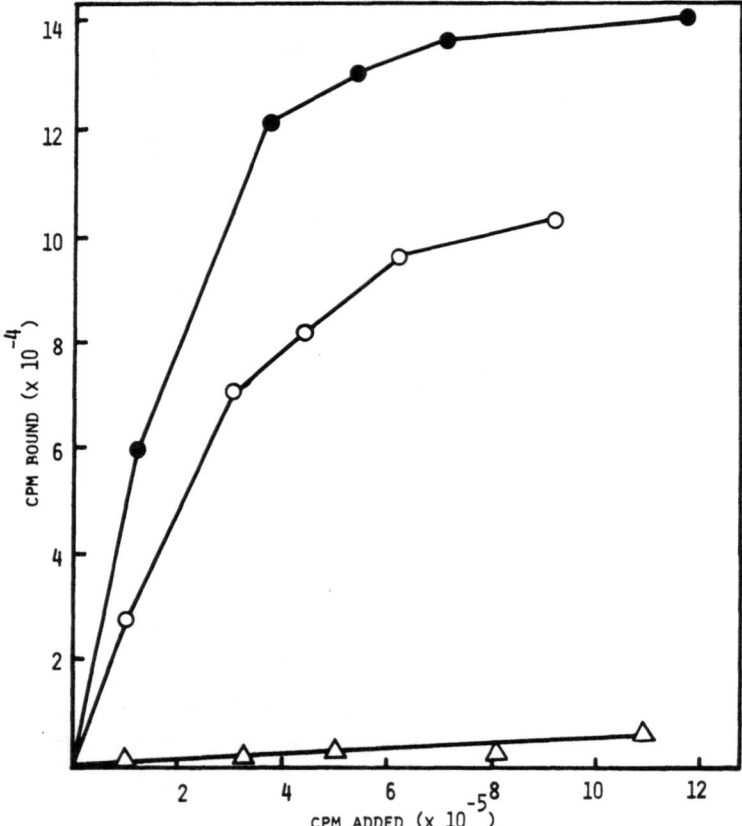

Figure 7. Saturation binding curves for ^{125}I-hCG (o—o—o) and asialo ^{125}I-hCG (•—•—•). Δ—Δ—Δ, ^{125}I-FSH.

low activity for the hormone binding sites or they interact non-specifically with the membranes, causing an overall conformational change which inhibits the binding.

The neuraminidase-galactosidase treated hCG (NG-hCG) had greater binding activity than the native hCG, but was less active than the asialo hCG. Subsequent removal of N-acetylglucosamine residues from NG-hCG by ß-N-acetylglucosaminidase did not alter the binding activity significantly from the native molecule. Thus, the data strongly suggest that sialic acid, galactose and N-acetyl-glucosamine are not at all or only weakly involved in the binding. This is further supported by the fact that the various monosac-charides and oligosaccharides failed to block the hormone binding

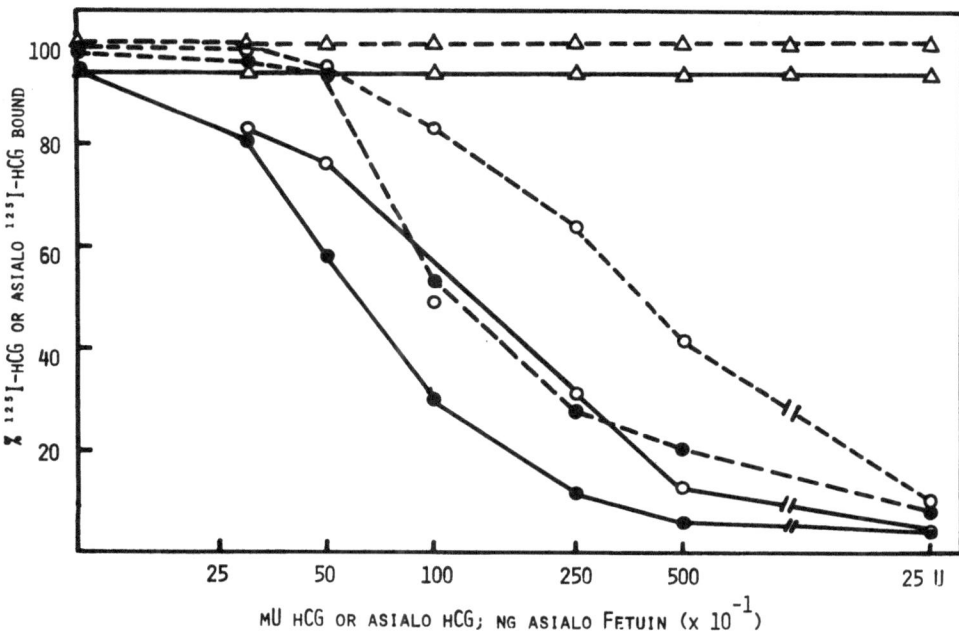

Figure 8. Competition for binding to membrane receptors:
o—o—o ^{125}I-hCG vs. hCG; •—•—• ^{125}I-hCG vs. asialo hCG;
o--o--o asialo ^{125}I-hCG vs. hCG; •··•--• asialo ^{125}I-hCG vs.
asialo hCG; Δ—Δ—Δ ^{125}I-hCG vs. asialo fetuin; Δ·-Δ·· Δ asialo
^{125}I-hCG vs. asialo fetuin.

sites. The hydrolysis of the mannose residues (20%) from NGA-
hCG drastically reduced the binding. This might be due to
either a drastic conformational change in hCG or mannose is
required for the binding because of the presence of a specific
binding site at the membranes. Also, the possibility of an artifact, introduced during enzymatic hydrolysis of NGA-hCG by
α-mannosidase such as oxidation of methionine or cystine residues can not be ruled out. It is surprising, however, that the
immunological activity of freshly prepared NGAM-hCG-1 is not
significantly different from that of NGA-hCG (Table III, Fig. 5).
This renders the possibility of a drastic conformational change
or an artifact less likely. As described above, on the removal
of mannose the molecule does become less stable. On the other
hand, the involvement of mannose in the interaction of macromolecules to the cell surfaces and in the intercellular interactions
has been observed recently. For example, the binding site of
phytoagglutinins of lentil and P. vulgaris on the red blood cell
involves mannose residues (25). Similarly, Yen and Ballou (30)

have recently reported the significance of mannose residues in the glycoproteins of the yeast cells in the intercellular agglutination. Therefore, the possibility of the mannose being involved in the binding is not inconceivable.

To test the possibility of the binding of the hormone being pre-ceeded by the hydrolysis of the carbohydrate by endogenous glyco-sidases, the appropriate inhibitors of the glycosidases such as sugar lactones were used in the binding assay. There was no effect of the lactones on the binding (Table IV).

Effect of the glycosidase treatment of the membranes on binding. The cleavage of almost all of sialic acid from the membranes by neuraminidase resulted in a greater binding. The hydrolysis of galactose residues, on the other hand, did not cause any change in the binding. It may be noted that the binding increases whether sialic acid is removed from the hormone or from the membranes.

The role of the carbohydrate in the stimulation of cyclic AMP accumulation and steroidogenesis. The various glycosidase-treated hCG derivatives were examined for their effect on the cyclic AMP accumulation and steroidogenesis. In the absence of theophylline, the asialo hCG partially stimulated cyclic AMP accumulation, the relative response being 40% that of hCG. The NG-hCG, NGA-hCG and NGAM-hCG-1 did not give any measurable response (Table V). However, all of these derivatives strongly inhibited competetively the stimulation of cyclic AMP accumulation by hCG indicating that they were active in binding (Table V). With the exception of NGAM-hCG-1, in all others, the ratio between the concentration of the derivative required for 50% inhibition and that of the hCG concentration for half-maximal stimulation was approximately 1:1. In the case of NGAM-hCG-1 this ratio was about 7:1 (Table V) again showing that the binding was drastically reduced as was found with the 2000 g pellet. NGAM-hG2 which was obtained by treating hCG with all of the glycosidases simultaneously, was quite a potent inhibitor of cyclic AMP accumulation although it, like NGAM-hCG-1, did not show high binding in the competition experiments with the 2000 g pellet (Fig. 6).

In the presence of theophylline, all of the above derivatives stimulated the cyclic AMP formation. The relative stimulation declined from 100 to 30% with the sequential removal of the sugars from the hormone (Table VI). Again, they were all potent inhibitors of adenyl cyclase indicating that they had high binding activity.

Table V

Stimulation of cyclic AMP accumulation by hCG
(in the absence of theophylline)

Hormone/ Derivative	Concentration for half-maximal stimulation ng/ml	Relative stimulation %	Relative[a] inhibition	
			Expt. 1	Expt. 2
hCG	300 (100-500)	100	-	-
N-hCG[b]	300 (100-400)	40	0.5:1	1.0:1
NG-hCG	n.d.	0	1.5:1	1.2:1
NGA-hCG	n.d.	0	2.0:1	1.0:1
NGAM-hCG-1	n.d.	0	3.5:1	7.5:1
NGAM-hCG-2[c]	300	20	1.0:1	1.0:1

[a]Ratio of the concentration of hCG derivative for 50% inhibition to the concentration of hCG for half-maximal stimulation.

[b]hCG treated sequentially with V. cholerae neuraminidase (N-hCG), then with A. niger β-galactosidase (NG-hCG), then with A. niger β-N-acetylglucosaminidase (NGA-hCG), and finally with A. niger α-D-mannosidase (NGAM-hCG-1).

The glycosidase-treated derivatives stimulatd steroidogenesis, The extent of the response in each case was similar to that of hCG (Table VII) although the concentration required for the maximal stimulation appreciably increased with the sequential removal of the carbohydrate implying a decrease in the affinity for the steroidogenic sites. Their relative potencies determined from the relative concentrations of the derivatives required for half-maximal stimulation ranged between 85 and 1% (Table VII).

In conclusion, the data clearly indicate that with the possible exception of mannose, the other monosaccharides are not or only weakly involved in the binding of the hormone. This is shown by the ability of the glycosidase-treated hCG derivatives to compete with 125I-hCG in the binding assay and by the fact that they are

Table VI

Stimulation of cyclic AMP accumulation by hCG
(in the presence of theophylline)

Hormone/ Derivative	Concentration for half-maximal stimulation ng/ml	Relative stimulation %	Relative[a] potency
hCG	300 - 1,000	100	-
N-hCG[b]	1,000	70	1:1
NG-hCG	300 - 1,000	55	1:1
NGA-hCG	1,000	30	1:1
NGAM-hCG-1	3,000 - 10,000	30	10:1
NGAM-hCG-2[c]	1,000	45	1:1

[a]Ratio of the concentration of hCG derivative for 50% stimulation to that of hCG for half-maximal stimulation.

[b]hCG treated sequentially with V. cholerae neuraminidase (N-hCG), then with A. niger β-D-galactosidase (NG-hCG), then with A. niger β-N-acetylglucosaminidase (NGA-hCG), and finally with A. niger α-D-mannosidase (NGAM-hCG-1).

[c]hCG treated with all of the glycosidases simultaneously.

all potent inhibitors of adenyl cyclase. Secondly, the removal of the carbohydrate from hCG alters its affinity for the sites which cause steroidogenesis without affecting its binding to the sites which induce cyclic AMP formation. Thus, there appears to be two types of sites on the plasma membranes, one for steroidogenesis and the other for cyclic AMP production. These results would support the idea of more than one type of receptor for hCG. It is interesting to note that, in the presence of excess

Table VII

Stimulation of steroidogenesis by hCG and
glycosidase-treated hCG derivatives

Hormone/ Derivative	Concentration for half-maximal stimulation ng/ml	Relative[a] stimulation %	Relative[a] potency %
hCG	0.1 - 0.3	100	100
N-hCG[b]	0.1 - 0.3	100	85
NG-hCG	0.3 - 1.0	100	33
NGA-hCG	1.0 - 3.0	100	13
NGAM-hCG-1	10.0 - 30.0	100	1
NGAM-hCG-2[c]	1.0 - 3.0	100	20

[a]Average of five experiments.

[b]hCG treated sequentially with V. cholerae neuraminidase
(N-hCG), then with A. niger β-galactosidase (NG-hCG), then with
A. niger β-N-acetylglucosaminidase (NGA-hCG), and finally with
A. niger α-D-mannosidase (NGAM-hCG-1).

[c]hCG treated with all of the glycosidases simultaneously.

of the derivatives, the cyclic AMP stimulation was completely
suppressed but the steroidogenic response was still maximal.
This would indicate that either there is a separate cyclic AMP
pool or there is an alternate pathway for steroidogenesis.
Obviously, the glycosidase-treated hCG derivatives provide
powerful tools for probing the molecular mechanisms of gonadotropin action.

Footnotes

Supported by research grants from U. S. P. H. S. , AM-10273, and from the Population Council of New York.

Abbreviations used: NANA, N-acetylneuraminic acid; GluNAc, N-acetylglucosamine; GalNAc, N-acetylgalactosamine; Man, mannose; Gal, galactose; Fuc, Fucose; hCG, human chorionic gonadotropin; N-hCG, neuraminidase treated; NG-hCG, neuraminidase-galactosidase treated; NGA-hCG, neuraminidase-galactosidase-acetylglucosaminidase-mannosidase treated hCG (stepwise); NGAM-hCG-2, hCG treated with all of the glycosidases simultaneously.

References

1. Cuatrecasas, P., Proc. Nat. Acad. Sci. 63: 450, 1969.

2. Rodbell, M., Krans, H. M. J., Pohl, S. L., and Birnbaumer, L., J. Biol. Chem. 246: 1861, 1971.

3. Lefkowitz, R. J., Roth, J., and Pastan, I., Science 170: 633, 1970.

4. Catt, K. J., Tsuruhara, T., and Dufau, M. L., Biochim. Biophys. Acta 279: 194, 1972.

5. Danzo, B. J., Biochim. Biophys. Acta 304: 560, 1973.

6. Saxena, B. B., and Rao, Ch. V., Biochim. Biophys. Acta 313: 372, 1973.

7. De Krester, D. M., Catt, K. J., and Paulsen, C. A., Endocrinology 80: 332, 1971.

8. Lee, C. Y. and Ryan, R. J., Endocrinology 89: 1515, 1971.

9. Lee, C. Y. and Ryan, R. J., Biochemistry 12: 4609, 1973.

10. Means, A. R. and Vaitukaitis, J. L., Endocrinology 90: 39, 1972.

11. Bhalla, V. K. and Reichert, L. E., J. Biol. Chem. 249: 43, 1974.

12. Moyle, W. R. and Ramachandran, J., Endocrinology 93: 127, 1973.

13. Dufau, M. L., Charreau, E. H., and Catt, K. J., J. Biol. Chem. 248: 6973, 1973.

14. Tsuruhara, T., Dufau, M. L., Hickman, J., and Catt, K. J., Endocrinology 91: 296, 1972.

15. Eylar, E. H., J. Theor. Biol. 10: 89, 1965.

16. Morell, A. G., Gregoriadis, G., Scheinberg, H. I., Hickman, J., and Ashwell, G., J. Biol. Chem. 246: 1461, 1971.

17. Van Hall, E. V., Vaitukaitis, J. L., Ross, G. T., Hickman, J. W., and Ashwell, G., Endocrinology 88: 456, 1971.

18. Bahl, O. P., J. Biol. Chem. 244: 565, 1969.

19. Bahl, O. P., in Hormonal Proteins and Peptides, Li, C. H. (ed.), Academic Press, p. 171-199, 1973.

20. Bellisario, R., Carlsen, R. B., and Bahl, O. P., J. Biol. Chem. 248: 6797, 1973.

21. Carlsen, R. B., Bahl, O. P., and Swaminathan, N., J. Biol. Chem. 248: 6810, 1973.

22. Bahl, O. P., J. Biol. Chem. 244: 575, 1969.

23. Greenwood, F. C., Hunter, W. M., and Glover, J. S., Biochem. J. 89: 114, 1963.

24. Ray, T. K., Biochim. Biophys. Acta 196: 1, 1970.

25. Kornfeld, S. and Kornfeld, R., in Glycoproteins of Blood Cells and Plasma, Gameison, G. A and Greenwalt, T. J. (eds.), J. B. Lippincott Co., p. 50-67, 1971.

26. Gilman, A. G., Proc. Nat. Acad. Sci. 67: 305, 1970.

27. Dufau, M. L., Catt, K. J., and Tsuruhara, T., Endocrinology 90: 1032, 1972.

28. Bahl, O. P. and Agrawal, K. M. L., J. Biol. Chem. 244: 2970, 1969.

29.   Matta, K. L. and Bahl, O. P., J. Biol. Chem.
247: 1780, 1972.

30.   Yen, P. S. and Ballou, C. E., J. Biol. Chem. 248:
8316, 1973.

COUPLED EVENTS IN THE EARLY BIOCHEMICAL ACTIONS

OF FSH ON THE SERTOLI CELLS OF THE TESTIS

Anthony R. Means and Claire Huckins

Department of Cell Biology
Baylor College of Medicine
Houston, Texas 77025

Over the past several years this laboratory has been concerned with attempting to define in chemically precise terms the
temporal sequence of events which occur upon the initial interaction of FSH with its testicular target cells. Previous studies
have revealed that a single injection of this gonadotropin to
immature male rats results in a rapid stimulation of RNA and
protein synthesis (1-3). It is well established that FSH is a
polypeptide hormone composed of two dissimilar subunits. Since
studies with other peptide hormones such as insulin, glucagon,
ACTH and LH have demonstrated that these hormones apparently
do not enter the cell but instead bind specific receptors present
on the surface of the target cell, we wished to investigate this
possibility with respect to FSH and the testis. Our initial
studies were made possible by the development of a procedure
by van Lenten and Ashwell (4) for the radio-labeling of glycoproteins with tritium. Vaitukaitis and colleagues applied this
procedure first to hCG (5) and then to FSH (6). Tritiation of
the FSH involved oxidation of the carbohydrate side chain with
periodate followed by reduction with tritiated borohydride. This
procedure results in more than 85% of the tritium attached to
the C^7 position of sialic acid which comprises the terminal carbohydrate residue of the FSH side chain. FSH, radiolabeled in
this fashion maintained a high biologic activity (1400 IU/mg)
although the specific radioactivity was only about 0.25 mCi/mc.

It was demonstrated that tritiated FSH would bind specifically
to testis (7). Although on a mass basis more hormone was bound
to immature tissue, demonstrable hormone binding could be found
when tritiated FSH was incubated with testis from rats of all
ages. Moreover this interaction exhibited all the properties

145

attributable to a biologically significant process. That is, it was dependent upon time and temperature of incubation as well as being a saturable process of high affinity and low capacity. (Recently, these studies have been confirmed by Bhalla and Reichert (8) used hFSH labeled with [125]I.) Examination of the subcellular distribution of the ^{3}H-FSH revealed it was primarily associated with plasma membrane fractions. Subsequently, plasma membranes were isolated from the testis and shown to bind FSH in a specific manner (7,9). Only when membranes were prepared from seminiferous epithelium was binding demonstrable (Fig. 1). Cells or membranes from the interstitial area of the testis or similar preparations from non-target tissues such as liver exhibited little or no specific binding for FSH.

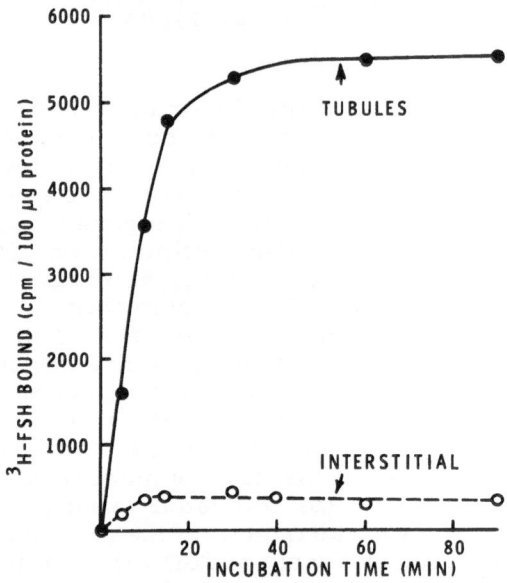

Figure 1. FSH binding to isolated testis membranes. Plasma membranes were prepared from tubules or interstitial tissue from 16 day-old rats as described by Neville (36) and incubated using the procedure of Rodbell et al. (37). Each tube contained membranes (200 μg protein) 2.5% ovalbumin, 1 mM EDTA, 20 mM HEPES (pH 7.2) and 3 x 10^{-9}M ^{3}H-FSH in a final volume of 200 μl. Separation of membrane-bound and free radioactivity was performed exactly as the Method B described by Rodbell et al. (37).

Several laboratories had reported that FSH stimulated adenylate cyclase when incubated with testis from several species of animals (10-12). If the action of this hormone were to prove similar to other peptide hormones one would expect the

interaction of FSH with its membrane binding sites to result in
the activation of adenylate cyclase. This in fact proved to be the
case. A precise temporal correlation was shown to exist between
the binding of FSH to isolated seminiferous epithelial membranes
on the one hand and activation of membrane bound adenylate cyclase on the other hand (9). Moreover, as shown in Table 1, an
8-fold enrichment of both FSH-receptors and adenylate cyclase
was achieved in plasma membranes prepared from isolated seminiferous tubules. In addition, the activation of cyclase resulted
in an increase in the intracellular concentration of cyclic AMP
(13). Again, the extent of this accumulation of cyclic AMP was
dependent upon the concentration of FSH and the time of incubation (14 and Fig. 2).

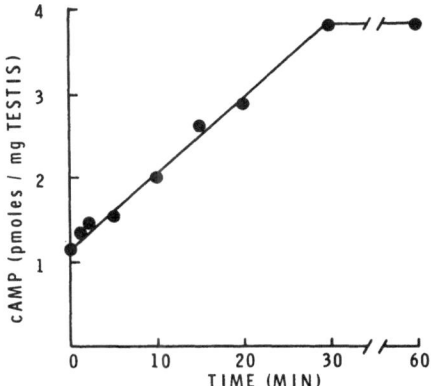

Figure 2. Cyclic AMP production in the presence of FSH.
Tubules were prepared from 16 day-old rats and incubated in
the presence of 50 ng/ml of FSH (Papkoff) and 0.2 mM 1-
methyl 3-isobutyl xanthine at 32°. Cyclic AMP was quantitia-
ted by the binding procedure as outlined by Gilman (38).

The next step was to provide evidence that the increase in
cyclic AMP could be correlated with the stimulation of some
intracellular event. The most logical candidate to bridge the
gap between increased levels of cyclic AMP and altered cellular function in response to peptide hormones appeared to be the
cyclic AMP-dependent protein kinase. It has been demonstrated that certain specific enzymes such as adipose tissue trigly-
ceride lipase are phosphorylated in the presence of stimulatory
hormones and this phosphorylation is mediated through the action
of a cyclic AMP-dependent protein kinase. Likewise, protein
kinase has been shown to play an important role in modulating
the activity of muscle phosphorylase kinase and glycogen synthe-
tase. Reddi et al (15) had shown the presence of a cyclic AMP-
dependent protein kinase in testis tissue. Therefore, we

Table I

Concomitant Enrichment of FSH-Receptors and
Adenylate Cyclase in Testis Tubule Membranes

	FSH-Receptor (moles x 10^{-14}/mg protein)	Adenylate Cyclase Activity (pmoles cAMP/mg protein)
Tubules	7	2.1
Membranes	55	17.8

All rats were 16 days old.

Specific binding of ^{3}H-FSH was measured as previously described
(7,9). Adenylate cyclase was assayed by a modification (13) of
the procedure described by Murad et al. (10). Plasma membranes
were prepared from isolated tubules as outlined in a previous
communication (7).

decided to determine whether FSH could affect the activity of this
enzyme and attempt to correlate changes in activity with binding
of FSH to its receptor and activation of adenylate cyclase.

The mechanism of activation of protein kinase by cyclic AMP
in vitro has been established using enzymes isolated from a
variety of mammalian tissues (16). This mechanism is illustrated by the following equation:

$$RC + cAMP \rightleftharpoons R \cdot cAMP + C$$

Binding of cyclic AMP to the regulatory subunit [R] of the inactive protein kinase [RC] allows dissociation of the enzyme into the
regulatory subunit-cyclic AMP complex (R·cAMP) and the active
catalytic subunit of the enzyme [C]. Extrapolation of this in
vitro mechanism to the regulation of cyclic AMP-dependent protein
kinase in vivo predicts that hormonal modulation of the intracellular concentration of cyclic AMP would affect the protein
kinase activity ratio, that is, the ratio of [C] to [RC+C]. Experimental verification of this hypothesis has recently been reported
by Soderling et al. (17) for the regulation of adipose tissue protein kinase by epinephrine and insulin. Therefore, we applied
these techniques to a study of the regulation of protein kinase
activity in testis by FSH. Incubation of seminiferous tubules
isolated from testis of immature rats with FSH results in a
very rapid activation of protein kinase (9,13). An effect is

demonstrable as early as 3-5 minutes and a maximal state of activation is achieved by 20 minutes at which point a 3-fold enhancement of activity is observed. In addition, the increased enzyme activity can be directly and positively correlated with increased intracellular accumulation of cyclic AMP (13). Activation of the testicular protein kinase is specific for FSH and is dependent upon time and temperature of incubation as well as the concentration of hormone. Increased kinase activity in response to the continued presence of FSH exhibits a half life time of 2-4 hours. Furthermore, bound FSH can be recovered following treatment of the tissue at acid pH and this hormone retains the ability to activate protein kinase in a fresh tissue preparation, suggesting that a significant portion of FSH may not be degraded while attached to testicular receptors.

Stimulation of protein kinase activity by FSH was shown to be dependent upon the age of the animal (13). FSH results in a marked stimulation of protein kinase in seminferous tubules isolated from rats 16 days of age. However, the magnitude of this response decreases with age until finally in rats 30 days old or older no stimulation of protein kinase can be demonstrated. On the other hand, if rats of any age are hypophysectomized, sensitivity of the protein kinase to FSH is again established within the first 10 days following the operation. The underlying mechanism which results in the loss of sensitivity to FSH with age of the animal has long been a mystery. All biochemical effects which have been reported to be stimulated by FSH in testis are age dependent (1, 2, 9, 13, 14). Moreover, these biochemical effects usually disappear between 21 and 26 days of age. On the other hand, we (7) and Bhalla and Reichert (8) have demonstrated that testes from mature animals contain receptor sites for FSH. These observations suggested that during the initial establishment of the spermatogenic process, some system or systems became active which resulted in a decreased biochemical response to exogenous FSH.

Kuehl et al. (11) had reported the presence in testis of a phosphodiesterase which specifically hydrolyzed cyclic AMP. More recently, the level of phosphodiesterase in testis during postnatal maturation has been studied by Monn et al. (18). Testes of immature animals were shown to have relatively low levels of phosphodiesterase. However, as the age of the animal increased, a specific isozyme of this enzyme appeared and reached maximal levels at approximately 35 days of age. If cyclic AMP was necessary to mediate subsequent effects of FSH on the testis, it was possible that the appearance of the phosphodiesterase isozyme would result in increased degradation of the newly synthesized cyclic AMP, thus causing a short circuit in the temporal sequence of biochemical events normally

mediated by FSH. These results led us to investigate the effect
of FSH on protein kinase activity in testis that was incubated in
the presence of a potent inhibitor of phosphodiesterase, 1-methyl-
3-isobutyl xanthine (MIX). Our initial studies revealed that addition of this inhibitor to the incubation medium at a final concentration of 1.0 mM resulted in a small but repeatable activation of
protein kinase in tubules isolated from 16 day old rats (13). On
the other hand, FSH produced a 3-fold stimulation of kinase activity. When FSH and MIX were included in the incubation medium
together, the activation of protein kinase appeared to be additive
compared to the effect of either compound alone. These experiments were next repeated using testes from adult animals which
had previously been shown not to respond to FSH. Addition of the
phosphodiesterase inhibitor resulted in a considerable activation
of protein kinase in a testis tubule preparation. Moreover, this
activation of protein kinase could again be correlated with an increase in the intracellular levels of cyclic AMP. When FSH and
MIX were added together a synergistic effect was demonstrated
with regard to the activity of protein kinase. Furthermore,
Christiansen and Desautel (19) have reported that the specific
phosphodiesterase isozyme disappears from testis following
hypophysectomy. Taken together, these data offer the possibility that phosphodiesterase may play a role in the regulation of
the action of FSH in mature rats.

Using metabolic inhibitors to disect the temporal sequence of
events in the action of a hormone can lead to considerable misin-
terpretation of data. This is because most inhibitors are not
uniquely specific for the reaction which one wishes to inhibit.
Thus, phosphodiesterase inhibitors such as MIX at a concentration of 1 mM inhibit protein synthesis, RNA synthesis (14) and
DNA synthesis (20). This compound also results in an abnor-
mally high production of cyclic AMP. In fact, intracellular
concentrations can reach 20-30 times the values found in the normal testicular cells. Because of these difficulties considerable
more experimentation is necessary before one can draw a
definite cause and effect relationship between phosphodiesterase
activity and the metabolic effects of FSH. However, utilization
of MIX has an interesting positive effect. That is, it lowers by
nearly two orders of magnitude the sensitivity of the testis
adenylate cyclase system to FSH. Thus, as shown in Figure 3
linear responses of cAMP production to FSH in the presence of
0.2 mM MIX can be seen between hormone concentration of
6×10^{-11} to 6×10^{-9} molar FSH. Finally, the sensitivity and specificity of this response suggests its possible use as an assay for
FSH activity.

As mentioned previously, excellent temporal correlation
exists between the binding of FSH and activation of adenylate
cyclase in membrane preparations. Moreover, the preparation

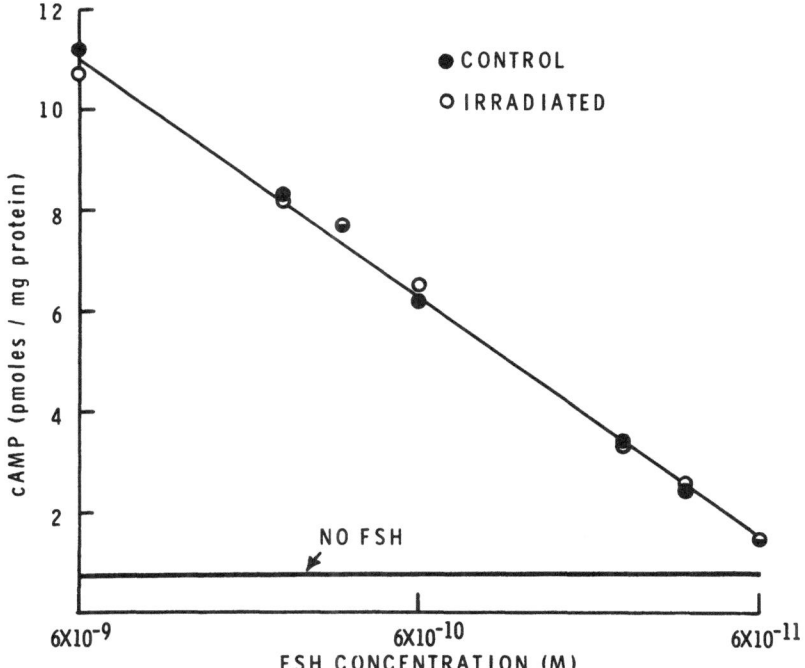

Figure 3. Comparison of cyclic AMP production of testis
tubules from normal and irradiated rats in response to FSH.
All animals were 16 days old and irradiation of pregnant females
was administered as described in the text. Tubules (~ 60 mg)
were incubated in Krebs-Ringers bicarbonate buffer (pH 7.2)
for 20 minutes at 32°. Cyclic AMP was measured by the Gilman
procedure (38).

of membranes results in an 8-fold enrichment of the testis for
FSH receptors when compared to tubules (Table I). This subcellular fractionation also results in an 8-fold enrichment for
adenylate cyclase when expressed on a mg of protein basis.
Thus, these data suggest an intimate physical relationship may
exist between the FSH receptor and hormone-sensitive adenylate
cyclase. Positive correlation also exists between the binding of
FSH and the activation of testicular protein kinase (9). On the
other hand, much less FSH is required to maximally activate
protein kinase than is required to result in maximal intracellular
levels of cyclic AMP (13). Again, less FSH is required to produce maximal cyclic AMP levels than is required to saturate
the binding sites for this hormone. In fact, protein kinase is
activated at concentrations of FSH which barely produce detectable increases in cyclic AMP (Fig. 4). Similar observations have
been reported by Beall and Sayers (21) for the ACTH system as

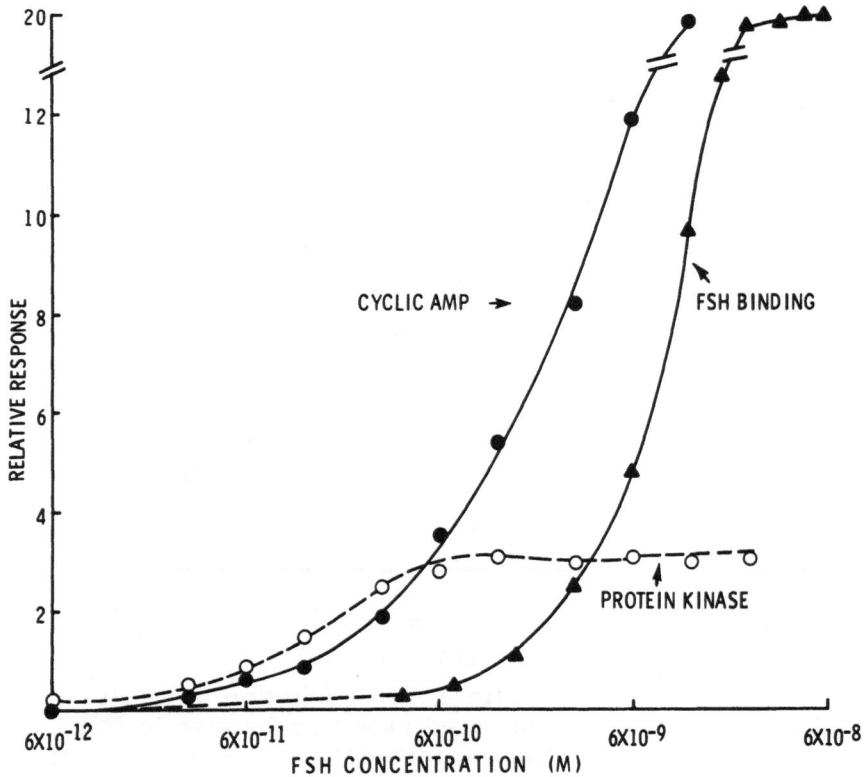

Figure 4.   Binding of FSH to testis tubules in relationship to
stimulation of cyclic AMP production and activation of protein
kinase.   Tubules were prepared from testes of 16 day-old rats
and incubated at 32° with various concentrations of ³H-FSH of
oFSH (Papkoff).   Binding reactions were incubated for 2 hours
whereas tubules for cyclic AMP and protein kinase were incubated for 20 minutes.   Methods have been previously detailed
(7, 9, 13).

well as by Catt and Dufau (22) for LH action upon the testis. · In
both of these systems less hormone seems to be required for
maximal steroid production than is necessary for saturation of
the receptors.   Again, maximal steroid production is achieved
at concentrations of peptide hormones which result in no demonstrable increase in cyclic AMP.   It has been suggested that these
effects may be due to the presence of spare receptors.   The
greater the receptor reserve, the greater the sensitivity of isolated adrenal cortical cells to ACTH.   Again, similar studies
have been reported for the action of glucagon on the liver by

Exton et al. (23) and for TSH action upon the thyroid by William-
son (24). Another more plausible explanation for these effects
of peptide hormones has been proposed by Rodbard (25). He has
theorized that the receptor site may be regarded as a quantal unit
so that a cell would respond in a maximal all-or-none fashion if
the number of sites filled exceed a given threshold. Mathematical treatment of this model reveals that it would be consistent with
the observations made by Catt and Dufau (22) in the hCG-testis
system and also by Beall and Sayers (21) in the ACTH-adrenal
system. Whichever of these theories proves to be true it is clear
that for several peptide hormones including FSH less concentration is necessary to maximally stimulate biological response than
is necessary to saturate the receptor sites.

Our data suggest that three of the earliest events following
administration of a single dose of FSH to immature rats are: 1)
the binding to receptors present on cells of seminiferous epithelium; 2) the resulting stimulation of membrane-bound adenylate
cyclase and an associated increase in the intracellular accumulation of cyclic AMP; and 3) the activation of cyclic AMP-dependent
protein kinase. Moreover, the kinetics of stimulation of these
three events strongly suggest a coupled system. What is now
required is to elucidate the relationship of these initial events to
subsequent effects of FSH on transcription and/or translation.

The type of cells in the seminiferous epithelium that constitute the targets for the initial actions of FSH have yet to be elucidated. Studies from our laboratory concerning the effect of FSH
on spermatogonial degeneration suggest that at least one of the
physiologic effects of this hormone may be manifest at the level
of the type A spermatogonia (14,26). Whether this is a direct
action or mediated by some other cell type such as the Sertoli
cells which immediately abut on the spermatogonial cells is not
known. In this regard, Dym and Fawcett (27) have demonstrated
that Sertoli cell membranes surround all of the spermatogonial
components of the testis and tight junctions between adjacent
Sertoli cells constitute a blood testis barrier. Thus, morphologically the Sertoli cell represents a logical candidate for the
primary target cell for FSH.

Several reports have appeared which suggest that the Sertoli
cell is affected by FSH. Murphy (23,29) has reported that injection of this gonadotropin into rats results in a change in the morphology of the Sertoli cell. Studies from Castro et al. (30) suggested that FSH labeled with electron-dense substances such as
ferritin was localized in or on the Sertoli cells and also in peritubular elements of the testis. However, the only definitive way
by which to answer the question of localization of target cells for
FSH is to obtain a preparation enriched in these cells which would
demonstrate the same temporal sequence of biochemical events

upon administration of FSH that is found in the normal intact animal. Thus, we and others have recently begun to investigate various preparations that are enriched in Sertoli cells. These have included long term hypophysectomy, animals rendered cryptorchid for long periods of time and adult animals exposed to X-radiation. Indeed, these animal models appear to respond to FSH (14, 31). However, all of these systems suffer from one drawback, that is, they represent situations in which the germinal epithelium has been damaged in order to provide an enrichment in Sertoli cells. We now believe we have a system in which it is valid to examine the biochemical effects of FSH in the absence of germ cells.

The primordial germ cells in fetal rat testes comprise a unique radiobiological system. Unlike somatic tissues which generally show increasing radiosensitivity with increasing mitotic activity the gonocytes are maximally sensitive to radiation at the time of mitotic dormancy. In male rats, gonocytes actively divide until the 17th day of embryonic life at which time they altogether cease to divide for a period of approximately 11 days (32, 33). This quiescent period terminates at the end of the first postnatal week when the gonocytes engage in a single final division to form definitive spermatogonia. When pregnant female rats are given whole body radiation at known times during the gestation period it has been shown that the gonocytes in male fetuses display increasing radiosensitivity up to 18 days of embryonic life (32). Between 19 and 21 days, they are acutely sensitive, but thereafter show a decreasing response to radiation into the first days of neonatal life. As little as 100-150 r administered between 19 and 21 days of fetal life is lethal to almost all gonocytes, and these cells subsequently degenerate when they attempt the definitive postnatal division. This results in a sterile testis (32, 34). On the other hand, the somatic supporting cells (Sertoli cells) are not adversely affected by such low doses of radiation and apparently continue their normal course of development in the germ cell-free environment.

This preferential sensitivity of germ cells versus somatic cells offers the unique opportunity to study Sertoli cells development both morphologically and biochemically in sterile seminiferous tubules, and thus allows us to probe the specific roles and activities of these cells. In the experiments to be described adult female rats were time-bred. On the 19th day of pregnancy, they were placed in wooden boxes which contained individual compartments and were roofed by plexiglass. These animals were exposed to 125 r whole body cobalt[60]-radiation. Animals were sexed and the female neonates discarded within 24 hours following parturition. Young male rats from irradiated and control litters were sacrificed at specific intervals timed from the day of conception. The testis from these animals were prepared for histological examination or used for biochemical experiments. The biochemical criteria examined were: 1) binding of tritiated FSH; 2) FSH activation of adenylate cyclase and intracellular accumulation of cyclic AMP; 3) stimulation of protein kinase and 4) phosphodiesterase activity.

In the days immediately following parturition there are no overt signs of radiation damage to testes of the young animals delivered by females which had received 125 r cobalt radiation. As in normal testes during the first postnatal week the gonocytes are mitotically quiescent and many of them degenerate, while supporting cells continue to actively proliferate. However, at the end of the first postnatal week, when gonocytes in the irradiated testis attempt to produce spermatogonia, they all degenerate. This results in sterile sex cords populated only by the still mitotically active supporting elements. As in nonirradiated control testes, mitotic activity gradually diminishes in the supporting cells to about 1% at 16 days of age and ceases all together by 18 days of birth. At this time, supporting cells in testes from irradiated rats are indistinguishable from those in normal testes which contain germinal elements (Plate 1). The presumptive seminiferous tubules in these sterile testes are populated by closely packed supporting cells whose immature nuclei are characteristically small and ovoid and contain numerous heterochromatin granules and flakes. The cytoplasm is scanty and compact. During the next 2 weeks the supporting elements mature into the typical adult Sertoli cell seen in nonirradiated control testes. The nucleus becomes pale and voluminous and displays the characteristic spherical nucleolus with 2 heterochromatin bodies (Plate 1). The cytoplasm becomes abundant and forms branching processes which extend into the center of the seminiferous tubule. Unlike the normal animal the onset of cytoplasmic branching is not coincident with lumen formation. Rather no definite lumen can be seen until after 30 days of age (Plates I and II). It has been suggested that in normally developing rat testis that lumen formation depends on and immediately follows the formation of Sertoli-Sertoli cell junctions and the establishment of the blood testis barrier between 16 and 20 days (35). This would indicate that in testes of irradiated animals, tight junctions between adjacent Sertoli cells appear even in the absence of the usual germ cell complement but such formations are temporarily delayed. Indeed, preliminary experiments by R. Vitale using horseradish peroxidase tracer confirms the early presence of a blood testis barrier. Finally, once the Sertoli cells have matured and the lumina have formed, the sterile seminiferous tubules remain unchanged in morphological appearance up to adulthood (Plate II). Lacking a full roster of germinal elements however, the Sertoli cell-only tubules are markedly smaller in diameter than those in normal adult testes.

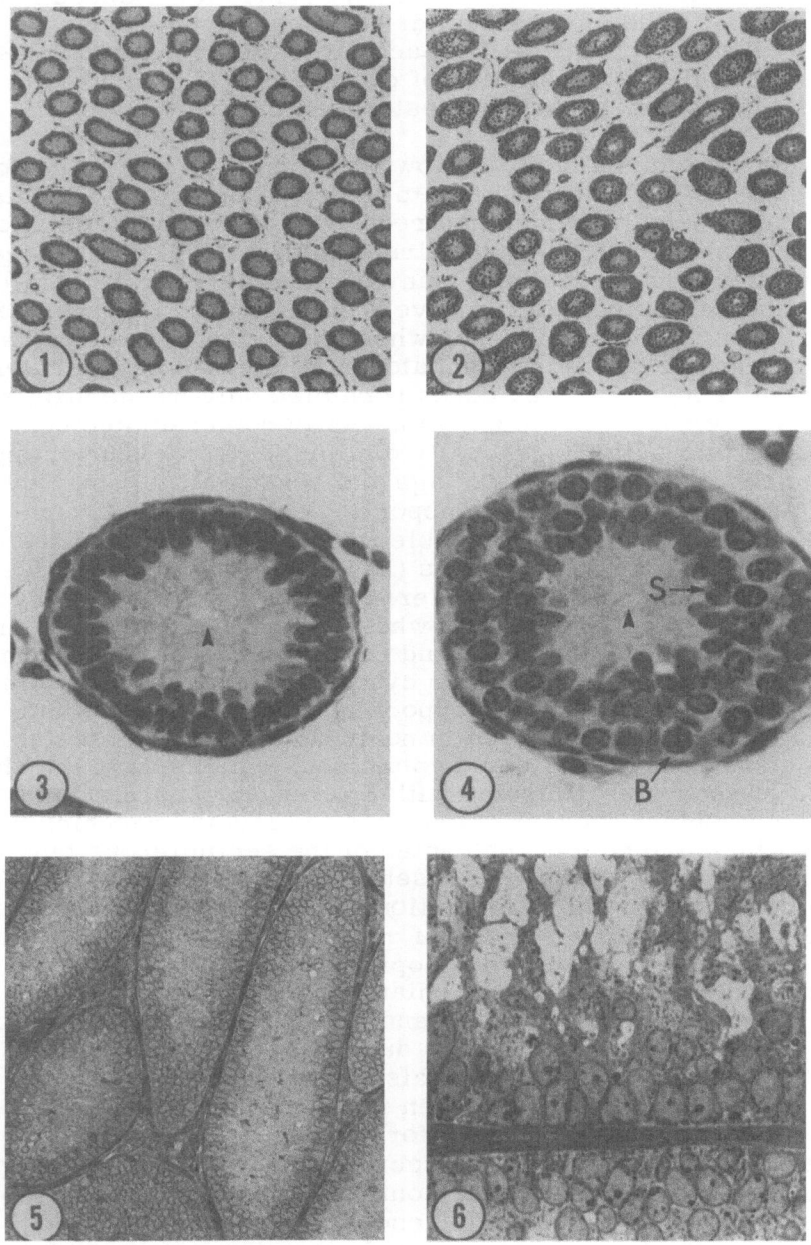

Plate I. 1. Sixteen day old irradiated testis, fixed in Zenker-
formol and stained by periodic acid - Schiff - hematoxylin technique. In this low power field, it can be seen that the seminiferous tubules are populated exclusively by Sertoli cells (62x).

It would appear then that this low dose of irradiation given to pregnant females has no adverse effect on the subsequent development of the Sertoli cell population in the fetal male animals. Since all morphological events occur at similar times in both control and irradiated animals we conclude that maturation of a competent Sertoli cell population is not dependent upon the presence of germinal elements and that this constitutes a valid model system for investigating the specific contribution of this population to spermatogenesis. We now report our initial attempt to characterize this model system with respect to the biochemical effects of FSH.

Testis seminiferous tubules from the Sertoli cell-only animals contained FSH specific receptors with properties similar to those previously described in normal animals. Thus, binding is a saturable process of high affinity (Kd $\sim 10^{-10}$ M) and low capacity. Table II shows that testes of normal rats 19 days of age have the capacity to bind 3.15×10^{-13} Moles of FSH per testis. Similarly, although testes from irradiated rats weighed less, the capacity to bind FSH is the same. Since the number of Sertoli cells is identical in the control and irradiated tubules this would suggest that most of the binding sites exist on Sertoli cells in both types of testis preparations. It can also be seen from Table II that the molar concentration of binding sites for FSH does not increase in the irradiated testis after approximately 19 days of age. Again, this would be compatible with the fact that the adult Sertoli cell concentration has been reached by 19 days of age.

Plate I. 2. Matching low power field in normal 16-day old testis. The tubules are heavily populated by developing germ cells, and many have begun to form lumina (62x).

Plate I. 3. Sertoli cell only tubule from 16-day old irradiated testis. Note the closely packed Sertoli cell nuclei (625x).

Plate I. 4. The matching control seminiferous tubule has a larger diameter. A peripheral ring of type B spermatogonia (B) has displaced the Sertoli cell nuclei (S) toward the center where a lumen is developing (625x).

Plate I. 5. Thick epon section of irradiated 16-day old testis which has been perfused with glutaraldehyde and stained with toluidine blue. The tubules only contain abundant Sertoli cells (156x).

Plate I. 6. Higher magnification of tubular walls in irradiated testis from Figure 5. The immature Sertoli cell nuclei are irregularly ovoid with scattered flakes of heterochromatin free and adherent to the nuclear membrane. The prominent dark circles are nucleoli. At this age, the Sertoli cell cytoplasm has begun to branch.

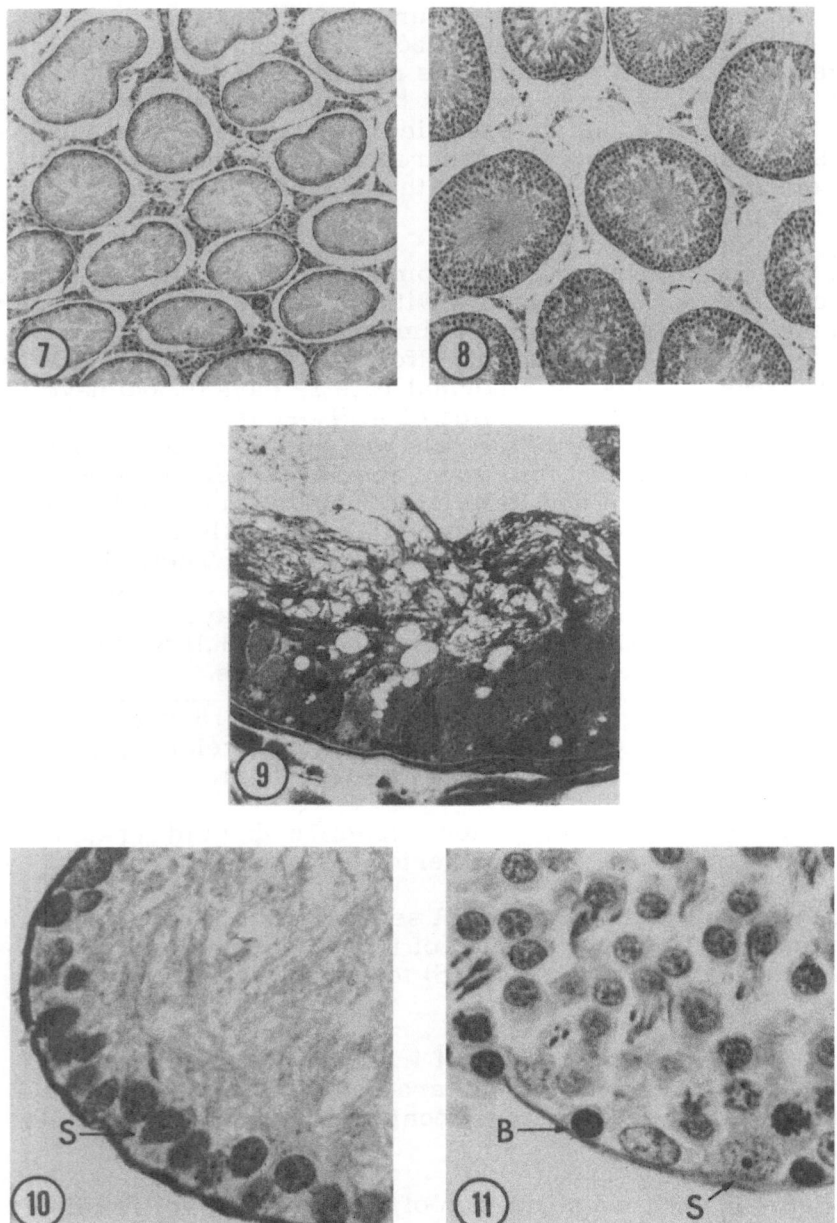

Plate II

Table II

Concentration of FSH-Binding Sites in Testes
from Normal and Irradiated Rats

Age (days)	Treatment	Testis Weight (mg)	FSH-Binding (moles x 10^{-13}/testis)
19	Normal	90	3.05
19	Irradiated	60	3.60
46	Normal	162	3.82
46	Irradiated	1042	3.90

Tubules were prepared from rat testes and 100mg portions incubated for 120 minutes at 32^0 with various amounts of ^{3}H-FSH. Previous studies have shown 120 minutes to represent apparent equilibrium conditions (9,13). The data were used to construct Scatchard plots. In all cases the Kd of the hormone-receptor complex was approximately 1×10^{-10}M. The concentration of binding sites was determined from the intercept with the abscissa (9).

Plate II. 7. Sterile seminiferous tubules from adult testis which was irradiated pre-natally. The tubules have grown markedly (compare with Figure 1), but are still smaller than those from normal testes (62x).

Plate II. 8. Seminiferous tubules from matching control adult testes (62x).

Plate II. 9. Epon section showing portion of seminiferous tubule from 32 day old irradiated testis which has been perfused with glutaraldehyde and stained with toluidine blue. Note the attenuated cytoplasmic branching of the Sertoli cells into the lumen (625 x).

Plate II. 10. High power of Sertoli cell only tubule. The Sertoli cell nuclei exhibit normal adult characteristics. The voluminous cytoplasm forms a frothy mass in the tubule lumen (625 x).

Plate II. 11. Part of seminiferous epithelium from control adult testes showing the full complement of germinal elements (B). Although the Sertoli cell nuclei (S) may be somewhat larger than in irradiated animals, they exhibit similar morphological features (625x).

As previously discussed for the normal animal the binding of FSH to testis of the Sertoli cell-only animals results in increased activity of adenylate cyclase which is expressed by an increased intracellular accumulation of cyclic AMP. The correlation of this effect of FSH on cyclic AMP accumulation is striking and can be seen in Figure 3. When tubules are incubated for 20 minutes in the presence of FSH concentrations between 6×10^{-11} and 6×10 M, linear increases in the intracellular content of the cyclic AMP can be seen when normal rats are used. The response of Sertoli cell-only animals to similar concentrations of FSH is not distinguishable from the normal situation. Again, these data would suggest that the Sertoli cell-only tubules contain the same number of FSH responsive cells as do testes of normal animals.

Soluble protein kinase activity was next measured during development of the Sertoli cell-only testes and compared to normal animals of the same age. It was found for the first 20 days the specific activity of protein kinase (U/mg protein) increased in concert in the two types of testis preparations (Figure 5). However, in the Sertoli cell-only animals maximal values of protein kinase were achieved at 20 days of age whereas

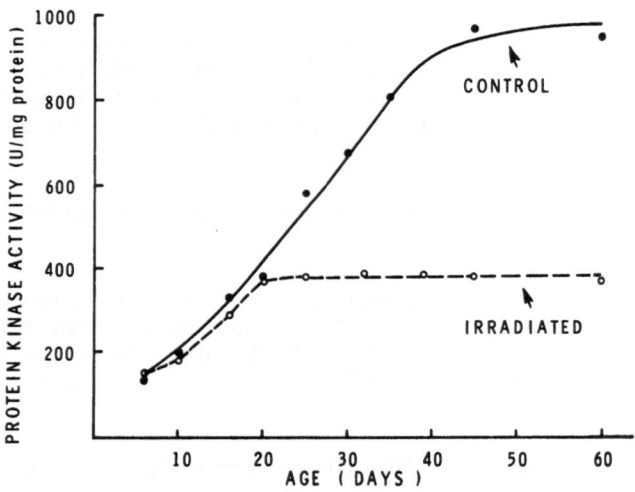

Figure 5. Protein kinase in testes of normal and irradiated rats during postnatal maturation. Pregnant females were exposed to 125 r whole body ^{60}Co-radiation as described in the text. Protein kinase was measured as previously described (9, 13) at various stages during development. Control animals were subjected to all experimental protocols except the actual exposure to radiation.

in the adult animal protein kinase continued to increase another
2-fold reaching adult values at approximately 45 days of age.
Similar data were seen with respect to phosphodiesterase activities in the two types of testes. FSH was shown to increase the
activity of protein kinase in Sertoli cell-only testis tubules.
The kinetics of this response were identical to those seen in the
normal animal. Surprisingly, the response to FSH in the Sertoli
cell-only testis was also found to be age dependent. Figure 6
shows that for the first 26 days of age, FSH caused a marked stimulation in protein kinase activity. By 32 days however, no stimulation was noted and this lack of response continued until at least
60 days of age. These data were identical to those found in the
control animals. Addition of an inhibitor of phosphodiesterase to

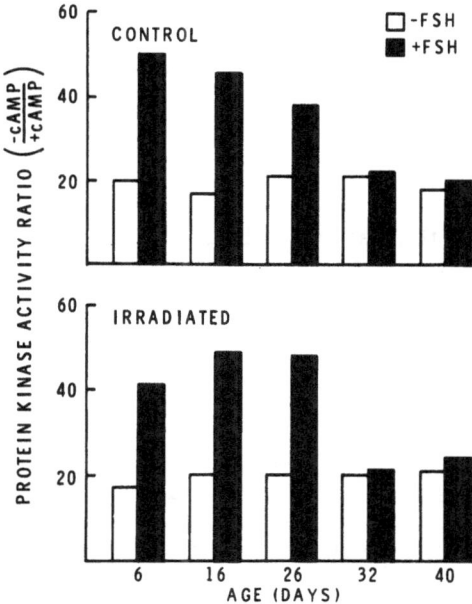

Figure 6. Effect of FSH on activation of protein kinase in testis
tubules from control or irradiated rats during development.
Methods were precisely as described by Means et al. (13).

the incubation medium restored the sensitivity of Sertoli cell-
only tubules to FSH (Figure 7). Again, this response was
indistinguishable from that which occurred in normal animals.

   These data provide the first direct evidence that the Sertoli
cell is a primary target for FSH and suggest that at least three
biochemical events can be coupled in the initial response to this
gonadotrophin. Thus, FSH first binds to receptors present on the

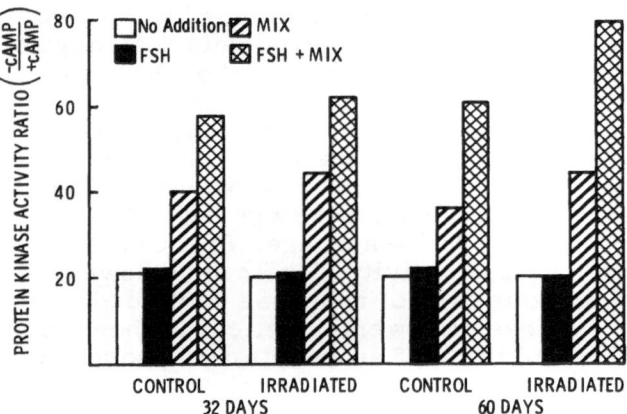

Figure 7. Synergistic effects of FSH and 1-methyl 3-isobutyl xanthine (MIX) on activation of protein kinase in testes of control and irradiated rats. Details of experimental procedures have been detailed (13).

plasma membranes of the target cells. This interaction results in the stimulation of membrane-bound adenylate cyclase which leads to an increase in the intracellular concentration of cyclic AMP. The newly synthesized cyclic AMP interacts with the regulatory subunit of inactive cyclic AMP-dependent protein kinase resulting in an increased catalytic activity. It now seems valid to assume that these events occur in the Sertoli cell. In the normal animal, subsequent to the membrane associated events discussed in this paper FSH results in the stimulation of both RNA and protein synthesis. Stimulation of transcription and translation appear to be of a general rather specific nature. We have hypothesized that FSH affects the number of degenerating spermatogonia in the differentiating compartment of the testis. If this theory proves correct this would explain the reason for a general effect on cell metabolism. Thus, since the overall effect would be to increase the number of spermatogonia of the same type, one would assume that the total compliment of RNA and protein would remain constant. At present, we have no evidence to suggest that the FSH-mediated events in the Sertoli cell are responsible for these biochemical effects on transcription and translation or lead to the changes seen in spermatogonial degeneration. It remains possible that the testes of normal animals contain more than one type of FSH-sensitive cells. However, just as plausible is the possibility that all of the effects of FSH are mediated through the Sertoli cell. What is now necessary is to design experiments which will link these seemingly unassociated events in a logical manner and in so doing define the mechanism by which FSH affects the testis.

References

1. Means, A. R. and Hall, P. F., Endocrinology 81: 1151, 1967.

2. Means, A. R. and Hall, P. F., Biochemistry 8: 4293, 1969.

3. Means, A. R., Endocrinology 89: 931, 1971.

4. van Lenten, L. and Ashwell, G., J. Biol. Chem. 246: 1889, 1971.

5. Vaitukaitis, J. L., Hammond, J., Ross, G. T., Hickman, J. and Ashwell, G., J. Clin. Endocr. 32: 290, 1971.

6. Vaitukaitis, J. L., Sherins, R., Ross, G. T., Hickman, J. and Ashwell, G., Endocrinology 89: 1356, 1971.

7. Means, A. R., and Vaitukaitis, J. L., Endocrinology 90; 39, 1972.

8. Bhalla, V. K., and Reichert, L. E., J. Biol. Chem. 249: 43, 1974.

9. Means, A. R., Adv. Exp. Med. Biol. 36: 431, 1973.

10. Murad, F., Strauch, B. S. and Vaughn, M., Biochim. Biophys. Acta 177: 591, 1969.

11. Kuehl, F., Patanelli, D. J., Tarnoff, J. and Humes, J. L., Biol. Reprod. 2: 154, 1970.

12. Dorrington, J. H., Vernon, R. G. and Fritz, I. B., Biochem. Biophys. Res. Commun. 46: 1523, 1972.

13. Means, A. R., MacDougall, E., Soderling, T. R. and Corbin, J. D., J. Biol. Chem., in press, 1974.

14. Means, A. R., In: Handbook of Physiology, Greep, R. O., and D. W. Hamilton (eds.), Amer. Phys. Soc. Bethesda, Md., (In Press).

15. Reddi, A. H., Ewing, L. L. and Williams-Ashman, H. G., Biochem. J. 122: 333, 1971.

16. Krebs, E. G., Current Topics in Cell Regulation 5: 99, 1972.

17. Soderling, T. R., Corbin, J. D., and Park, C. R., J. Biol. Chem. 248: 1822, 1973.

18. Monn, E., Desautel, M. and Christiansen, R. O., Endocrinology 91: 716, 1972.

19. Christiansen, R. O. and Desautel, M., Endocrinology 92: A-100, 1973.

20. Hollinger, M. A., and Hwang, F., Endocrinology 94: 444, 1974.

21. Beall, R. J. and Sayers, G., Arch. Biochem. Biophys. 148: 70, 1972.

22. Catt, K. J. and Dufau, M. L., Adv. Exp. Med. Biol. 36: 379, 1973.

23. Exton, J. H., Lewis, S. B., Ho, R. J., Robison, G. A. and Park, C. R., Annals N. Y. Acad. Sci. 185: 85, 1971.

24. Williams, J. A., Endocrinology 91: 1411, 1972.

25. Rodbard, D., Adv. Exp. Med. Biol. 36: 342, 1973.

26. Huckins, C., Mills, N., Besch, P. and Means, A. R., Endocrinology 92: A-94, 1973.

27. Dym, M. and Fawcett, D. W., Biol. Reprod. 3: 308, 1970.

28. Murphy, H. D., Proc. Soc. Exp. Biol. Med. 118: 1202, 1965.

29. Murphy, H. D., Proc. Soc. Exp. Biol. Med. 120: 671, 1965.

30. Castro, A. E., Alonso, A. and Mancini, R. E., J. Endocr. 52: 129, 1972.

31. Dorrington, J. H. and Fritz, I. B., Endocrinology 94: 395, 1974.

32. Beaumont, H. M., Int. J. Rad. Biol. 2: 247, 1960.

33. Huckins, C. and Clermont, Y., Arch. Anat. Hist. Embry. 51: 343, 1968.

34. Hughes, G., Int. J. Rad. Biol. 4: 511, 1962.

35. Vitale, R., Fawcett, D. W. and Dym, M., Anat. Rec. 176: 333, 1973.

36. Neville, D. M., Biochim. Biophys. Acta. 154: 540, 1968.

37. Rodbell, M., Krans, H.M.J., Pohl, S. L. and Birnbaumer, L., J. Biol. Chem. 246: 1861, 1971.

38. Gilman, A. G., Proc. Natl. Acad. Sci. U.S.A. 67: 305, 1970.

THE PRODUCTION OF ANDROGEN BINDING

PROTEIN BY SERTOLI CELLS

Donald J. Tindall, William T. Schrader
and Anthony R. Means

Department of Cell Biology
Baylor College of Medicine
Houston, Texas 77025

Studies designed to elucidate the biochemical mechanism of action of FSH in the testis have long been hampered by two major problems. First, the precise target cell affected by this gonadotrophin was difficult to pinpoint because of the heterogeneity of cells within the germinal epithelium. Secondly, no specific endpoint for the acute effect of FSH was available.

As described in the preceeding chapter of this book (1), the first problem has now been resolved in studies of rat testis containing no germinal cells. Irradiation of pregnant female rats causes the male offspring to develop testis with tubules consisting solely of Sertoli cells. These testes bind FSH and respond to this hormone in a normal fashion. Such studies showed clearly that the primary target cell for FSH is the Sertoli cell. With this Sertoli cell-only (SCO) model available, it seemed appropriate to study the second problem stated above. Since our initial studies in 1967 (2), it has been known that FSH stimulates testicular protein synthesis. Thus a Sertoli cell-specific protein would be a logical candidate for regulation by FSH.

Androgen binding protein (ABP) is a 90,000 molecular weight substance that is produced in the testis (3-6). This protein specifically binds androgen and is transported via the tubule lumina through the efferent ducts into the caput epididymis (3,7,8). French and co-workers have presented indirect evidence that this molecule is synthesized in the Sertoli cell (9). Moreover, ABP disappears following hypophysectomy and replenishment requires injection of FSH (10). Thus, demonstration of ABP in the SCO testis would provide direct evidence of the cellular site of synthesis of this protein. Furthermore, if ABP were made in the Sertoli cell in response to FSH, ABP synthesis could then serve as a molecular marker for the action of FSH on the Sertoli cell.

In order to measure ABP, the steady-state polyacrylamide gel electrophoresis system described by French et al. was utilized (9). In each experiment the complete absence of germ cells was determined by examining histological sections from one testis of each rat. Cytosol from the other testis was prepared by homogenizing the tissue in 4 volumes of 0.25 M sucrose in 50 mM Tris-HCl buffer (pH 7.4) containing 1 mM EDTA and centrifuging for 1 hour at 105,000 g. The cytosol was treated with a charcoal suspension in buffer for 2 hours to remove endogenous androgen and incubated with ^{3}H-dihydrotestosterone (^{3}H-DHT). The samples were then electrophoresed for 3 hours at 3 mA per tube on 6.5% polyacrylamide gels containing 2.3 nM ^{3}H-DHT. Figure 1C shows that a major peak of radioactivity exists which co-migrates with ABP from normal testis (R_f - 0.5). Since ABP is transported from the testis via the efferent ducts and is concentrated within the caput epididymis, the caput epididymal cytosol from SCO rats was analyzed for ABP. Like the normal rat, SCO rats had much higher concentrations of androgen binding protein in the caput than in the testis or the cauda epididymis (Fig. 1).

In addition to ABP, both testis (11,12) and epididymis (13-16) have been shown to contain a cytoplasmic receptor for androgen. Therefore, it was necessary to rule out the possibility that the DHT binding protein detected in SCO-rats might be an intracellular receptor. First, the binding protein from these organs did not appear to be a cytoplasmic receptor since DHT-binding was stable to charcoal treatment whereas such treatment will destroy binding of cytoplasmic receptor from these organs. Moreover, the cytoplasmic receptor from both the epididymis and testis had an R_f of 0.4 (17) as compared to 0.5 for the ABP (7). A striking characteristic of ABP is the rapid rate of dissociation from DHT (17). When the ABP-^{3}H-DHT complex was incubated at 0° with 100-fold excess cold DHT its half-life of dissociation was 3 minutes. The cytoplasmic androgen receptors from both the testis and epididymis, on the other hand, have characteristic half-lives of many days at 0° (12,17). Therefore, a preparation of ^{3}H-DHT labeled ABP from SCO caput epididymis was treated with excess unlabeled DHT. Binding to ^{3}H-DHT was again examined after 1 hour incubation at 0°. As can be seen from Figure 2A-B, the labeled DHT was completely displaced by the unlabeled DHT within 1 hour. These data indicate that the binding component isolated from the SCO-rat epididymis cytosol has the same

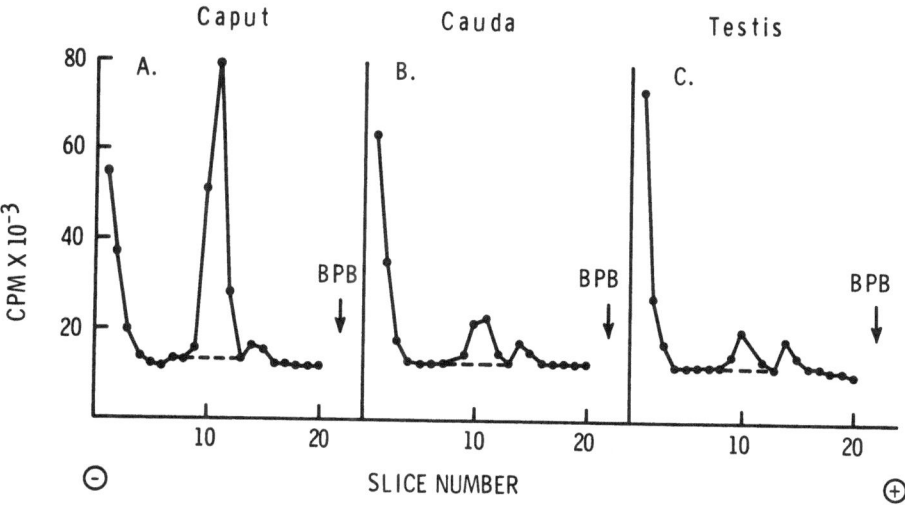

Figure 1. Steady-state polyacrylamide gel electrophoresis of
caput and cauda epididymis and testis cytosols from 40 day old
Sertoli cell-only rats. 105,000 g supernatants were prepared
from A: caput epididymis; B: cauda epididymis and C: testis.
Steady-state polyacrylamide gel electrophoresis was performed
as described by French et al. (9). After treatment with dextran-
coated charcoal (0.5% Norite A, 0.05% Dextran 80 w/v) for 2
hours the cytosols were labeled with ^{3}H-DHT. Gels were
electrophoresed for 3 hours at 3 mAMP per tube, sliced into
2 mm cross sections, extracted for 16-18 hours with toluene-
liquifluor scintillation mixture and counted for radioactivity.
The dotted line represents the base line of radioactivity from
which subsequent calculations were made in quantifying ABP.

characteristics as ABP from the normal rat. Furthermore,
binding of ^{3}H-DHT to the androgen binding proteins from both
the SCO and normal rats was unaffected by treatment with the
sulfhydryl reagent, n-ethylmaleimide (Fig. 2-C,D). This is
another characteristic feature of ABP since binding ability
of cytoplasmic androgen receptors of both testis and epididymis
is destroyed by treatment with sulfhydryl reagents (15).
Finally, in data not shown here, both normal and SCO ABP's
were found to be stable at 50° for 30 minutes whereas intracellular receptors for androgen are destroyed at temperatures
between 25° and 50° (12,15).

It is well established that ABP is a secretory product of
the testis and exits through the tubule lumina (3-6). It was

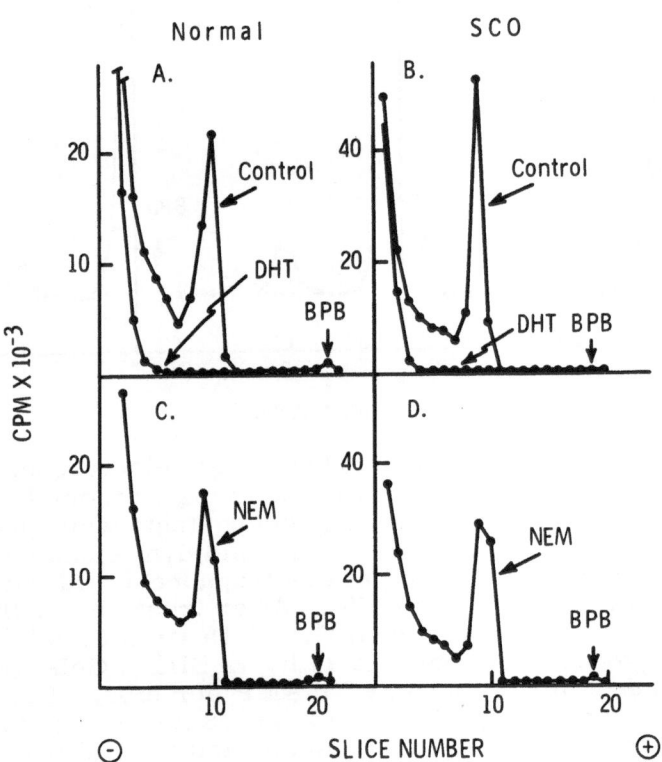

Figure 2. Polyacrylamide gel electrophoresis of caput epididymal cytosols from Sertoli cell-only and normal rats after treatment with unlabeled DHT or N-ethyl maleimide. Cytosols were
treated with charcoal and labeled with ^{3}H-DHT before treatment.

A, B: Treatment of cytosol for 1 hour at 0° alone or in the presence of 100-fold excess unlabeled DHT.

C, D: Treatment of cytosol for 1 hour at 0° in the presence of
1 mM N-ethyl maleimide. Aliquots of 100 μl were electrophoresed on 6.5% nonlabeled polyacrylamide gels for 3 hours at
3 mAMP per tube and extracted as described in Figure 1.

Table 1

Androgen Binding Protein Concentrations in Testis,
Caput and Cauda Epididymis at Different
Ages of SCO and Normal Rats

Age (days)	Tissue	SCO	Normal
		ABP$\left(\dfrac{\text{pmoles}}{\text{mg prot}}\right)$	
15	Testis	0.25[a]	0.31
	Epid	ND[b]	ND
18	Testis	0.68	0.82
	Epid	ND	1.00
21	Testis	1.18	1.08
	Epid	ND	3.50
24	Testis	1.73	0.92
	Epid	ND	3.48
29	Testis	2.77	0.65
	Epid	0.10	6.71
30	Testis	1.79	0.36
	Caput	3.09	4.51
	Cauda	1.24	1.92
40	Testis	1.43	0.39
	Caput	9.17	7.41
	Cauda	1.78	1.76
47	Testis	0.75	1.59
	Caput	7.78	13.31
	Cauda	0.42	2.74
57	Testis	0.49	0.90
	Caput	7.01	14.91
	Cauda	0.42	3.76

a) Concentrations of ABP were measured using the steady-state polyacrylamide gel electrophoresis method described by French (9). Pregnant Sprague Dawly rats were obtained from Holtzmann and irradiated as described by Means and Huckins (1) on day 19 of gestation. b) ND = none detectable.

of interest, therefore, to determine whether ABP could be
detected in testes before lumina had formed and if so whether
appearance in the epididymis was dependent on the presence of a
lumen. Vitale et al. (18) have shown that tight junctions form
between adjacent Sertoli cells at 16-18 days of age in normal
rat testis. Moreover, formation of this blood-testis barrier is a
prerequisite for establishment of lumina within the seminiferous
tubules (18). Table 1 shows ABP concentrations in the testis of
normal and SCO-rats of various ages. In the 15 day normal rats,
ABP was present in the testis but not in the epididymis. Since
lumina are not present in these tubules, this suggests that no
transport occurs until formation of this passage. By 18 days of
age in the normal rat the lumina have formed, and ABP can be
detected in the epididymis. As development proceeds, ABP
titers decrese in testis and increase in epididymis, reaching
maximal values in this organ and at about 57 days of age
(Table 1).

A different picture emerged when postnatal development of the
SCO-animals was investigated. Androgen binding protein was
detected in testis as early as 15 days and the testicular concentration continued to increase until 29 days of age. Between 29 and
30 days, ABP decreased dramatically in the testis. Concomitant
with this decrease was an increase in epididymal ABP from undetectable levels at 29 days to 1.8 pmoles per mg protein at 30
days. Epididymal ABP increased thereafter reaching maximal
concentrations at appproximately 40 days. These data suggest
that the delay in transport of ABP from testis to epididymis in
SCO-rats might be reflected by a similar delay in lumen formation. Indeed, histological studies have shown that the blood-testis
barrier formation (and associated tubule lumina) in the SCO-rat
testis is delayed until 29 to 30 days of age (R. Vitale, et al.,
manuscript in preparation). Thus, ABP is formed in the Sertoli
cells of the testis, and transport of the secreted ABP is dependent
upon formation of the blood-testis barrier.

The biosynthesis of ABP in normal rats has been shown to
be dependent on FSH and not directly affected by LH or testosterone (10). In order to see if the Sertoli-cell only testes
would respond to exogenous FSH, SCO rats 21 days of age were
hypophysectomized and 6 days later given two injections of
either FSH or LH 8 hours apart. Eighteen hours following the
last injection the rats were killed and cytosols prepared from
testis and epididymis. As can be seen from Table 2 the concentration of ABP was much higher in the SCO testis than in the
epididymis at 29 days of age. This agrees with the earlier
observation that transport of ABP into the epididymis was just
beginning at this age in SCO rats. Six days after hypophysectomy there was an almost complete disappearance of ABP
from the SCO testis. These observations correspond to

Table 2

Effect of FSH and LH on ABP Production
in Testis from Hypophysectomized Rats

Treatment	Testis	Epididymis
	dpm/mg protein	
Intact	110,000	650
Hypophysectomized Control	550	110
Hypophysectomized + FSH	8,350	520
Hypophysectomized + LH	4,310	1,320

SCO rats were hypophysectomized at 22 days of age and 6 days later treatment begun. FSH and LH (50 mg/50 g body weight) were administered subcutaneously in two doses 8 hours apart and the animals were sacrificed 18 hours later. Cytosols were prepared from testis and epididymis and electrophoresed on nonlabeled 6.5% polyacrylamide gels. Radioactivity was calculated by subtracting background counts from peak counts. Animals were 29-30 days at the time of the experiment.

similar observtions made by French et al. (10) in normal rats. The acute treatment with FSH resulted in significantly increased concentrations of ABP within the SCO testis compared to the level observed in the 6 day hypophysectomized SCO control. However, FSH treatment did not restore ABP concentrations to their non-hypophysectomized values. This is as expected since the sensitivity of normal testis to FSH decreases with time after hypophysectomy (19). Treatment of the hypophysectomized SCO rats with LH resulted in a small but significant increase in ABP levels within the testis. It is not yet apparent whether this effect is due to FSH contamination in the LH preparation or due to an actual induction of ABP by LH. Sensitivity of the testis to FSH following hypophysectomy has been shown (19) to be restored by priming with high doses of testosterone propionate (2 mg/day/90 g body weight). Therefore there is the possibility of a synergistic effect from LH through testosterone in initiating synthesis of ABP. Both the FSH and LH treatments appeared to result in the appearance of a small amount of ABP in the epididymis. Since these animals were 29 to 30 days old at the time of the experiment, the data may represent the formation of the blood testis barrier in only a few tubules. Indeed a few such formations were observed by Dr. Vitale using the peroxidase histology technique.

Our results demonstrate directly that ABP is produced by the Sertoli cell of the testis. Furthermore, the confinement of ABP to the testis prior to lumen formation demonstrates that development of the blood testis barrier is a prerequisite for transport of these macromolecules from testis to epididymis. Finally, the fact that ABP disappears following hypophysectomy and reappears following administration by FSH suggests that this protein may be useful as an endpoint marker for assessing the temporal biochemical sequence of events which occur in the Sertoli cell in response to FSH.

The function of ABP in the male reproductive system is not yet understood. It is likely that one role may be to transport testosterone from testis to epididymis. Indeed, the differentiation of the epididymis is regulated by testosterone as is the maturation of spermatozoa which occurs in this organ. However, it is also possible that ABP may play a role in providing testosterone to androgen-sensitive cells within the seminiferous epithelium. At first glance this might seem an unlikely concentrating mechanism since ABP appears to be rapidly secreted into the lumen following synthesis in the Sertoli cell cytoplasm. Closer scrutiny of the androgen-dependent steps in spermatogenesis reveals a close analogy between ABP and steroid binding globulins in the blood. It is well recognized that the meiotic process requires testosterone. The pacytene primary spermatocytes undergo reduction division in close proximity not to the basement membrane but instead to the lumen. Androgen binding protein could therefore provide a vehicle for the transfer of testosterone from tubule lumina to a cytoplasmic androgen receptor protein present in the meiotic cell similar to the transfer of steroid from the blood capillaries to surrounding target epithelial cells. Such interesting possibilities should provide the impetus for many future studies involving both the function of ABP and the use of the Sertoli-cell only rat for the study of the mechanism of FSH action.

References

1. Means, A. R., and Huckins, C., This volume, p. 143.

2. Means, A. R., and Hall, P. F., Endocrinology 81, 1151, 1967.

3. French, F. S., and Ritzen, E. M., Endocrinology 93, 88, 1973.

4. French, F. S., and Ritzen, E. M., J. Reprod. Fert. 32, 479, 1973.

5. Hansson, V., Djoseland, O., Reusch, E., Attramadal, A., and Torgersen, O., Steroids 21, 457, 1973.

6. Ritzen, E. M., Dobbins, M. C., Tindall, D. J., French, F. S., and Neyfeh, S. N., Steroids 21, 593, 1973.

7. Ritzen, E. M., Nayfeh, S. N., French, F. S., and Dobbins, M. C., Endocrinology 89, 143, 1971.

8. Hansson, V., Steroids 20, 575, 1972.

9. French, F. S., McLean, W. S., Smith, A. A., Tindall, D. J., Weddington, S. C., Petrusz, P., Sar, M., Stumpf, W. E., Nayfeh, S. N., Hansson, V., Trygstad, O., and Ritzen, E. M., this volume, p. 258.

10. Hansson, V., Reusch, E., Trygstad, O., Torgersen, O., Ritzen, E. M., and French, F. S., Nature New Biol. 246, 56, 1973.

11. Mainwaring, W.I.P., and Mangan, F. R., J. Endocrinol. 59, 121, 1973.

12. Hansson, V., McLean, W. S., Smith, A. A., Tindall, D. J., Weddington, S. C., Nayfeh, S. N., and French F. S., Steroids 23, 823, 1974.

13. Blaquier, J. A., Biochem. Biophys. Res. Comm. 45, 1076, 1971.

14. Tindall, D. J., French, F. S., and Nayfeh, S. N., Biochem. Biophys. Res. Comm. 49, 1391, 1972.

15. Hansson, V., Djoseland, O., Reusch, E., Attramadal, A., and Torgersen, O., Steroids 22, 19, 1973.

16. Blaquier, J. A., and Calandra, R. S., Endocrinology 93, 51, 1973.

17. Tindall, D. J., Hansson, V., Sar, M., Stumpf, W. E., French, F. S., and Nayfeh, S. N., Endocrinology (in press).

18. Vitale, R., Fawcett, D. W., and Dym, M., Anat. Rec. 176, 333, 1973.

19. Hansson, V., Weddington, S. C., Ritzen, E. M., Nayfeh, S. N., and French, F. S., Endocrinology 94A, 200, 1974.

FSH BINDING IN RAT TESTES DURING MATURATION AND FOLLOWING HYPOPHYSECTOMY. CELLULAR LOCALIZATION OF FSH RECEPTORS

Anna Steinberger, K. H. Thanki, and B. Siegal

Program in Reproductive Biology and Endocrinology
University of Texas Medical School at Houston
Houston, Texas

Introduction

Follicle stimulating hormone (FSH) has been recognized to play a paramount role in the regulation of spermatogenesis. However, its precise function and cellular site of action in the testis have not been clarified (1). Several morphologic and biochemical parameters are known to be affected by FSH. These effects have been more readily demonstrable in testes of immature or hypophysectomized animals compared to intact adults.

Steinberger and Duckett (2) showed that FSH is required for final steps of spermiogenesis in the mature rat. Addition of FSH to organ culture of neonatal rat testes induced morphologic changes in the Sertoli cells compatible with maturation (3). FSH was also shown to stimulate protein and RNA synthesis (4) in rat testes and to increase the level of endogenous c-AMP in isolated seminiferous tubules incubated in vitro (5,6).

Cytochemical (7,8) and radioautographic studies with labeled FSH demonstrated localization of the hormone in the seminiferous tubules, primarily in the Sertoli cells but also in some spermatogonia and spermatocytes.

Means and Vaitukaitis (9) using ^{3}H-FSH showed presence of specific FSH-binding receptors in testes of 20 day old rats.

In our study, we investigated binding of 125I-FSH to rat testes during different stages of development and to mature testes at various time periods following hypophysectomy. In an attempt to identify the cells which possess FSH receptors, different cell types were isolated from the testes and tested for FSH binding ability.

Materials and Methods

Rats of the Long-Evans strain at various stages of maturation were supplied by our own breeding colony. Hypophysectomized rats (Sprague Dawley strain) were purchased from Hormone Assay Laboratories, Chicago, Ill.

Carrier-free 125I for hormone iodination was purchased from Cambridge Nuclear Corp., Boston, Mass. Human FSH (LER-1366), porcine FSH (NIH-FSH-P-1), ovine FSH (NIH-FSH-S3 and S11), ovine LH (NIH-LH-S5 and S11), bovine LH (NIH-LH-B5) and human LH (LER-960), were gifts from NIH.

Plastic carrier dishes (Falcon) and culture media were obtained from Bio Quest (Cockeyville, Md).

Iodination procedure

Iodination of human FSH (LER 1366, containing 2782 IU FSH and 92 IU LH activity, bioassay, 2nd IRP standard) was carried out by a modified procedure of Greenwood et al (10). The ratio of chloramine-T to hormone was 1:1 (wt/wt) and the reaction was carried out at 0° C for 20 sec. After addition of sodium meta-bisulfate to stop the reaction, the iodinated hormone was separated from free iodine by passage through a 1 x 20 cm column of Biogel P-60 (Bio Rad Laboratories). A typical elution pattern of 125I-FSH is shown in Figure 1. Each fraction within the peak was tested for specific binding to rat testes and those showing high specific binding were pooled, diluted with Tris-HCl buffer containing 1% bovine serum albumin, and stored in small aliquots at -20° C. The specific activity of the iodinated hormone ranged from 7-20 μCi/μg. The labeled hormone was used within several weeks following iodination.

Hormone binding

Animals were sacrificed by overdose of chloroform and the testes or other tissues removed and kept on ice. 250 mg of whole tissue or isolated seminiferous tubules were homogenized in a glass homogenizer (Curtin Sci. Cat. 072-835) with 2 ml

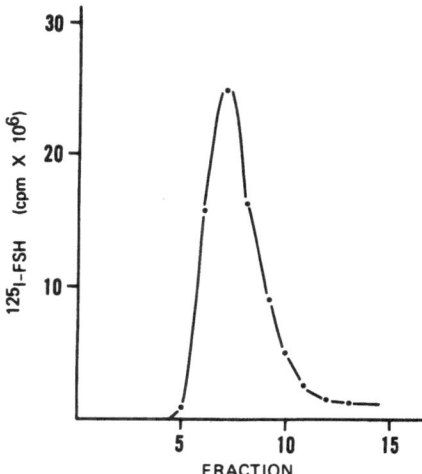

Figure 1. Typical elution pattern of ^{125}I-FSH iodinated by a modified procedure of Greenwood et al. (10) using 1:1 ratio of chloramine T/hormone, 20 sec reaction time at 0° C.

of 0.1 M Tris/HCl buffer (5 mM Mg Cl$_2$, 0.1 M sucrose and 1% bovine serum albumin) pH 7.4. The homogenization was carried out in a bath of crushed ice using 20 manual strokes. The homogenate was diluted with 2 ml of same buffer and 0.4 ml aliquots, containing 25 mg equivalent of tissue, were distributed to assay tubes. When isolated cells were used for hormone binding approximately 1 million cells were used per assay tube. All tubes then received 100 μl of ^{125}I-FSH (approximately 1 x 10^5 cpm) and either 20 μl (10 μg) of unlabeled hormone or buffer. Each sample was always assayed in two or more replicate tubes.

After total radioactivity per tube was measured in a well-type gamma spectrometer (Nuclear Chicago, 56% counting efficiency for ^{125}I) the tubes were incubated in a shaker water bath (120 oscillations/min) at 37° C for 2 hr. Following incubation the tubes were spun at 1200 x g for 15 min at 4° C. The supernatant was aspirated, the pellet resuspended in 2 ml of cold buffer and spun as before. The "washing" procedure was repeated once more and the pellet-associated radioactivity measured in the gamma spectrometer.

The counts obtained from replicate tubes were averaged and corrected for background radioactivity. That amount of ^{125}I-FSH which could be competitively inhibited by excess amounts of unlabeled FSH was considered to represent specific binding.

Separation of interstitial cells and seminiferous tubules

The interstitial cells and seminiferous tubules were separated
by a previously described method (11). Briefly, the decapsulated
testes were placed over a stainless steel grid (70-100 μ mesh
size) and the tubules gently separated with fine-point forceps.
Care was taken not to break the tubules and release the germ
cells. A large volume of chilled Tris-HCl buffer was poured over
the tissues in a forceful stream causing the interstitial cells to
become dislodged from the tubules and pass through the grid. The
interstitial cells were then recovered from the filtrate by mild
centrifugation, resuspended in a small volume of fresh buffer
and counted in a hemacytometer. Approximately 1×10^6 cells
were used per assay tube for hormone binding.

The seminiferous tubules were cut with scissors, completely
teased apart and washed thoroughly with additional 300-400 ml
of buffer. Parts of tissue which resisted separating into individual tubules were discarded. The tubules were then weighed and
handled in the same manner as whole tissue for hormone binding.

Germ cells

The germ cells (predominantly spermatids and spermatocytes)
were obtained by mincing seminiferous tubules which had been
separated from the interstitial cells (see above). The germ cells
"spilling" out from the cut tubules into the surrounding buffer
were recovered by mild centrifugation and used for hormone binding.

Peritubular cells

The peritubular cells were isolated by a culture method (11).
Individual seminiferous tubules, separated from the interstitial
cells, were placed into culture dishes (10-15 pieces/60 mm dish)
containing 0.1 ml of culture medium (Eagle's minimum essential
medium supplemented with 1.0 M Na-pyruvate, 0.1 M of non-
essential amino acids, 4 mM glutamine and 10% fetal calf serum
(Bio Quest Lab). A strip of cellophane was placed over the
tubules, to prevent them from floating, and the dishes incubated
at 37° C in an atmosphere of 5% CO /95% air. After significant
cell outgrowth had occurred along the tubule (24-48 hrs) the
cellophane and the tubules were discarded and the remaining
peritubular cells were allowed to proliferate for an additional

8-12 days. The monolayers were composed of endothelial and myoid cells. For hormone binding, the cells were dislodged from the culture dish by a teflon spatula.

Protein determination

The protein content of tissues or isolated cell fractions, used for hormone binding, was determined by the method of Lowry et al. (12). Protein concentration/mg tissue or 1×10^6 cells - provided a basis for comparing hormone binding of the various cell suspensions to that of whole testes or seminiferous tubules.

Testis organ culture

Four-week organ cultures of testis were used to obtain testicular tissue which was depleted of germ cells and Leydig cells. The culture method was the same previously described (13). Such cultures were shown previously to contain morphologically intact Sertoli and peritubular cells but no germ cells, except occasional primitive type A spermatogonia and no functional Leydig cells (3, 14, 15).

Results

Binding of ^{125}I-FSH to testis homogenates is a time dependent process reaching a plateau after 60 min incubation at 37° C. Figure 2 shows the amount of hormone bound after various incubation intervals. Up to 3% of total added radioactivity was bound at 60 min. Incubation of 25 mg tissue with increasing concentrations of ^{125}I-FSH results in saturation of the receptors at hormone concentration of 40 ng per 0.5 ml (Fig. 3). Binding of ^{125}I-FSH increased linearly when increasing amounts of tissue were incubated with 100,000 cpm of hormone (Fig. 4). All values in Figures 2-4 represent specific binding of the hormone.

That the binding of ^{125}I-FSH was tissue specific is evident from Figure 5 showing no significant specific binding of the hormone to homogenized spleen, muscle or lung, while up to 85% of the hormone bound to homogenized testis was specific. Only unlabeled FSH preparations significantly inhibited the binding of ^{125}I—FSH. LH preparations and hCG had a slight or no inhibitory effect.

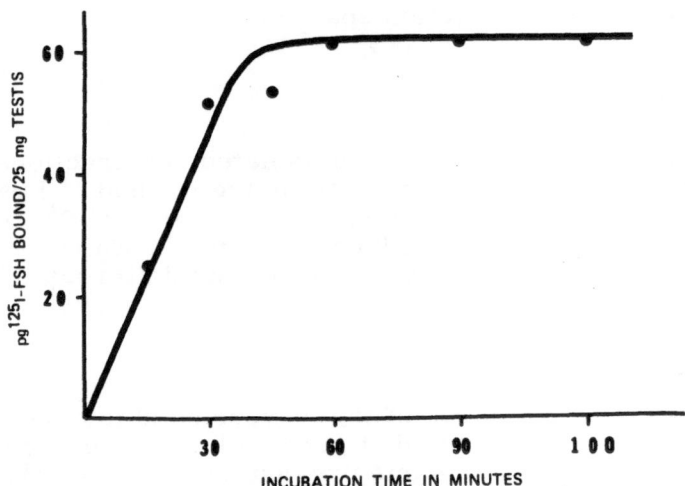

Figure 2. Time course of 125I-FSH binding by testis homogenate
at 37° C. All values are means of four samples and represent
specific binding. Maximum binding is reached after 60 min incubation.

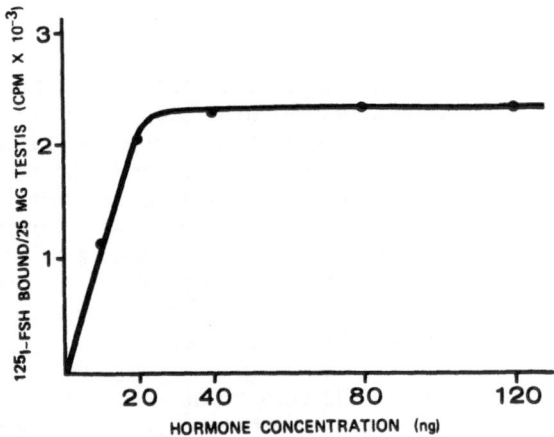

Figure 3. Specific binding of 125I-FSH to 25 mg of testis homogenate incubated with increasing concentrations of the labeled
hormone. Each point on the graph represents mean value of
four samples. Under the employed experimental conditions,
saturation binding sites occurs at hormone concentration of
40 ng/0.5 ml.

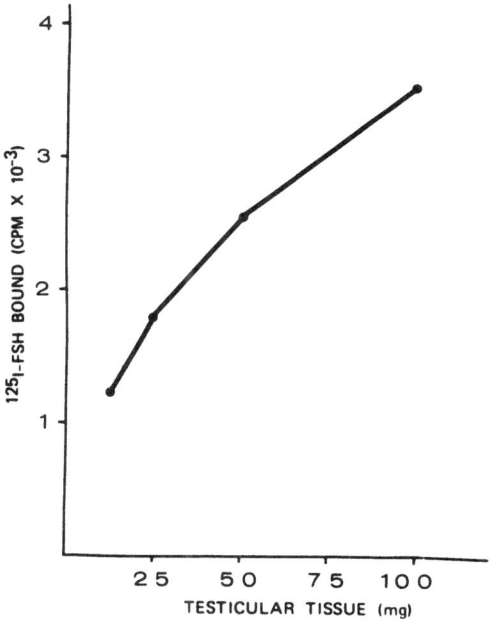

Figure 4. Effect of increasing receptor concentration on the specific binding of ^{125}I-FSH by testis homogenate. Varying amounts
(10-100 mg) of testis were incubated for 60 min at 37° C with
82,000 cpm ^{125}I-FSH (η = 4).

FSH binding to testes at different stages of maturation

Testes from rats ranging in age from 10 to 90 days were compared for their ability to bind ^{125}I-FSH. The results are shown
in Figure 6 as cpm ^{125}I-FSH specifically bound by 25 mg of homogenized tissue. Serum FSH levels in animals of various ages (16)
are also plotted in Figure 6 for comparison with hormone binding
in the testes. The amount of bound ^{125}I-FSH increased from 2100
cpm on the 10th day to 2500 cpm on the 15th day, then declined to
1000 cpm by the 25th day. An additional drop to 500 cpm was observed by day 40. No change in binding occurred between days
40 and 90.

The serum level of FSH, on the other hand, rose between the
20th and 35th day and then decreased to a value below that of 20
day old animals by day 63, and became slightly lower in 77 day old
animals. Thus, no correlation could be established between the
degree of FSH binding by the testis and the circulating levels of
FSH.

Scatchard plots (17) of ^{125}I-FSH binding to testes from 16,

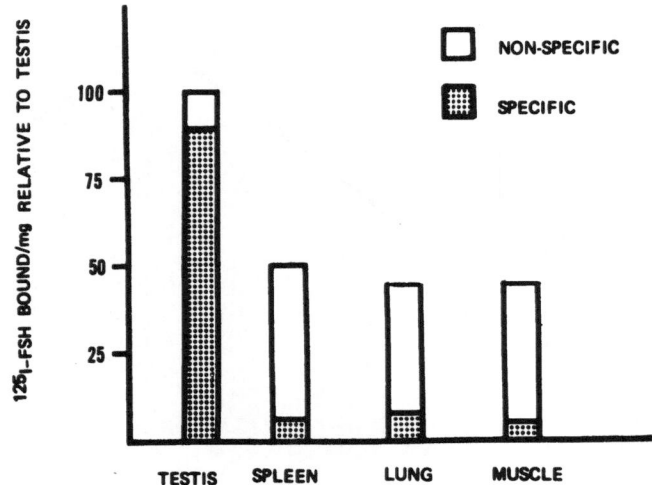

Figure 5. Binding of ^{125}I-FSH to different tissues. 25 mg of homogenized testes, spleen, lung and muscle were incubated with 100,000 cpm of ^{125}I-FSH for 60 min at 37° C. The ^{125}I-FSH binding in the spleen, lung and muscle represents a small fraction of the specific binding observed in the testes.

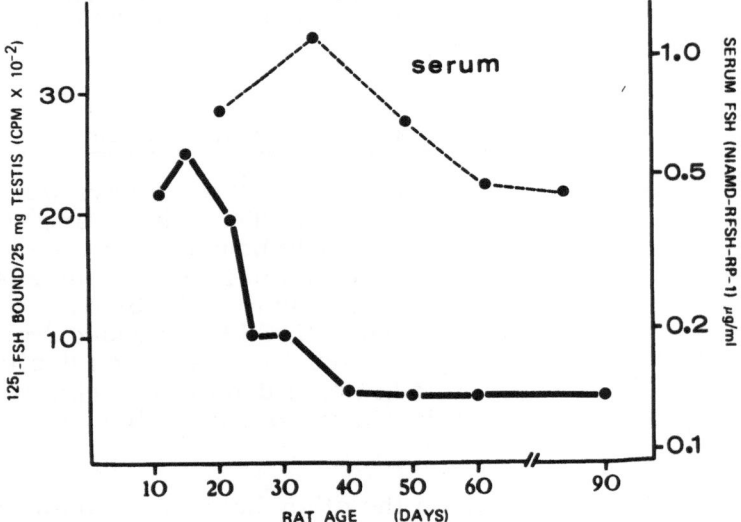

Figure 6. Serum FSH levels from Swerdloff et al. (16). o——o specific binding of ^{125}I-FSH to testes at different stages of maturation. At all ages, 25 mg of homogenized testes were incubated with ^{125}I-FSH for 60 min at 37° C. N=4.
o - - - o serum FSH levels (16). There is no correlation between the degree of ^{125}I-FSH binding in the testis and level of circulating FSH.

25 and 90 day rats are shown in Figures 7-9. The association constant (K_a) for the hormone-receptor interaction was calculated form the slope of the line, analyzed by least squares. The

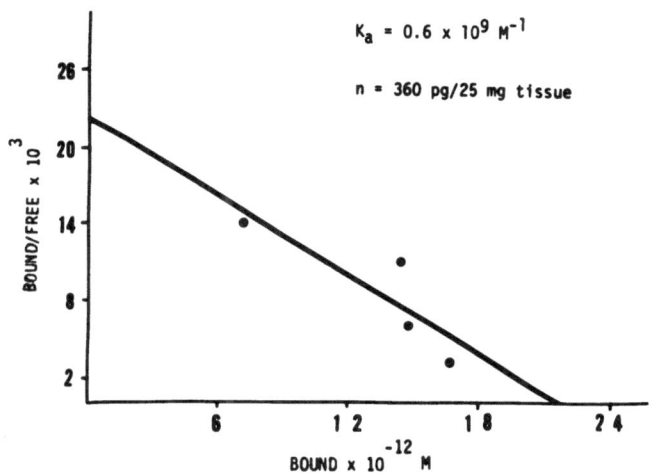

Figure 7. Scatchard plot for ^{125}I-FSH binding by 25 mg testes from 16-day rats. The association constant $(K_a) = 0.6 \times 10^9$ M^{-1}. Receptor concentrations = 364 pg/25 mg tissue.

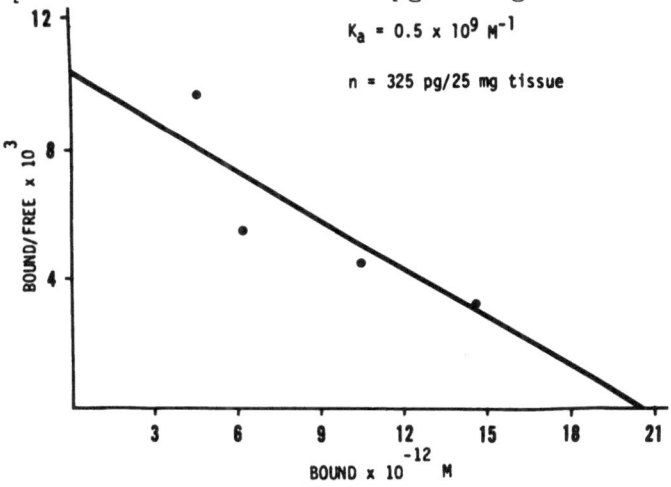

Figure 8. Scatchard plot for ^{125}I-FSH binding by 25 mg testes from 25-day rats. $K_a = 0.5 \times 10^9$ M^{-1}, receptor concentration - 325 pg/25 mg tissue.

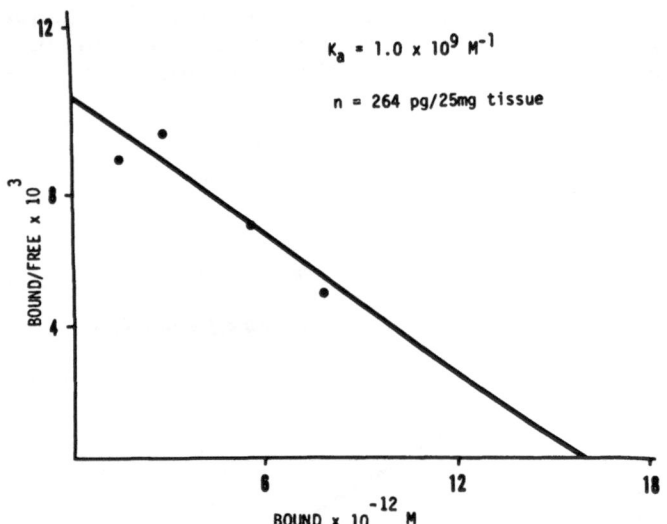

Figure 9. Scatchard plot for ^{125}I-FSH binding by 25 mg testes from 90 day rat K_a = 1.0 x 10^9 M^{-1}, receptor concentration - 266 pg/25 mg tissue.

intercept on the abscissa gave a measure of receptor concentration. Assuming the molecular weight of FSH as 33,000 (18), the number of binding sites per 25 mg testis was 360 pg in 16-day old animals, 325 in 25-day, and 264 in 90-day old animals. The K_a values were 0.6 x 10^9 M^{-1}, 0.5 x 10^9 M^{-1} and 1.0 x 10^9 M^{-1} for the 16, 25 and 90-day age groups respectively.

FSH binding to testes of hypophysectomized rats

Sprague Dawley rats hypophysectomized at 60 days of age were sacrificed at various time intervals following the operation and the testes used for hormone binding. The results are summarized in Figure 10. No significant changes in ^{125}I-FSH binding was observed up to 37 days following hypophysectomy.

FSH binding to various cell fractions

Seminiferous tubules isolated from interstitial cells bound

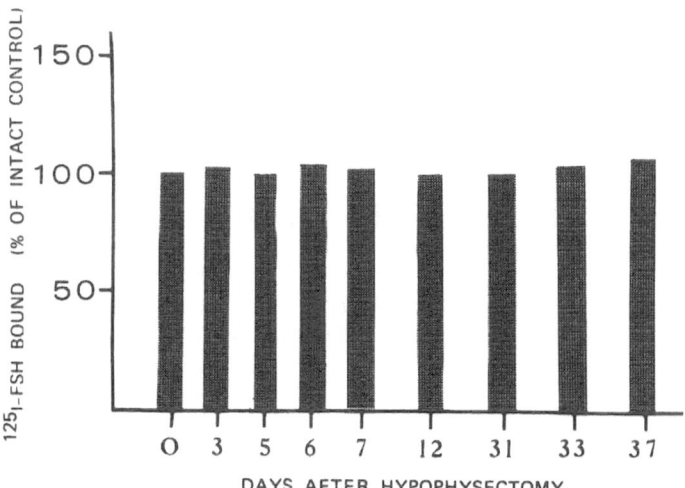

Figure 10. Effect of hypophysectomy on testicular binding of ^{125}I-FSH. Testes were obtained from mature animals at various time periods following hypophysectomy. The height of each bar represents specific binding relative to ^{125}I-FSH binding in intact mature animals. N=2.

^{125}I-FSH to the same extent as did whole tissue. No specific binding of the hormone was observed to either interstitial cells, germ cells or peritubular cells. All of these cell types bound small amounts of hormone in a non-specific fashion. It seems pertinent to mention that isolated interstitial cells bound significant amounts of ^{125}I-LH (19).

Discussion

Previous studies on FSH binding to testicular receptors have been performed using H-FSH (9). Labeling with ^{125}I has been successful with a number of peptide hormones such as LH (20), ACTH (21) and several others. It has been difficult, however, to prepare ^{125}I tagged FSH without significant loss of biological activity (22). Using a modified method of iodination, we obtained ^{125}I-FSH which retained approximately 80% of its biological activity and proved suitable for in vitro study of the hormone-receptor interaction in rat testes. Recently, ^{125}I-labeled human FSH was shown by several physical parameters to react as a single molecular species, similar to ^{3}H-labeled or native hormone (23).

The binding of ^{125}I-FSH to testis was shown to be 85% specific in contrast to non-target tissues such as spleen, lung or muscle which bound the hormone in a non-specific fashion. The specificity of ^{125}I-FSH binding in the testis was further verified by obtaining significant competitive inhibition with various FSH preparations (NIH-FSH-S3; NIH-FSH-P1) but not with HCG (Ayerst) or LH (NIH-LH-S5; NIH-LH-S-11; NIH-LH-B5; LER 960).

The binding of ^{125}I-FSH to testis was time dependent reaching maximum after 60 min incubation at 37° C. The dissociation of the bound hormone, however, was a slow process with only 20% of the hormone being released from the receptor after 2 hr at 37° C. This is comparable to the slow dissociation of LH bound by granulosa cells (24).

The amount of bound ^{125}I-FSH was linear to hormone concentration until the available receptors became saturated at hormone concentration of 40 ng/0.5 ml. The association constant for ^{125}I-FSH binding by testes homogenate was similar to that obtained with ^{3}H-FSH binding by testicular mince (9). In our experience, homogenized tissue proved superior to minced tissue, in that it bound greater amounts of ^{125}I-FSH and yielded more reproducible results.

The more readily demonstrable effects of FSH in testis of immature or adult hypophysectomized animals compared to testes of intact adults, has been interpreted by some investigators (5, 6) as being due to higher endogenous levels of FSH in the intact adult animals. In our studies, testes of 10-25 day rats bound considerably more FSH/mg tissue than did testes of animals that were older than 40 days. Means and Vaitukaitis (9) also reported greater binding of ^{3}H-FSH to testes of 20 day rats compared to mature animals. However when binding of ^{125}I-FSH to testis of different age animals was compared with levels of circulating FSH, no correlation was found between these two parameters. If one assumes that endogenous concentration of FSH in the testes parallels serum FSH level, then the changes in ^{125}I-FSH binding in testes with age, cannot be explained by the changes in endogenous FSH. Serum FSH level in 21 day rats is about twice that found in a mature animal and coincides with higher binding of ^{125}I-FSH in the testes, while binding to testes of mature animals is lowest in spite of also lowest FSH concentration in the serum. This is quite opposite to what one would expect if the differences in FSH binding by the testes were primarily due to changes in endogenous hormone concentrations. Moreover, we found no significant difference in the amount of ^{125}I-FSH bound by testes of adult hypophysectomized animals, tested up to 37 days following pituitary removal.

Scatchard plots of ^{125}I-FSH binding to testes of 16, 25 and

90-day old rats revealed a slight but progressive decrease in receptor concentration with age which coincide with declining ^{125}I-FSH binding. The association constant in the three age groups, however, did not differ significantly indicating a similar nature of hormone-receptor binding between the 16th and 90th day.

The changes in receptor concentration with age could have been due to changes in cell composition of the testis during maturation. It is tempting to postulate, that FSH receptors in the testes may be located in the Sertoli cells. Since these cells replicate only until the 15th postnatal day their relative number (thus the receptor concentration) decreases after the 15th day due to appearance of differentiating germ cells.

So far, there is only indirect evidence suggesting presence of FSH binding receptors in Sertoli cells. It has been previously reported and demonstrated in this study, that the receptors are associated with cells of the seminiferous tubules and not the interstitial cells. Of the cell types which compose the seminiferous tubules neither the spermatocytes, spermatids or the peritubular cells bind ^{125}I-FSH. While isolated spermatogonia have not been tested directly for their ability to bind FSH, organ cultured testes which contained no other germ cells, except occasional primitive type A spermatogonia, bound significant amounts of ^{125}I-FSH. The specific binding of ^{125}I-FSH in the organ cultured testes would seem to be due to the Sertoli cells, which retain their viability and morphologic integrity in culture for prolonged periods of time (2, 3, 13).

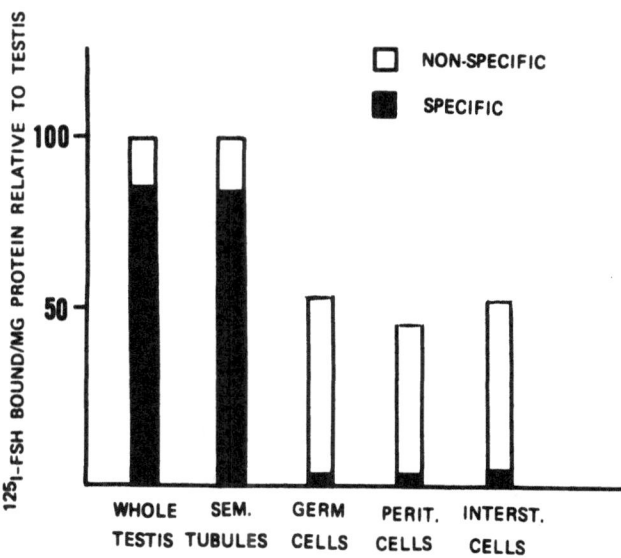

Figure 11. Binding of ^{125}I-FSH to various testes components.

It appears, from all available indications, that the FSH binding receptors in the testes are located in the Sertoli cells which may represent the primary target site for FSH activity in the seminiferous tubules.

The peritubular cells were isolated by a culture method and the other components by mechanical means. Homogenates of 25 mg whole testis or seminiferous tubules and 1×10^6 cells were used for hormone binding. ^{125}I-FSH/mg protein bound by individual components are compared with ^{125}I-FSH/mg protein bound by the whole testes. The hormone binds specifically to a seminiferous tubule component but not to germ or peritubular cells.

Acknowledgments

This work was supported in part by NICHD grand HD06319.

The authors express their gratitude to NIAMD and National Pituitary Agency for the generous gift of LH and FSH preparation.

References

1. Steinberger, A., and Steinberger, E., Biology of Reprod. 4, 484, 1971.

2. Steinberger, A., and Steinberger, E., J. Reprod. Fertil. Suppl. 2: 117, 1967.

3. Steinberger, E., Steinberger, A., and Perloff, W. H., Endocrinology 74: 788, 1964.

4. Means, A. R., and Hall, P. F., Endocrinology 81: 1151, 1967.

5. Kuehl, F. A., Patanelli, D. J., Tarnoff, J., and Humes, J. L., Biology of Reprod. 2: 154, 1970.

6. Dorrington, J. H., Vernon, R. G., and Fritz, I. B., Biochem. Biophys. Res. Comm. 46:1523, 1972.

7. Mancini, R. E., Castro, A., and Seiguer, A. C., J. Histochem. Cytochem. 15: 516, 1967.

8. Castro, A. E., Alonso, A., and Mancini, R. E., J. Endocrinology 52: 129, 1972.

9. Means, A. R., and Vaitukaitis, J., Endocrinology 90: 39, 1972.

10. Greenwood, F. C., Hunter, W. M., and Glover, J. S., Biochem. J. 89: 114, 1963.

11. Steinberger, A., In "Methods in Enzymology", O'Malley, B. W., and Hardman, J. G. (eds.), Academic Press, New York, in press.

12. Lowry, O. H., Rosebrough, N. J., Farr, A. L., and Randall, R. J., J. Biol. Chem. 193: 265, 1951.

13. Steinberger, E., Steinberger, A., and Perloff, W. H., Anat. Record. 148: 581, 1964.

14. Steinberger, E., and Ducket, G. E., J. Reprod. Fertility (Suppl. 2) 75: 715, 1967.

15. Vilar, O., and Steinberger, E., Zeitschr. fur Zellforsh. 78: 221, 1967.

16. Swerdloff, R. S., Walsh, P. C., Jacobs, H. S., and O'Dell, W. D., Endocrinology 88: 120, 1971.

17. Scatchard, G., Ann. N. Y. Acad. Sci. 51: 660, 1949.

18. Sherwood, A., In Methods in Enzymology", O'Malley, B. W., J., and Hardman, J. G. (eds.), Academic Press, New York (in press).

19. Steinberger, A., Yang, K. P., and Ward, D. H. Abstract 447, 55th Annual Meeting of the Endocrine Society, 1973.

20. Catt, K. J., Dufau, M. L., and Tsuruhara, T., J. Clin. Endocr. Metab. 32: 860, 1971.

21. Lefkowitz, r. J., Roth, J., Pricer, W., and Pastan, I., Proc. Natl. Acad. Sci. U.S.A. 65: 745, 1970.

22. Butt, W. R., In Immunoassays of Gonadotropins, Dichfalusy, E. (ed.), Stockholm, p. 24, 1969.

23. Sherins, R. J., Vaitukaitis, J. L., and Chrambach, A., Endocrinology 92: 1135, 1973.

24. Channing, C. P., and Kammerman, S., Endocrinology 92: 531, 1973.

BINDING OF HUMAN FSH AND ITS SUBUNITS TO RAT TESTIS

David Rabin

Department of Chemical Endocrinology
Hadassah University Hospital, Jerusalem, Israel

Diabetes Section, Clinical Endocrinology Branch
National Institute of Arthritis, Metabolism, and Digestive
Diseses, National Institutes of Health, Bethesda, Maryland 20014

Introduction

It has long been recognized that for a hormone to activate a target tissue, it must bind to some element of the cell. Roth and his colleagues (1) and Goodfriend and Lin (2) introduced appropriate techniques for directly studying the binding of a hormone to its target cell. Catt, Dufau and their colleagues (3, 4) and Reichert et al. (5) have characterized the binding of labeled human Luteinizing Hormone (hLH) and of human Chorionic Gonadotropin (hCG) to rat testis in vitro and impressive advances have been made in the isolation of the specific receptor hCG.

Means and Vaitukaitis have pioneered the studies on specific binding of hFSH to testis (6, 7). These authors employed tritiated hFSH, using initially a mince of rat testis and later isolated testicular cells.

We were stimulated by these reports to explore the possibility of binding ^{125}I-labeled hFSH to rat testis. We have developed a binding assay employing an homogenate of rat testis. The method of iodination, and the subsequent preparation of the tracer are of critical importance in obtaining ^{125}I-hFSH which exhibits specific binding to gonadal tissues (8-10).

Procedures

Iodination: We have iodinated two pituitary hFSH preparations: LER-1366 and LER-869-2. Iodination was performed by the Chloramine T method of Greenwood et al. (11) as modified by Roth (12). In our original studies we iodinated gently to achieve specific activities of between 1.2-36 $\mu C/\mu g$. Free iodine was separated from protein on a short column of Sephadex G-75. The protein fractions from the latter were then passed over a long 90 x 2.5 cm Sephadex G-100 column. The fractionation patterns of four representative iodinations are shown in Figure 1.

More recently we have employed only 1% or less of the amounts of Chloramine T we had previously used, and have dispensed with subsequent addition of sodium metabisulfite. A typical reaction mixture would be

hFSH	4 μg in 20 μl
0.3 $\underline{M}$ PO$_4$ buffer	10 μl
Na- ^{125}Iodide	5 μl (100 μC/μl)
0.2 $\underline{M}$ NaH$_2$PO$_4$	5 μl
Chloramine T	5 μl (30 μg/ml)

Testicular homogenate: Young rats (15-21 days) were sacrificed by cervical dislocation. The testes were removed and decapsulated. Homogenization was performed with an electric blender. The homogenate was centrifuged at 600 x g and the supernatant ("tissue fraction" was decanted and used in the receptor binding studies.

Receptor Assay: 0.2 ml of tissue fraction containing 1.5-2.0 mg of protein was incubated with tracer FSH for six hours at 20° C. The tubes were then centrifuged at 38,000 x g for 30 min at 4° C. Both the pellet and the supernatant were counted in a Packard autogamma counter. Samples were counted for a sufficient length of time to ensure no more than a 2% counting error.

RESULTS

I. Binding of ^{125}I-hFSH

Labeled hFSH preparations differed markedly in their ability to bind "specifically" to gonadal tissue. This is illustrated in

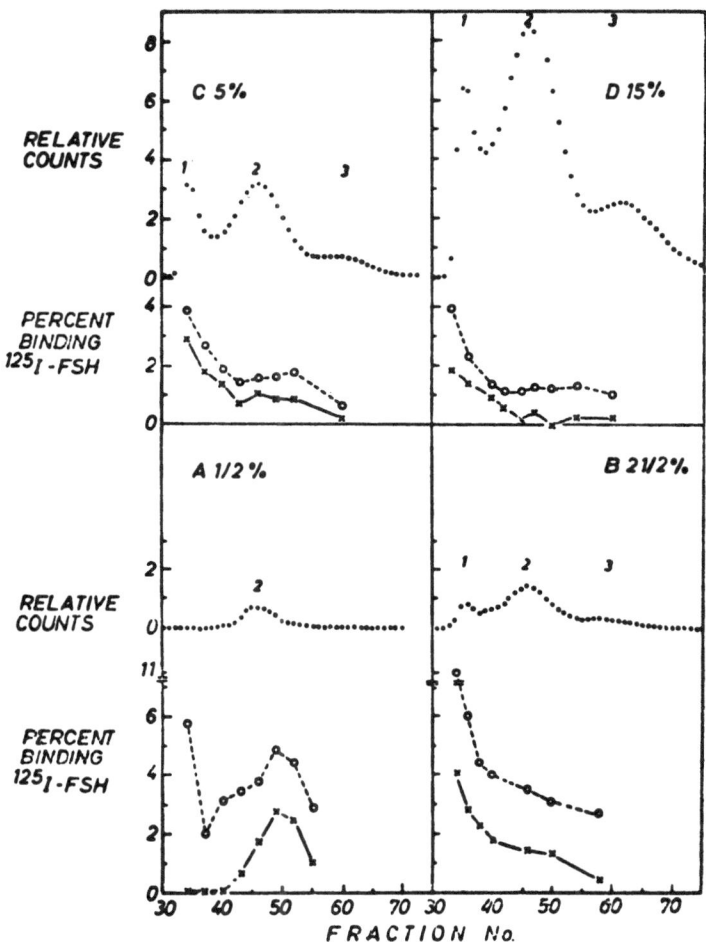

Figure 1.   Comparison of the testicular receptor binding of different fractions of ^{125}I-FSH obtained by G-100 Sephadex gel
filtration of iodinated FSH from four separate iodinations, A-D,
with degrees of iodination of 1/2%, 2 1/2%, 5% and 15%, respectively.   The dots represent the relative number of counts in each
fraction after gel filtration, the same scale being used for A, B,
C and D.   The open circles represent the percentage of added
counts bound to the testicular tissue in the absence of cold FSH.
The crosses represent the percentage of added counts which were
displaced from the testicular tissue when cold FSH (200 mIU of
HMG) competed with the iodinated FSH for the "receptor".   The
numbers 1, 2 and 3 above the peaks in the gel filtration pattern
(dots) indicate Peaks 1, 2 and 3.

Figure 1. In general, the best binding was achieved by using
as tracer, fractions which eluted with a K_{av} = 0.10 (Peak 1
in Fig. 1). We have suggested elswhere (9) that Peak 1 may
represent aggregates of FSH. Specific binding was not as good
in Peak 2 (associated hFSH) and was negligible with Peak 3 (which
probably reflects free subunits of hFSH).

Specific binding was observed only with testis. Spleen, heart,
liver and kidney showed little total binding, and the latter was
not displaceable with hMG (Pergonal, Serono). By contrast,
binding of hFSH to testis was readily observed, which binding was
readily displaced by 200 mIU of hMG (Fig. 2).

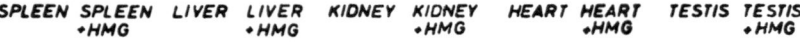
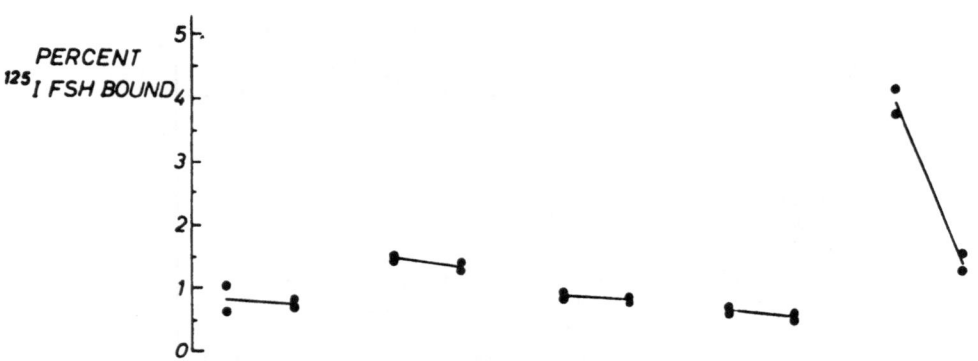

Figure 2. Comparison of total binding of ^{125}I-FSH and binding
of ^{125}I-FSH in the presence of competition by cold FSH (200 mIU
of HMG) in different tissues.

II.   Studies with hFSH, hMG, and α and ß subunits of hFSH

We have compared LER-1366, LER-869-2 and 2nd IRP-hMG
as competitors with labeled FSH for binding to tissue fractions
of rat testis. There did not appear to be substantial differences
between FSH of pituitary and of urinary origin when the latter
were expressed in terms of their stated biologic potencies. By
contrast, competition by the ß subunit of hFSH was only 1/50th
that of hFSH, and that α chain was even weaker (Fig. 3).

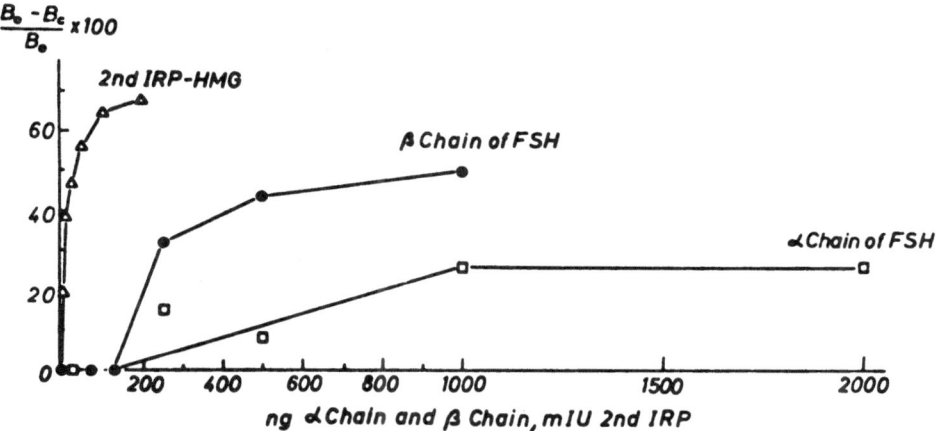

Figure 3. Comparison of the competition for the testicular FSH "receptor" by 2nd IRP-HMG, α chain of FSH and ß chain of FSH. The Y axis shows percent displaceable binding. The scale of the abscissa is in mIU/tube for 2nd IRP-HMG and in ng/tube for the α and ß chains of FSH.

III. Competition studies with hCG

In our original studies we noticed that hCG competed with labeled hFSH at concentrations of 1 Unit and displacement was maximal with 100 Units of hCG (Organon hCG, "Pregnyl") (Figure 4).

In more recent studies, in collaboration with Drs. J. Roth and B. Weintraub, we have extended these observations. Competition was observed with each of four preparations of hCG tested: hCG Organon (Pregnyl), hCG Ayerst (APL), hCG Hickman and hCG Canfield. Under conditions where maximal competition was observed with 5 Units of Pergonal (or 2 μg of LER-136, stated potency of 6 Units of FSH) we required up to 500 Units of hCG to achieve similar displacement. No significant inhibition of binding was observed with either hCG α or hCGß.

Discussion

Iodinated hFSH is bound specifically by an homogenate of rat testis. Even under conditions in which substantially less than one atom of iodine was introduced per molecule of FSH, different fractions of the hormone displayed disparate binding activity.

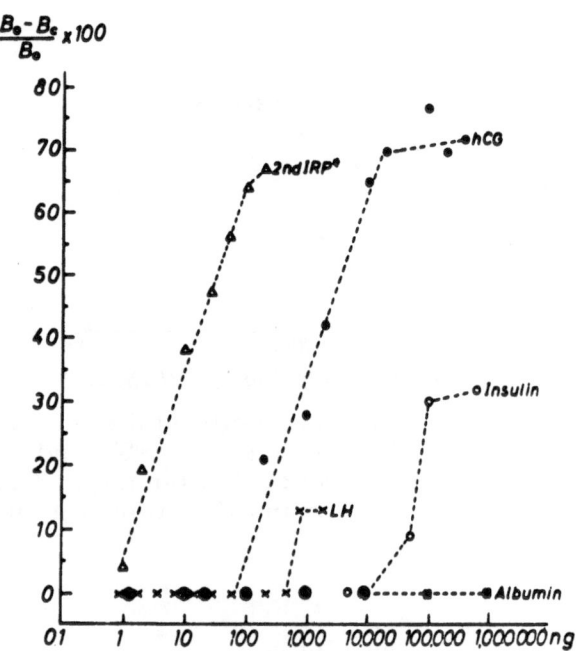

Figure 4. Comparison of competition for the testicular FSH
"receptor" by 2nd IRP-HMG (triangles), hCG (closed circles),
LH (LER 960, crosses), insulin (open circles) and albumin
(solid squares).

The FSH molecule appears to be particularly susceptible to
damage and thus gentle iodination becomes a critical prerequisite for binding studies. Even so, we have succeeded in
achieving binding of only 5% or so of tracer hFSH. Several factors probably contribute to this: the system we have used
appears to result in degradation of FSH receptors and there also
appears to be partial destruction of tracer. Thus, binding may
be enhanced by using a more purified testicular preparation.
Also, we have succeeded in reducing degradation, by shortening
incubation time to 3 hours or less. Until we can fully resolve
the above technical questions, we will be unable to establish
whether a relatively small number of receptors contributes to
the low degree of binding observed.

Despite these strictures, useful and reproducible data have
been collected with the present assay. We have shown

considerable specificity of the receptor: whereas hFSH of pituitary and of urinary origin compete equally, neither the α nor the ß subunit of hFSH displaced labeled hFSH significantly. The receptor assay differs in this respect from many anti-FSH antisera which readily recognize the ß subunit of FSH (8). Conversely, an human anti-hFSH antiserum which we observed in an individual with isolated FSH deficiency after Pergonal therapy, behaved in a manner similar to the Receptor Assay. That is, the antiserum recognized native hFSH much more avidly than either of the subunits (8).

In our early studies we made the interesting observation that hCG competed for binding to the FSH receptor. We have confirmed this with four different hCG preparations which varied widely in potency and purity. The hCG preparations were much less potent that hFSH when comparison was made in terms of mass or or units (2nd IRP-hMG and 2nd International Standard of hCG are of course not comparable). This theoretically may provide a partial explanation for the so-called FSH-like action of hCG (13). We are presently exploring other systems for their potential to bind hFSH. Thus far we have not succeeded in our attempts to show binding to either peripheral or culture lymphocytes.

Summary

Specific binding of ^{125}I-hFSH to rat testicular tissue has been demonstrated. Methods of labeling hFSH are critical in ensuring label suitable for binding studies. Three dissimilar hFSH-containing preparations displaced tracer from testicular tissue in a relationship proportional to the stated biologic activity of the preparation. Subunits of hFSH and of hCG showed negligible competition. However, hCG competed for binding at concentrations 100 times that of hFSH.

Acknowledgments

We thank Dr. R. E. Canfield for hCG, hCG and hCGß and Dr. L. E. Reichert for hFSH   (LER-1661 (8-10)) and hFSHß (LER-1679-82). Original work was supported in Dr. R.'s laboratory by the Israel Cancer Association, The Population Council and the Joint Fund, Hebrew University-Hadassah Medical School.

References

1. Lefkowitz, R. J., Roth, J., and Pastan, I., Science 170: 633, 1970.

2. Lin, S-Y., and Goodfriend, T. L., Amer. J. Physiol. 218: 1319, 1970.

3. Catt, K. J., Dufau, M. L., and Tsuruhara, T., J. Clin. Endocr. 34: 123, 1972.

4. Catt, K. J., Tsuruhara, T., and Dufau, M. L., Biochim. Biophys. Acta (Amst.) 279: 194, 1972.

5. Liedenberger, F., and Reichert, L. E., Jr., Endocrinology 91: 901, 1972.

6. Means, A. R., and Vaitukaitis, J., Endocrinology 90: 39, 1972.

7. Means, A. R., Adv. Exp. Med. Biol. 36: 431, 1973.

8. Rabinowitz, D., Bell, J., Benveniste, R., and Schwartz, S., Nature New Biol. 245: 245, 1973.

9. Bell, J., Benveniste, R., Schwartz, S., and Rabinowitz, D., Endocrinology, in press.

10. Schwartz, S., Bell, J., Rechnitz, S., and Rabinowitz, D., Europ. J. Clin. Invest., Dec. 1973.

11. Greenwood, F. C., Hunter, W. M., and Glover, J. S., Biochem. J. 89: 1214, 1963.

12. Roth, J., Metabolism 22: 1059, 1973.

13. Albert, A., J. Clin. Endocr. 29: 1504, 1969.

FSH RECEPTORS IN RAT TESTES: CHEMICAL PROPERTIES AND SOLUBILIZATION STUDIIES

V. K. Bhalla and Leo E. Reichert, Jr.

Division of Basic Health Sciences, Emory University
Atlanta, Georgia 30322

Introduction

The interaction of protein hormones with specific receptors is believed to initiate a series of events at the molecular level leading ultimately to a physiologically significant response. We have previously demonstrated the presence luteinizing hormone (LH) specific receptors in Leydig cell homogenates (1, 2) and follicle stimulating hormone (FSH) specific receptors in seminiferous tubule homogenate (3) of mature rat testes. These studies allowed development of tissue receptor assays for hLH (2, 4) and hFSH (5) suitable for measurement of gonadotropin activities in pituitary fractions as well as for various types of structure-function studies. We have extended our earlier binding studies with FSH (3) and in this report describe our recent observations on the interaction of ^{125}I-hFSH with testicular receptors as well as preliminary studies on the chemical properties of the receptor and attempts directed towards its solubilization.

Materials and Methods

Mature rats (250-300 g) of the Sprague-Dawley strain were utilized. Triton X-100 and Hyamine 2389 were purchased from J. T. Baker & Co., N.Y.; Lubrol PX and WX and Sepharose 6B-100 from Sigma Chemical Co., Mo.; trypsin (TPCK) and soy bean trypsin inhibitor are from Worthington Biochemical Corp., N.J.; and carbowax 400 and 6000 from Schwarz/Mann, N. Y.

Iodination of hFSH and hLH were carried out as described earlier (2, 3, 5). The methods utilized for preparation of Leydig

Table 1

Conditions for Iodination of hFSH by Chloramine-T Method

Method	FSH (μmoles)[a]	Molar Ratio hFSH/Chl.T.	T(C)	Time[b] (sec)	^{125}I-Na mCi	pH	SA μCi/μg	Activity	Non-Specific Binding
Butt (7)[c]	1.5×10^{-4}	1:2372	not rep.	60	2-4	7.5	not rep.	-	-
Miyachi et al. (9)	6.0×10^{-5}	1:1482	room T.	60	1	7.8[d]	not rep.	-	-
This report									
Modification A	1.5×10^{-3}	1:15.8	4	30	1	7.5	9.5 ± 2	100	20
Modification B	1.5×10^{-3}	1:15.8	4	120	2	7.5	35 ± 2	46	30

[a] Estimated on basis of MW of 33,000 for hFSH.
[b] Reaction time before addition of metabisulfite.
[c] These conditions developed for iodination of GH (6) are also generally utilized for radioimmunoassay of hFSH.
[d] Iodination carried out in presence of 0.15 M NaCl.
[e] For details see reference (5).
[f] For definition see Material and Methods. For details see reference (3).

cell homogenate and seminiferous tubule homogenate have already been described (3, 5). Seminiferous tubule homogenates were prepared as described in (3). The homogenate was filtered through a single layer of cheese cloth which permits the separation of the tubules from larger tissue fragments. In practice, smooth and fast filtration is achieved by "see-sawing" the cheesecloth onto which the homogenate is poured. When this is done, larger tissue fragments do not clog the pores and smaller tubules fragments easily pass through the cheesecloth. Binding studies were carried out as described earlier (3). Homogenates of intact testes were prepared as follows: rat testes were weighed to the nearest milligram, the tunica albuginea removed and the remaining tissue chilled and homogenized in a teflon pestle tissue grinder (Arthur H. Thomas, Philadelphia). Further processing of the homogenate for use in receptor studies was described elsewhere (3).

Results and Discussion

Iodination of hFSH[1]. Our procedure for iodination of hFSH (5) differs in various details from the classical chloramine-T method as described by Greenwood et al. (6) (Table 1). It was reported by other laboratories (7-9) that the chloramine-T procedure for iodination of proteins results in pronounced loss of biological activity when applied to FSH. We have since demonstrated that careful control of experimental conditions can result in the preparation of ^{125}I-hFSH that retains biological activity (Table 1). A variable of particular importance is the hormone to chloramine-T ratio utilized for the preparation of ^{125}I-hFSH. Our mild experimental conditions, using hormone: chloramine-T ratio of 1:16, resulted in the preparation of ^{125}I-hFSH which gave an acceptable 20% non-specific binding in the tissue receptor assay under our standard conditions (3, 5).

Specific binding is calculated as

$$\frac{B_t - B_n}{B_t} \times 100$$

where B_t is total counts bound to the homogenate in the absence of excess unlabeled hormone and B_n is total counts bound to the homogenate in the presence of excess cold hormone. Six hundred fold molar excess of hormone is usually selected for the estimation of non-specific binding. We feel that in studies relating to membrane bound and soluble receptor assays a common system

---

[1] The abbreviations used are: FSH, follicle-stimulating hormone; hFSH, human follicle-stimulating hormone; LH, luteinizing hormone; hLH, human luteinizing hormone; PEG, polyethylene glycol.

Table 2

Influence of Tissue Preparation on Binding ^{125}I-hLH and ^{125}I-FSH

4.5 mg Leydig cell homogenate and 45 mg of seminiferous tubule and intact homogenate was taken per tube for binding studies in a total volume of 1 ml containing 5 ng of 125I-hLH and 125I-hFSH with and without excess cold hormone. Binding studies were described earlier (3).

	^{125}I-LH Binding % specific binding[a]	^{125}I-FSH Binding % specific binding[a]
Leydig cell homogenate[a]	70.5	25.5
Seminiferous tubule homogenate[a]	65.5	68.2
Intact fresh homogenate	89.5	78
Leydig cell[b]	85	68.8
Seminiferous tubule[b]	60	81

[a]Preparations of homogenate are described in detail elsewhere (3,5). Values are mean of duplicate determinations.

[b]Leydig cells and seminiferous tubules were prepared according to the method of Christensen and Mason (12).

of defining specific and non-specific binding should be adapted to avoid the confusion which occasionally arises in the literature when discussing these parameters. It is also desirable to check the non-specific binding for each new iodinated preparation by running an assay with increasing doses of unlabeled hormone, and selecting the level which gives the least non-specific binding.

Site of action of LH and FSH in rat testes. The site of action of
LH and FSH in rat testes has long been a subject of debate. Mancini
et al. (10) reported accumulation of LH and FSH in the Leydig cells
and the Sertoli cells respectively. Kuehl et al. (11) described stimulation of adenyl cyclase by LH in isolated seminiferous tubules.
Christensen and Mason (12) found that both tissues, i.e., Leydig
cells and seminiferous tubules, are capable of converting progesterone to testosterone, though seminiferous tubules were less effective in this regard. Our initial justification for using seminiferous
tubule homogenate for ^{125}I-hFSH binding studies has been described
elsewhere (3). These and further studies (Table 2) suggest the presence of LH and FSH receptors in both the Leydig cells and seminiferous tubules. In order to rule out the possibility of Leydig cell
contamination in the seminiferous tubule homogenate and vice versa,
more highly purified Leydig cell and seminiferous tubule fractions
were prepared by the method of Christensen and Mason (12). The
results are in accordance with our earlier findings (Table 2).

Furthermore, specific binding of ^{125}I-hFSH to Leydig cells and
to seminiferous tubules can only be inhibited to a significant extent
by unlabeled FSH (Fig. 1). The % specific binding of ^{125}I-hFSH to
Leydig cell homogenate though quantitatively less than for ^{125}I-hLH,
clearly reveals a dose response relationship (Fig. 1A). Other hormones like insulin, ACTH, growth hormone and prolactin had no
effect (data not shown). Similar results were obtained utilizing
^{125}I-hLH and ^{125}I-hFSH using seminiferous tubules (Fig. 1B).
Thus, separate receptors for LH and FSH would seem to be present
in the Leydig cells as well as in seminiferous tubule homogenates.
Though the presence of LH receptors in seminiferous tubules support the contention of Christensen and Mason (12) and Kuehl et al.
(11) which suggests a role of LH in conjunction with FSH in steroidogenesis in rat seminiferous tubules, the role of FSH in Leydig cell
physiology is not yet clear. Final proof awaits the availability of
more effective techniques for separation of Leydig cells and seminiferous tubules and rigorous evaluation of the purity of each type of
preparation. We recognize the argument that some of our results
may be partially explained by LH contamination in the FSH preparation used for iodination and vice versa, but the extent of cross contamination of these gonadotropin with one another is estimated to
be less than 5% on a mass basis. This would not be enough to
account for our results. The caveat that our Leydig cell or seminiferous tubule preparation may be contaminated one with the other,
is also recognized. However, we do feel that the presence of a
large percentage of seminiferous tubule fragments in the Leydig
cell homogenate is not a likely possibility due to the method used
for its preparation (12). The possibility that the tubular preparation is contaminated with Leydig cells cannot be completely ruled
out at present, as discussed elsewhere (3).

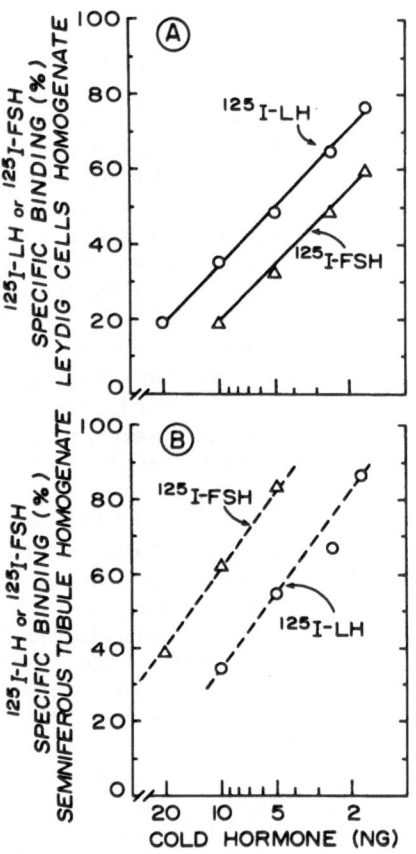

Figure 1. Binding of ^{125}I-LH and its displacement by unlabeled LH
(o-o) and binding of ^{125}I-FSH and its displacement by unlabeled FSH
(-$\triangle$-$\triangle$-$\triangle$) utilizing Leydig cell homogenate (Fig. 1A) and seminiferous
tubule homogenate (Fig. 1B). Hormones utilized were LER-960 for
LH and LER-1575-C for FSH. Leydig cell homogenate (4.5 mg
weight) and seminiferous tubule homogenate (45 mg weight) were
used in a total incubation volume of 1 ml. The non-specific binding
was corrected and specific binding was calculated as described in
Table 1. The values are the mean of two determinations. For
experimental details see reference (3).

Effects of EDTA, trypsin and sulfhydryl reagent upon ^{125}I-hFSH
binding. Specific binding of ^{125}I-hFSH, unlike insulin, is very
much dependent upon the ionic strength of the medium (3). Chelating
agents such as EDTA inhibit binding (Table 3) suggesting a requirement for divalent cations or metal ions for binding. N-ethyl maleimide (NEM), a sulfhydryl reagent, also inhibits the ability of the

Table 3

Effect of Chelating Agent and Trypsin Upon ^{125}I-hFSH Binding

Seminiferous tubule homogenate is suspended in 0.01 M phosphate buffer, pH 7.5 and triplicate tubes containing 45 mg/tube were centrifuged at 1500 x g for 10 min to discard supernatant. Indicated molar concentration of EDTA is present during the entire incubation time in a total volume of 1 ml containing homogenate, buffer and ^{125}I-hFSH (5 ng). Each set has tubes for non-specific determinations. Trypsin digestion, the fresh homogenate in tubes was centrifuged as described above and resuspended in 1 ml of buffer containing 0.005 M MgCl$_2$, 0.1 M sucrose, 0.0115 M CaCl$_2$ at 37° and trypsin. Incubation time and levels of trypsin are used as indicated. After digestion, one wash with 1 ml buffer was given followed by centrifugation. The pellet in triplicate tubes were then used to binding assay as described earlier (3) with tubes designated for non-specific determinations. Each tube contained 100 mg of soybean trypsin inhibitor which is present during the entire period of incubation (3). Trypsin inhibitor alone at a concentration used has no detectable effect upon binding.

Agent Added	Specific Binding	Specific Counts (cpm)[1] Bound
a) EDTA (M)		
None	100 + 2	
0.001	80 + 2	
0.001	75 + 2	
0.005	72 + 2	
0.025	51.6 + 3	
0.05	37.5 ∓ 3	
0.25	fluffy mass	
b) Trypsin[2] Treatment (μg)		
None		900 + 49
200		+
300		634 + 30
400		600 + 4
600		750 + 46
800		728 + 28
1000		792 + 8
c) Trypsin[3] Treatment (Minutes)		
30		630 + 20
60		482 + 4
90		730 + 32

[1] 5 ng of ^{125}I-hFSH contains 43,296 cpm.

[2] Trypsin used was TPCK treated and had 216 IU/mg activity. Trypsin incubation was for 30 min at 37°C. [3] Digestion was carried out at 37°C with 300 μg trypsin in each tube (45 mg homogenate).

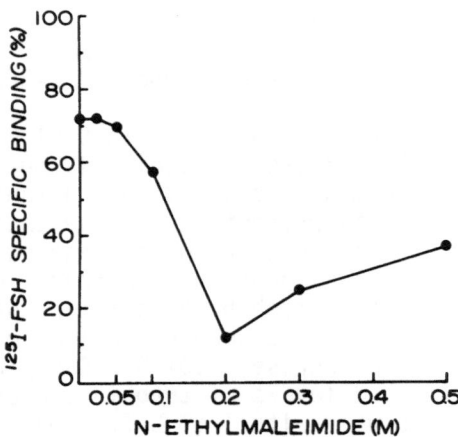

Figure 2. Effect of N-ethylmaleimide upon the ^{125}I-FSH binding ability of seminiferous tubule homogenate. Seminiferous tubules (45 mg/tube) were incubated with 1 ml of N-ethylmaleimide at concentrations as indicated for 45 min at room temperature and centrifuged at 1500 x g. The pellet was then washed with 3 ml buffer and recentrifuged. Control tubes were similarly treated with buffer instead of reagent. Binding assay was then carried out with and without excess cold hormone and each point represents the mean of triplicate experiments. The variation in replicate determinations was not more than 5%. For details of binding assays, see reference (3).

intact testicular homogenate to bind ^{125}I-hFSH (Fig. 2). The retention or slight elevation of specific binding of FSH at higher concentration of NEM may preclude a dependence of binding upon free-SH groups. The FSH-binding ability of the homogenate, when incubated with TPCK-treated trypsin, showed remarkable resistance to proteolysis, even when very high ratios of enzyme to substrates (1:45) were utilized (Table 3). Similarly, LH binding under the same experimental conditions show only 30-40% reduction in specific binding (data not shown).

Reduction in FSH binding as a result of treatment with N-ethyl maleimide or trypsin does not necessarily imply deactivation or digestion of the receptor since modification or disruption of membrane bound proteins could result in release of the functional receptor or "factor" (vide infra) into the supernatant. It has not been possible to measure FSH binding activity in such supernatants because of the availability of a reliable assay for the measurement of solubilized receptors or "factors" (vide infra). In our hands, procedures for measurement of soluble receptor (13, 19) activity

Table 4

Effects of Different Treatments Upon Binding of
$125I$-hFSH by Intact Testes Homogenate

Intact testes homogenate (45 mg/tube) was treated with 1 ml of detergent containing buffer to 1 hr at 4°C (except for freeze and
thaw). The pellet was washed and recentrifuged. The resulting
pellet was then used for binding studies with and without excess
cold hormone as described (3).

Treatment	Reduction in Binding of Homogenate after Treatment[a] % of untreated control
Freeze and thaw (5 times)	25-30 ± 2
Lubrol PX 0.12%	70 ± 2
Lubrol WX 0.09%	75.4 ± 3
Triton X-100 0.4%	73 ± 2
Hyamine	-
Ethanol 40%	80 ± 2

[a]Based upon inhibition of specific counts.

have not proven effective, for reasons not completely understood at
present (vide infra).

Solubilization of FSH receptors from rat testes. Attempts were
made to solubilize FSH receptors/factors by several different techniques (Table 4). Generally, the deliberate use of the term "receptors" has been confined to the hormone binding moiety which displays specificity with respect to FSH when in membrane bound as
well as "soluble form". In Rodbell's three component model systems of hormone responsive-membrane bound adenyl cylcase complex (14) the regulatory subunit of cyclase is a receptor which binds
to hormone while the catalytic subunit has access to ATP for generation of cAMP. As a consequence of the binding event, a coupler,
possibly a phospholipid, serves to transmit a signal causing activation of the cyclase and resulting in an increase of intracellular
levels of cAMP. It has also been suggested (15) that binding and
activation are separate events which are experimentally dissociable.
Although the presence of phospholipid is reported to be essential for
activation of adenyl cyclase, the lipid components are not required
for the initial interaction of norepinephrine with cardiac ß-receptors
(15). Although we have not yet studied the FSH responsive adenyl
cyclase, we do have preliminary evidence regarding the existence

of a functionally important factor which seems to be essential for
FSH binding. In subsequent discussion, therefore, we use the term
"receptors" for solubilization studies utilizing detergents and "factor" for studies utilizing ethanol and briefly report our preliminary
attempts to develop assays for measurement of the soluble receptor
and factor.

A.   Use of non-ionic detergent in solubilization of receptors.
The non-ionic detergents such as Triton X-100 or Lubrol PX have
greatly facilitated progress in the area of solubilization of membrane bound proteins (16), but they are usually difficult to remove
due to their binding to proteins. The binding occurs by possible
disruption of lipid protein interactions when detergent competes
for lipid binding sites of the protein (16). Detergents can restore
(17) or enhance the activity of adenyl cyclase (18). In the field
of soluble receptors, use of detergent either in buffers for chromatography or in polyethylene glycol assays have routinely been
recommended (13, 19). The presence of detergents, however,
can cause difficulty in interpretation of data because of the like-
lihood that they induce conformational changes in solubilized
receptor proteins (13).

We have, nevertheless, utilized non-ionic detergents for solubilization of FSH receptors (Table 4). Although detergent treated
homogenates lack ability to bind ^{125}I-FSH (Fig. 3) depending on the
amount of detergent used, we were unable to demonstrate the receptor activity in the supernatant to an acceptable degree. Detergent
extract was prepared utilizing 1 ml of 0.12% Lubrol PX per 45 mg
homogenate in a total volume of 1 ml and incubations were carrried
out as described under Figure 3. After detergent treatment the
homogenate was centrifuged at 20,000 x g for 1/2 hr followed by
recentrifugation of the supernatant at 150,000 x g for 1/2 hr. The
supernatant was then utilized as the receptor preparation in all subsequent studies relating to the development of soluble receptor assay.
Two methods utilized for the separation of bound from free were
gel filtration and selective separation of bound ^{125}I-hFSH from free
hormone by precipitation of the former with polyethylene glycol.
Gel filtration of putative ^{125}I-hFSH receptor complexes on sepharose 6B showed two peaks, the first peak being coincident with the
void volume (blue dextran) and the second peak representing free
^{125}I-hFSH. The first peak, which presumably represents a hormone receptor complex, when re-incubated with 600-fold excess
of unlabeled hormone and refiltered through the same column was
not decreased by more than 25% compared to the original pattern,
thus indicating high non-specific absorption. Results with Lubrol
WX or Triton X-100 were very similar. Polyethylene glycol
assays, when standardized with respect to volume, incubation time
and temperature, and % of PEG, with and without excess cold hormone, also displayed high non-specific binding (50-60%). Carbowax 6000 (25% w/v) was used to separate the bound ^{125}I-hFSH

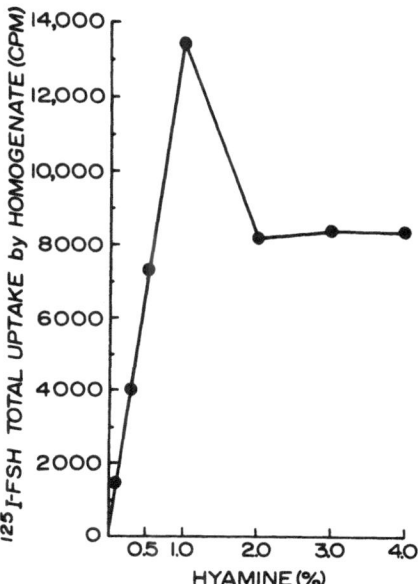

Figure 3.   Effect of detergent upon ^{125}I-hFSH binding.   Each tube contained 45 mg of intact testes homogenate and was treated with 1 ml of varying concentrations of Lubrol PX.   Incubations were carried out at 4° C for 1 hr followed by centrifugation at 1500 x g. The pellet was treated with 1 ml of buffer and recentrifuged.   The control tubes contained 1 ml of buffer.   Binding assay was then performed with and without excess hormone.   The results are the mean of triplicate determinations.   For details of binding assay see reference (3).

from the free.   Specific binding was defined in these studies as

$$\frac{B_t - B_n}{B_t} \times 100$$

and our results were expressed at saturating protein concentrations with respect to 5 ng of ^{125}I-hFSH.

When the cationic detergent Hyamine 2389* (20) was used in our solubilization studies, unusual effects of binding were noted.   Treatment of testicular homogenates with Hyamine 2389 resulted in an increased binding of ^{125}I-hFSH by the homogenate (Fig. 4).   The

---

Hyamine 2389 contains methyl dodecyl benzyl trimethyl ammonium chloride and methyl dodecyl xylene-bis trimethyl ammonium chloride.

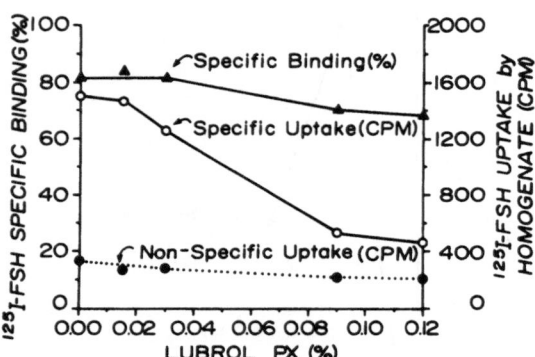

Figure 4. Effect of hyamine upon total binding of ^{125}I-FSH.
Experiment was essentially done as described under Fig. 3. Intact
testes homogenate (45 mg/tube) was treated with 1 ml of hyamine
solution at the concentration indicated and incubation was carried
out at 4° C for 1 hr followed by centrifugation and one wash. Binding assay was then performed with and without excess cold hormone
as described (3). Results are the mean of triplicate determinations.

total uptake was increased to 20% as compared to 2-4% with untreated homogenate, which probably reflects an ionic effect similar to
that seen in other studies (21) where the effects of reactants containing a quaternary ammonium moiety enhanced the magnitude of
binding of 3-fold.

B. Use of ethanol in solubilization of FSH-binding factor(s).
After removal of the tunica albuginea, the intact rat testes were
homogenized as described earlier (see Materials and Methods)
except that 30% ethanol containing buffer (v/v; 0.01 M phosphate
buffer with 0.1 M sucrose and 0.005 M MgCl) was used. The
homogenate (99 g of intact testes in a total volume of 200 ml of 30%
EtOH) was incubated at 37° C for 1 hr followed by centrifugation at
12,000 x g for 30 min. Supernatant was then recentrifuged at 48,000
x g for 30 min and diluted to a total volume of 800 ml of buffer. The
buffer utilized for this dilution was 0.01 M phosphate buffer containing 0.1 M sucrose and 0.005 M MgCl (but did not contain ethanol).
The final ethanol concentration after dilution was 10% (v/v). The
protein concentration as determined by the method of Lowry (22)
was 100 μg of protein per 100 μl with bovine serum albumin used as
standard. The data with "Factor" is expressed in terms of volume
since we do not have any information about its chemical nature and
100 μl of the final solution as prepared (vide supra) is equivalent
to that extracted from 12.3 mg intact testes, wet tissue weight.

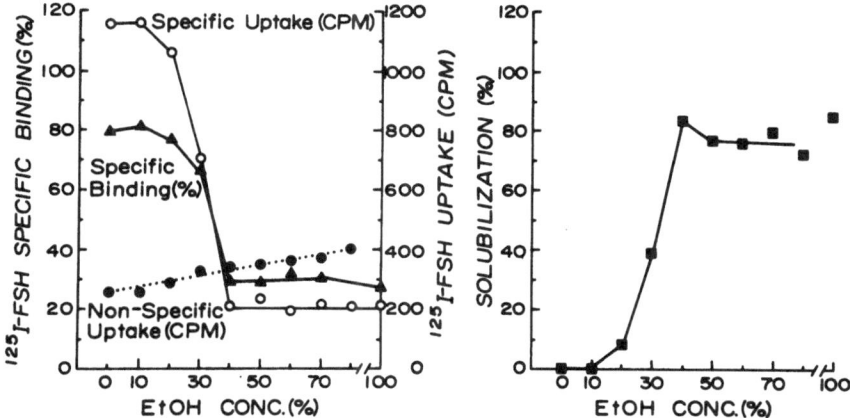

Figure 5. Effects of different concentrations of ethanol upon the
^{125}I-FSH binding ability of intact testes homogenate. Intact testes homogenate (45 mg/tube) was treated with 1 ml of indicated
concentrations of ethanol and incubations were carried out at 4° C
for 1 hr. After centrifugation and one wash, the treated pellet
was used for binding studies with and without excess hormone as
described earlier (3). % solubilization (right-hand plate) is calculated as

$$\frac{B_{un} - B_{tr}}{B_{un}} \times 100$$

where B_{un} is the specific counts in the untreated pellet and B_{tr}
is the treated pellet at any given EtOH concentration. Therefore
% solubilization is a reflection of a decreased specific binding of
^{125}I-FSH by the homogenate pellet.

Effect of ethanol extract upon ^{125}I-hFSH binding. The effects of
ethanol extraction of testicular homogenates (Fig. 5) are very similar to those seen after treatment with Lubrol PX (Fig. 3). Ethanol
seems to cause a solubilization of a "factor" essential for hormone
binding as reflected by loss of binding ability of the homogenate.
This loss of binding ability is temperature dependent (Fig. 6),
being maximum at 37° C and volume dependent (data not shown).
A simple delipidation of tissue homogenates by extraction with
ethanol would lead to similar effects but the chemical nature of this
factor has not yet been established. This observation is in direct
contrast to insulin binding to rat liver and fat cells where organic
solvent extractions of membrane (ethanol and ether) leads to an
increase in binding of hormone to the membrane preparation (23,
24). Loss of binding ability by the homogenate cannot be unequivo-
cally related to solubilization of an essential binding factor unless
hormone binding is demonstrable in the soluble supernate fraction.

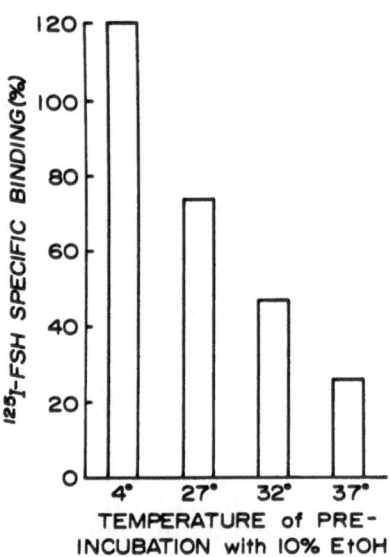

Figure 6. Effect of temperatures upon loss of ^{125}I-FSH binding ability of homogenate after pretreatment with a given concentration fo ethanol: The intact testes homogenate (45 mg/tube) were treated with 1 ml of 10% ethanol at various temperatures indicated for 1 hr. The respective control tubes contained 1 ml of buffer (without ethanol). After incubation, the tubes were centrifuged and supernatant was discarded. The pellet was washed with 2 ml of buffer and recentrifuged. The binding assay was then carried out as described earlier (3) with and without excess cold hormone. The specific binding at each temperature is represented as % of control and values are the mean of three determinations.

Several attempts were made to develop assays for measurement of a specific FSH binding factor in the ethanol supernatant. Column experiments using sepharose 6B in a manner similar to that described earlier (vide supra) revealed only one retarded peak, essentially indicating no substantial difference in molecular size of the free hormone compared to the presumed hormone-receptor complex. Application of a standard polyethylene glycol assay for detection of a hormone-receptor complex (vide supra) was also not successful. Two additional approaches were, therefore, used in an attempt to measure this "factor".

1) New polyethylene glycol assay method. The classical polyethylene glycol method originally proposed by Cuatrecasas for insulin (19) and modified by Dufau et al. (13) for application to hCG,

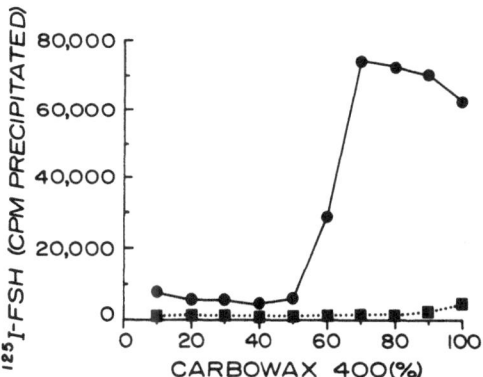

Figure 7. Effects of different concentrations of carbowax 400 upon
^{125}I-hFSH precipitation. ^{125}I-FSH (10 ng in 100 μl) was precipitated in the presence of (●——●) and the absence of (■···■) 100 μl of
ethanol soluble factor in a total volume of 500 μl containing 10%
ethanol in buffer.   Incubations were carried out at 27° C for 1 hr.
After incubations, 1 ml of different concentrations of polyethlyene
glycol were added in each tube as indicated.   Each determination
at a given polyethylene glycol concentration was run in triplicate
and the mean values are represented.   After addition of 1 ml of
polyethylene glycol, the tubes were kept in freezer (-20° C) for 30
min, followed by centrifugation at 1500 x g for 15 min. The supernatant was decanted and the tubes kept in inverted position on a
stand with adsorbent paper at the base for 2 hr at 4° C.   The tips
of the tubes were then wiped off with Kimwipes and tubes counted.
10 ng of ^{125}I-hFSh contained 98,242 cpm.

is based upon selective precipitation of the hormone receptor complex by polyethylene glycol, using gammaglobulin as a carrier protein.   The free hormone in the supernatant is separated by centrifugation and the pellet is counted.   Utilizing a different approach,
we developed a method which precipitates all the label as (free)
hormone, but leaves the "receptor-complex" in solution. We
utilized carbowax (70%; v/v) to precipitate ^{125}I-hFSH (Fig. 7).
Under these conditions 76% of all ^{125}I-hFSh was precipitable.
Carbowax 6000 even at saturated levels (50-55% w/v) did not precipitate more than 8-10% of ^{125}I-hFSH.   Precipitation of ^{125}I-
hFSH was inhibited in the presence of 100 μl of receptor (100 μg
of ethanol soluble protein) (Fig. 7).   This finding was utilized for
development of a receptor assay where a progressive decrease in
precipitated radioactivity was related to increasing concentrations
of ethanol solubilized extract.   The results of a typical experiment
are described in Figure 8.   Loss of precipitable counts in the presence of progressively increasing amounts of receptor could be

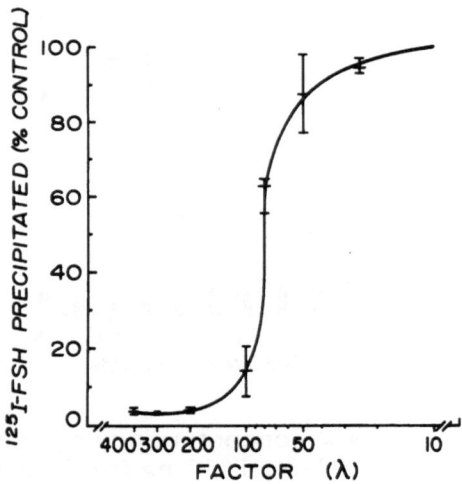

Figure 8. Effect of ethanol soluble factor concentrations upon inhibition of ^{125}I-hFSH precipitation. Ethanol soluble factor was incubated with ^{125}I-hFSH (10 ng) at 27° C for 1 hr in a total volume 0.5
ml. After incubation 1 ml of 70% polyethylene glycol was added in
each tube followed by the procedure described under Fig. 7. Control tubes did not contain any receptor and constituted 100% precipitation. Each estimation was run in triplicate. 10 ng of ^{125}I-hFSH
contained 90,342 cpm. 70% ^{125}I-hFSH was precipitated without
factor.

explained by binding of ^{125}I-hFSH with factor thus rendering the
complex more soluble in the upper PEG phase.

    2) Studies with ^{125}I-hFSH equilibrated sepharose column.
Another approach utilized a sepharose 6B column, equilibrated
with ^{125}I-hFSH (Fig. 9). Ethanol soluble extract was applied on
the column and eluted with buffer containing ^{125}I-hFSH. Thus,
a constant amount of ^{125}I-hFSH/ml was maintained during the
equilibration and elution. We expected to observe a peak of radioactivity, reflecting concentration of the labeled FSH by the factor,
followed by a trough. Instead, we observed only an intense peak
of radioactivity. Subsequent experiments revealed that [125]I-
hFSH binds to sepharose 6B. Therefore, we interpret the single
peak of radioactivity seen in Figure 9 to reflect elution of bound
[125]I-hFSH by the ethanol soluble factor. Ethanol or buffer without
factor produced no such effect when applied to the column in a similar fashion. The soluble factor was calculated to have a specific
binding of 1.7×10^{-15} moles of FSH/μg ethanol soluble protein which

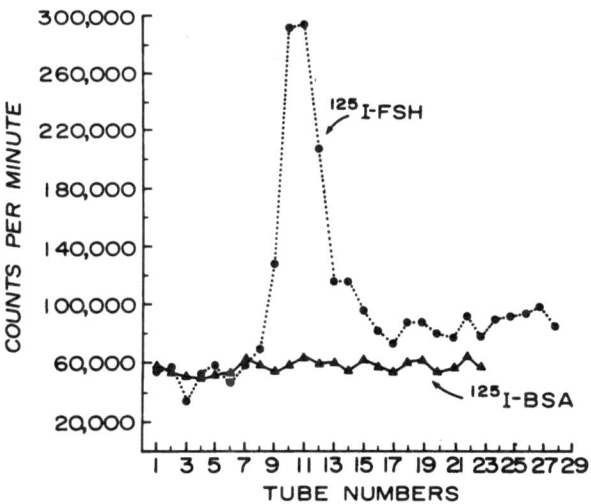

Figure 9. Binding of ^{125}I-hFSH with ethanol soluble factor. Ethanol extract (150,000 x g supernatant; 1.5 ml containing 1000 μg protein) was applied to a sepharose 6B column (26 x 0.9 cm) previously equilibrated by washing with 100 ml of ^{125}I-hFSH containing approximately 5 ng of ^{125}I-hFSH per ml in phosphate buffer (0.01 M containing 5 mM MgCl) containing 10% absolute ethanol (v/v). After equilibration with ^{125}I-hFSH solution, each ml eluted from column contained 60,000 cpm. Fractions of 1 ml were collected and counted (•·····•). Flow rate was maintained at 0.122 ml/min. After application of the factor, the same buffer was used for subsequent elution. Similarly another column chromatography on sepharose 6B, pre-equilibrated with ^{125}I-BSA was performed under similar conditions (▲———▲). In each column experiment, a total of 70 fractions were collected. No other peak was eluted.

is in close agreement with our PEG assay (Fig. 8: 1.1 x 10^{-15} moles/μg protein). A heat treated factor preparation had a specific activity of 2.2 x 10^{-15} moles/μg protein by column experiment. As judged by both assays, the ethanol soluble "factor" seems to be stable to boiling at 100° C for 5 min and can be stored at 4° C for one month without any detectable loss of activity. Significantly, when passed through a column of sepharose 6B pre-equilibrated with ^{125}I-BSA, the ethanol soluble factor did not elute any peak of radioactivity nor did it solubilize ^{125}I-BSA polyethylene glycol assay at the concentrations that inhibited the precipitation of ^{125}I-hFSH (Fig. 9).

Summary

Since the general utility of currently available detergent soluble and ethanol soluble receptor-factor assays have not yet been confirmed, it is difficult to comment on the similarities in properties between the proposed FSH receptor and the ethanol soluble "factor". The points of concern about soluble receptor assay are the apparent high non-specific binding and lack of tissue specificity we have encountered. In our hands, the degree of specific binding of ^{125}I-hFSH to detergent soluble extracts of liver and lung is comparable to testicular detergent extracts, and if confirmed this casts serious doubts on the usefulness of such assays for studies on detergent extracts of testicular or ovarian tissue. Nevertheless, the specific activity of the binding data obtained by us for the factor, using ^{125}I-hFSH equilibrated sepharose columns and our variation of the PEG assay (1.7 x 10^{-15} moles/μg protein; 1.1 x 10^{-15} moles of FSH/μg protein) is in agreement with the receptor preparation of Lee et al. (25) for LH-hCG receptors from rat luteal tissue. Extrapolation of the binding data for the soluble factor in terms of the binding capacity of intact testes, per mg wet weight of tissue, is 8.94 x 10^{-15} moles of FSH/mg. This is 55-fold greater than found on the basis of binding studies with the non-ethanol treated homogenate (Table 2: 0.16 x 10^{-15} moles of ^{125}I-hFSH/mg). Such a result might be explained on the basis of buried binding sites that are inaccessible to hFSH due to steric hindrance. This factor also seems to be present in liver, kidney and much less in muscle reflecting its role in binding of I-hFSH to a variety of tissues in a non-specific manner. This binding might as well be labile since accumulation of ^{125}I-hFSH after a single in vivo injection by several rat tissues have been reported (26). It is possible that such a factor could function to concentrate the hormone at or near the membrane till the hormone specific-response can be generated. Clearly, further studies will be required to conclusively identify the nature and significance of what we are presently terming the FSH binding "factor" in rat testes.

Acknowledgments

Appreciation is extended to Mrs. Eloise B. Carter for her excellent assistance. This study was supported in part by USPHS grant AM 3598. This is publication no. 1182 from the Division of Basic Health Sciences.

References

1. Leidenberger, F., and Reichert, L. E., Jr. Endocrinology 91: 135, 1972.

2. Reichert, L. E., Jr., Leidenberger, F., and Trowbridge, C. G. Recent Progr. Horm. Res. 29: 497, 1973.

3. Bhalla, Vinod K., and Reichert, L. E., Jr., J. Biol. Chem. 249: 43, 1973.

4. Leidenberger, F., and Reichert, L. E., Jr., Endocrinology 91: 901, 1972.

5. Reichert, L. E., Jr., and Bhalla, Vinod K., Endocrinology in press.

6. Greenwood, F. C., Hunter, W. M., and Glover, J. S., Biochem. J. 89: 114, 1963.

7. Butt, W. R., Acta Endocr. Suppl. 142: 13, 1969.

8. Miyachi, Y., Vaitukaitis, J., Nieschlag, E., and Lipsett, M. B., J. Clin. Endocrinol. Metab. 34: 23, 1972.

9. Miyachi, Y., and Chrambach, A., Biochem. Biophys. Res. Comm. 46: 1213, 1972.

10. Mancini, R. E., Costra, A., and Seiguer, A. C., Histochem. Cytochem. 15: 516, 1967.

11. Kuehl, F. A., Jr., Patanelli, D. J., Tarnoff, J., and Humes, J. L., Biol. Rep. 2: 154, 1970.

12. Christensen, A. K., and Mason, N. R., Endocrinology 76: 646, 1965.

13. Dufau, M. L., Charreau, E. H., and Catt, K. J., J. Biol. Chem. 248: 6973, 1973.

14. Rodbell, M., Birnbaumer, L., and Pohl, S. L., in "The Role of Adenyl Cyclase and cAMP in Biological Systems", Rall, T. M., Rodbell, M., and Condliffe, P. (eds.), U. S. Govt. Printing Office, Washington, D. C., p. 59, 1969.

15. Lefkowitz, R. J., and Levey, G. S., Life Sciences 11: 821, 1972.

16. Makino, S., Reynolds, J. A., and Tanford, C., J. Biol. Chem. 248: 4926, 1973.

17. Neer, E. J., J. Biol. Chem. 248: 3742, 1973.

18. Johnson, R. A., and Sutherland, E., J. Biol. Chem. 248: 5114, 1973.

19. Cuatrecasas, P., Proc. Nat. Acad. Sci. US 69: 318, 1972.

20. Allison, A. C., and Hartree, E. F., J. Reprod. Fert. 21: 501, 1970.

21. Karlin, A., Fed. Proceedings 32: 1847, 1973.

22. Lowry, O. H., Rosebrough, N. J., Farr, A. L., and Randall, R. J., J. Biol. Chem. 193: 265, 1951.

23. Cuatrecasas, P., Fed. Proceedings 32: 1838, 1973.

24. Cuatrecasas, P., J. Biol. Chem. 246: 6532, 1971.

25. Lee, C. Y., and Ryan, R. J., Fifth Annual Meeting of the Endocrine Society 280 (Abstract), 1972.

26. Butt, W. R., Ryle, M., and Shirley, A., J. Endocr. 58: 275, 1973.

IN VITRO BINDING AND AUTORADIOGRAPHIC LOCALIZATION OF HUMAN CHORIONIC GONADOTROPIN AND FOLLICLE STIMULATING HORMONE IN RAT TESTES DURING DEVELOPMENT

Claude Desjardins

Department of Zoology, The University of Texas
Austin, Texas

Anthony J. Zeleznik and A. Rees Midgley, Jr.

Reproductive Endocrinology Program, Department of Pathology
University of Michigan, Ann Arbor, Michigan

Leo E. Reichert, Jr.

Department of Biochemistry, Division of Basic Health Sciences
Emory University, Atlanta, Georgia

Introduction

The concept that certain target tissues contain specific receptors for peptide hormones has been widely recognized (1). In almost all instances the cellular attachment of peptide hormones to the cell surface has been correlated with the activation of membrane bound adenylate cyclase and the production of 3', 5' cyclic adenosine monophosphate, the presumed intracellular mediator of hormone action (1). A similar sequence of events has been postulated to occur after testicular interstitial tissue was exposed to human chorionic gonadotropin (hCG) or lutenizing hormone (LH) (2, 3), or seminiferous epithelial cells were exposed to follicle stimulating hormone (FSH) (4). While these results support the notion that hCG/LH and FSH exert their effects on cells in the interstitial and tubular compartments of the testis, positive

---

The term hCG/LH will be used interchangeably throughout this text since binding studies reveal that both hormones interact with similar receptor sites in gonadal tissue.

identification of the specific sites of high-affinity hCG/LH and FSH binding have not been defined at the tissue level in the same testis. Within this framework, it should be recognized that radioactive LH was localized selectively to Leydig cells (5-7) and that ferritin-labeled FSH appeared in the tubule wall and cytoplasm of Sertoli cells in rat testes (8). However, the latter findings may be questioned in view of the possibility that metabolites of the labeled hormone were localized rather than the labeled hormone per se , since the hormone used was highly impure and massive amounts (i.e., 5 to 10 mg) were injected (8). Recent advances in the autoradiographic localization of peptide hormones in target tissues circumvent the problems associated with hormone metabolites (9) and prompted us to reinvestigate the localization of gonadotrophic hormones in the testis.

The purpose of the present report is to summarize our findings concerning the in vitro binding and autoradiographic localization of ^{125}I-hCG and ^{125}I-rat FSH (rFSH) in rat testis during development. The evidence indicates that the maturational status of the testis influences the ability of testicular gonadotropin receptor preparations to bind ^{125}I-hCG and ^{125}I-rFSH in vitro and that ^{125}I-hCG and ^{125}I-rFSH were localized differentially in the interstitial and tubular compartments of the testis throughout development.

Procedures

Rats were puchased from the Holtzman Company, Madison, Wisconsin and killed between 5 and 90 days of age. Testes were removed immediately after death and handled in one of three ways: 1) placed in ice-cold 0.154 M potassium chloride, 2) quick-frozen in a mixture of ethanol and solid carbon dioxide in a small aluminum foil vessel containing buffer, or 3) fixed in Bouin's solution.

Highly purified hCG (10) and rFSH (11) were labeled with ^{125}I in the presence of lactoperoxidase and hydrogen peroxide at pH 7.0 using a modification (12) of the procedure of Miyachi, et al. (13) and repurified after iodination by polyacrylamide gel electrophoresis (14). Iodinated hormones were eluted from appropriate gel segments and diluted in 0.01 M sodium phosphate, pH 7.0 containing 0.14 M sodium chloride and 0.1% pig skin gelatin (12). The fraction of labeled hormone capable of being bound (determined as the fraction of ^{125}I-hormone capable of binding specifically to excess receptor) was 57% for ^{125}I-hCG and 30-35% for ^{125}I-rFSH. The specific activity of ^{125}I-hCG (15 μCi/ug) and ^{125}I-rFSH (3 μCi/ug) was assessed by radioreceptor assay using ^{125}I-hormone as tracer. Varying concentrations of the following unlabeled hormones were used to assess the specificity of ^{125}I-hCG and ^{125}I-rFSH binding: hCG (0. P. Bahl), rLH (LER-1484-1E), rFSH (LER-1422 76-90), rat thyroid stimulating hormone (rTSH) (LER-1101-B2), rat prolactin (rPRL) (NIAMD-rPRL-RP-1), and rat growth hormone (rGH) (NIAMD-rGH-B-1). Specific details regarding the potency and purity of these preparations have been described previously (12).

Testes placed in 0.154 M potassium chloride were decapsulated, weighed, homogenized in 0.01 M sodium phosphate, pH 7.0, containing 5 mM magnesium chloride, 0.1 M sucrose and 0.1% ovalbumin (RTH buffer) and centrifuged at 1500X g at 5 C (12,15). The supernatant was removed and the sedimentable material was resuspended in 2.5 ml of RTH buffer per gram of starting tissue. This suspension will hereafter be referred to as testicular gonadotropin receptor which is meant to signify a saturable, high-affinity binding component that is presumed, but not necessarily proven, to be coupled to responsive systems. In vitro binding analyses utilized 50 to 300 μl of the testicular gonadotropin receptor suspension in the presence of ^{125}I-hCG (2 ng) or ^{125}I-rFSH (15 ng) either alone or with a 100-fold excess of unlabeled tropic hormone (12). Sufficient radioactivity was present in each tube such that a 2-fold increase in the testicular receptor resulted in a corresponding increase in the amount of radioactivity bound.

The incubation mixture was adjusted to a final volume of 1 ml with RTH buffer, incubated for 3 hr at 37 C, and 1.5 ml of ice-cold RTH buffer was added at the end of the incubation. The tubes were centrifuged at 10,000X g and the sedimentable material was resuspended in 1.5 ml of RTH buffer and recentrifuged as described. Assay tubes were transferred to a Nuclear Chicago gamma counter with 45% counting efficiency to determine the amount of hormone bound. Specific hormone binding was determined as the difference between binding in the presence and absence of excess unlabeled hormone and was expressed as cpm bound per 100 μg of DNA (12).

Frozen testes were cut at 8 μ and sections were transferred to glass microscope slides. Labeled gonadotropic hormones (ca 1 x 10 cpm per 50 μl) were applied either alone or in combination with a 1000-fold excess of unlabeled hormone to surface of sections and incubated for 2 hr at 37 C (16). After incubation, sections were washed, air-dried, dipped in Kodak NTB-3 emulsion and processed for autoradiography (16,17). Sections were developed after 3-6 weeks, examined under phase-contrast and/or bright field microscopy and photographed without further preparation. Fixed testes were washed, dehydrated, embedded in paraffin, sectioned at 4 μ and stained with hematoxylin and eosin for comparison with fresh-frozen sections.

Statistical analyses were performed, when appropriate, by analysis of variance to determine the significance level of treatment differences. The significance level of specific treatments was evaluated by using the Newman-Keuls sequential range test (18).

Table 1

Comparison of ^{125}I-hCG and ^{125}I-rFSH binding to 1500X g
sedimentable material prepared from homogentates of
testicular, splenic, hepatic and cardiac tissue

Source of	cpm bound per 100 μg DNA	
1500X g pellet	^{125}I-hCG	^{125}I-rFSH
Testis	13,065 + 422	550 + 23.4
Spleen	253 + 21	62 + 8.5
Liver	177 + 19	81 + 9.7
Heart	158 + 20	36 + 4.1

Each value represents the mean + standard error of five determinations made after *in vitro* incubation at 37°C for 3 hr. Tissues
were obtained from 300-350 g rats and homogenized in the same manner as that described for testes.

Results

Sedimentable material (1500X g) bound approximately 40-
times more ^{125}I-hCG than that obtained from other tested somatic
tissues of adult rats (Table 1). Similarly, sedimentable material
obtained from testes bound about 8-times more ^{125}I-rFSH than
that prepared from spleen, liver or heart (Table 1).

Following demonstration that ^{125}I-hCG and ^{125}I-rFSH binding
exhibited high tissue specificity, subsequent studies were performed to determine the extent to which homologous and heterologous gonadotropins and other pituitary hormones of rat origin
interferred with the capacity of ^{125}I-hCG and ^{125}I-rFSH to interact
with gonadotropin binding sites in testicular pellets of adult rats.
Full symmetrical and parallel inhibition curves were obtained by
plotting log amounts of added unlabeled hormone versus the observed binding as a percent of hormone bound in the absence of
unlabeled hormone (Fig. 1). The slight degree of inhibition seen
with other pituitary hormones may be attributed to their known

Figure 1. Competitive inhibition curves obtained with gonadotropic and pituitary hormones in the presence of ^{125}I-hCG and a 100
μl suspension of testicular gonadotropin receptor (92.8 μg of DNA
per tube) prepared from adult rats. Each value represents the
mean of duplicate assays expressed as the percentage of the total
amount of radioactivity bound in the presence of unlabeled hormone
to that bound in the absence of the indicated unlabeled hormone.

Table 2

^{125}I-hCG and ^{125}I-rFSH binding to testicular gonadotropic
receptors after preincubation with enzymes

Enzyme Pretreatment	Amount of enzyme present (μg/ml)	cpm bound per 100 μg DNA	
		^{125}I-hCG	^{125}I-rFSH
None	--	12,467	2,062
DNase	5	13,920	1,963
RNase	5	12,796	2,281
Pepsin	10	0	0
Trypsin	10	0	99.7
Pronase	10	0	0
Phospholipase A	10	473	0

Each value represents the average of duplicate determinations performed with 200 μl of testicular gonadotropin receptor preparation
(328 μg DNA per tube). The receptor preparation was incubated in
the presence of the indicated enzymes for 30 min at 37°C in 1 ml,
centrifuged and washed twice with excess buffer before adding
labeled hormones in a final volume of 1 ml and reincubation at 37°C
for 3 hr.

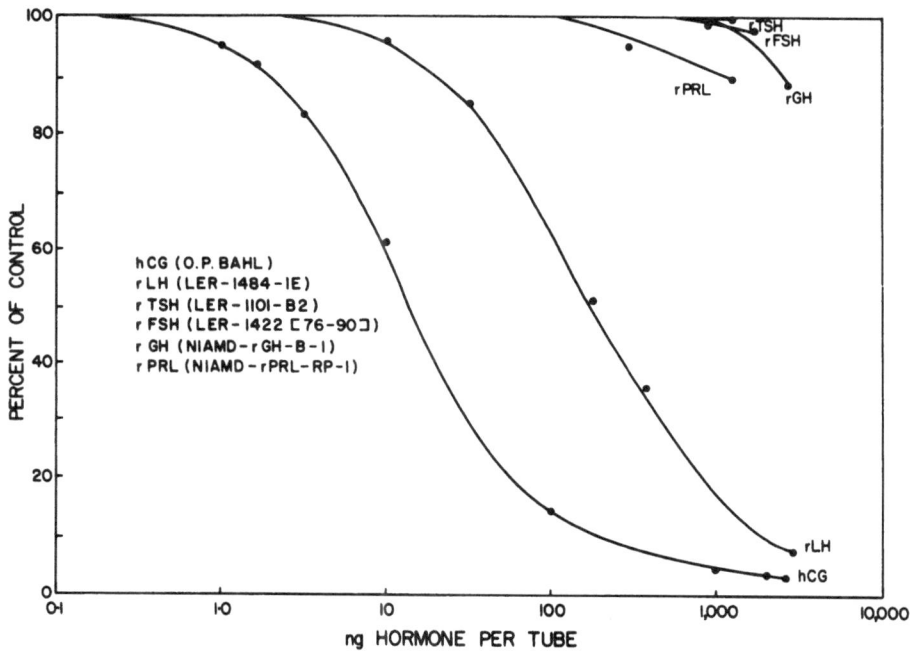

hCG (O.P. BAHL)
rLH (LER-1484-IE)
rTSH (LER-1101-B2)
rFSH (LER-1422 [76-90])
rGH (NIAMD-rGH-B-1)
rPRL (NIAMD-rPRL-RP-1)

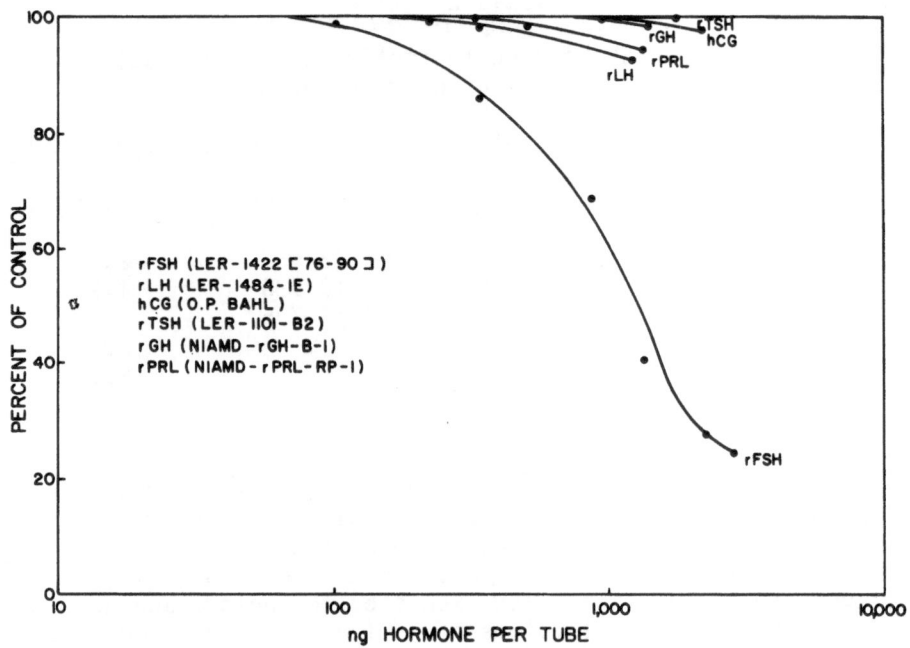

Figure 2. Competitive inhibition curves obtained with gonadotropic and pituitary hormones in the presence of 125I-rFSH and a
100 µl suspension of testicular gonadotropin receptor (92.8 µg of
DNA per tube) prepared from adult rats. Each value represents
the mean of duplicate assays expressed as the percentage of the
total amount of radioactivity bound in the presence of unlabeled
hormone to that bound in the absence of the indicated unlabeled
hormone.

contamination with LH (12). The inhibition curves shown in Figure
2 indicate that unlabeled rFSH was the primary hormone capable
of displacing 125I-rFSH from testicular gonadotropin receptors.
Other pituitary hormones exhibited only slight activity and this
may be attributed to the presence of FSH contaminants (12).

The hormone binding reaction was further characterized by incubating sedimentable material prepared from testes of adult rats
in the presence of various enzymes for 30 min at 37 C (Table 2).
The results demonstrate that the binding of 125I-hCG and 125I-
rFSH was not influenced by preincubation with either deoxyribo-
nuclease (DNase) or ribonuclease (RNase) (P > 0.25). However,
125I-hCG and 125I-rFSH binding was abolished or markedly

inhibited by pretreatment of the testicular gonadotropin receptor preparation with several proteolytic enzymes and phospholipase A.

The present results, indicating tissue and hormone specificity and observations indicating that binding was inhibited by preincubation with proteolytic enzymes, minimizes the possibility that the interaction of these hormones with receptors present in the 1500X g pellet of homogenates of adult rat testes could be artifactual. Additional studies, in our laboratory, have shown that the binding of ^{125}I-hCG and ^{125}I-rFSH to testicular gonadotropin receptor preparations was time and temperature dependent exhibiting maxima 37 C and 3 hr, respectively (12).

We next undertook experiments to determine whether or not gonadotropin receptors from testes of developing rats exhibited the same binding capacity as that found in adult testicular tissue. The results depicted in Figure 3 demonstrate that both gonadotropins bound to testicular pellets prepared from rats between 5 and 90 days of age. The amount of ^{125}I-hCG that was bound increased 25-fold between 5 and 55 days of age when expressed as cpm of ^{125}I-hCG bound per 100 μg of DNA. The increase in ^{125}I-hCG binding was characterized by small but gradual increments

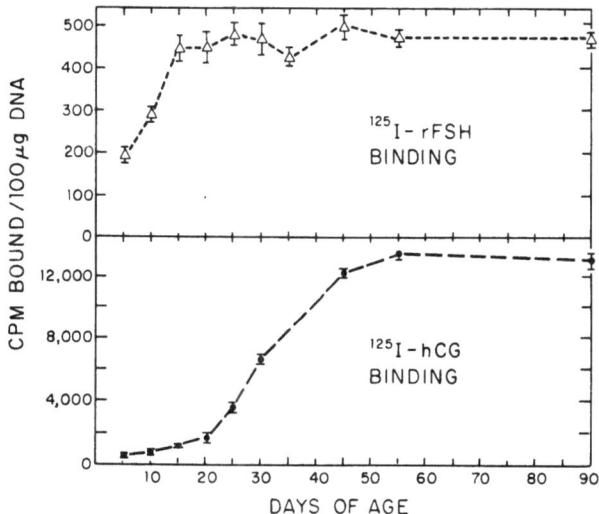

Figure 3. Relationship between ^{125}I-hCG (lower panel) and ^{125}I-rFSH (upper panel) binding to gonadotropin receptors prepared from rat testes at various stages of development. Each value represents the mean + standard error (vertical bars) made on three different pools of tissue per each age category. Sufficient radiolabeled hormone was present in each tube to result in a 2-fold increase in binding when the amount of testicular receptor preparation was doubled.

between 5 and 20 days with particularly pronounced and dramatic changes noted between 25 and 55 days. Following the peak observed at 55 days, ^{125}I-hCG binding appeared to plateau since equivalent amounts of hormone were bound at 55 and 90 days of age ($P > 0.25$). The capacity of ^{125}I-rFSH to bind to testicular gonadotropin receptors differed markedly from that observed for ^{125}I-hCG. ^{125}I-rFSH binding increased 2.5-fold between 5 and 15 days and remained unchanged ($P > 0.25$) throughout testicular development.

Autoradiographs prepared after ^{125}I-hCG was applied topically to the surface of fresh-frozen sections of testes consistently contained reduced silver grains in the intertubular areas of the testis (Figs. 8,9). Importantly, the number of silver grains localized over the interstitial elements of the testis increased during testicular maturation and appeared to correspond with increments in ^{125}I-hCG binding noted in vitro. Autoradiographs treated with ^{125}I-hCG in the presence of 1000-fold excess of unlabeled hCG or rLH were similar to buffer controls (Figs. 6,7), whereas those incubated with ^{125}I-hCG and 1000-fold excess of rFSH resembled those receiving ^{125}I-hCG alone (Figs. 8,9).

Autoradiographs developed after topical application of ^{125}I-rFSH contained reduced silver grains that were consistently localized over seminiferous tubules (Figs. 10,11). The greatest density of silver grains appeared over the seminiferous tubules of

---

Figures 4-11.   Histological (Fig. 4,5) and fresh-frozen sections (= 100X) of testes from 15 (Figs. 4,6,8,10) and 45 (Figs. 5,7,9, 11) day old rats processed for topical autoradiographic localization of ^{125}I-hCG and ^{125}I-rFSH. Figures 4 and 5. Cross section of Bouin's fixed testicular tissue from 15 (Fig. 4) and 45 (Fig. 5) day old rats for comparison with corresponding photomicrographs of fresh-frozen tissues. Figures 6 and 7. Fresh-frozen sections of testes from 15 (Fig. 6) and 45 (Fig. 7) day old rats treated with buffer alone and processed for autoradiography as control sections for comparison with (Figs. 8-11). Figures 8 and 9. Same area of testes shown in (Figs. 6 and 7) but treated with ^{125}I-hCG. Note localization of reduced silver grains in the intertubular areas of both figures as well as the marked increase in grain density seen in sections of mature (Fig. 9) as compared to immature testes (Fig. 8). Figures 10 and 11. Similar regions of immature and mature testes as shown above after exposure to ^{125}I-rFSH. Note localization of reduced silver grains over the seminiferous tubules of 15 day testes which contain Sertoli cells and all classes of spermatogonia (Fig. 10). Reduced silver grains attributed to ^{125}I-rFSH were confined to the seminiferous tubules of 45 day testes with appreciably greater grain density over the basal rather than the apical regions of tubules.

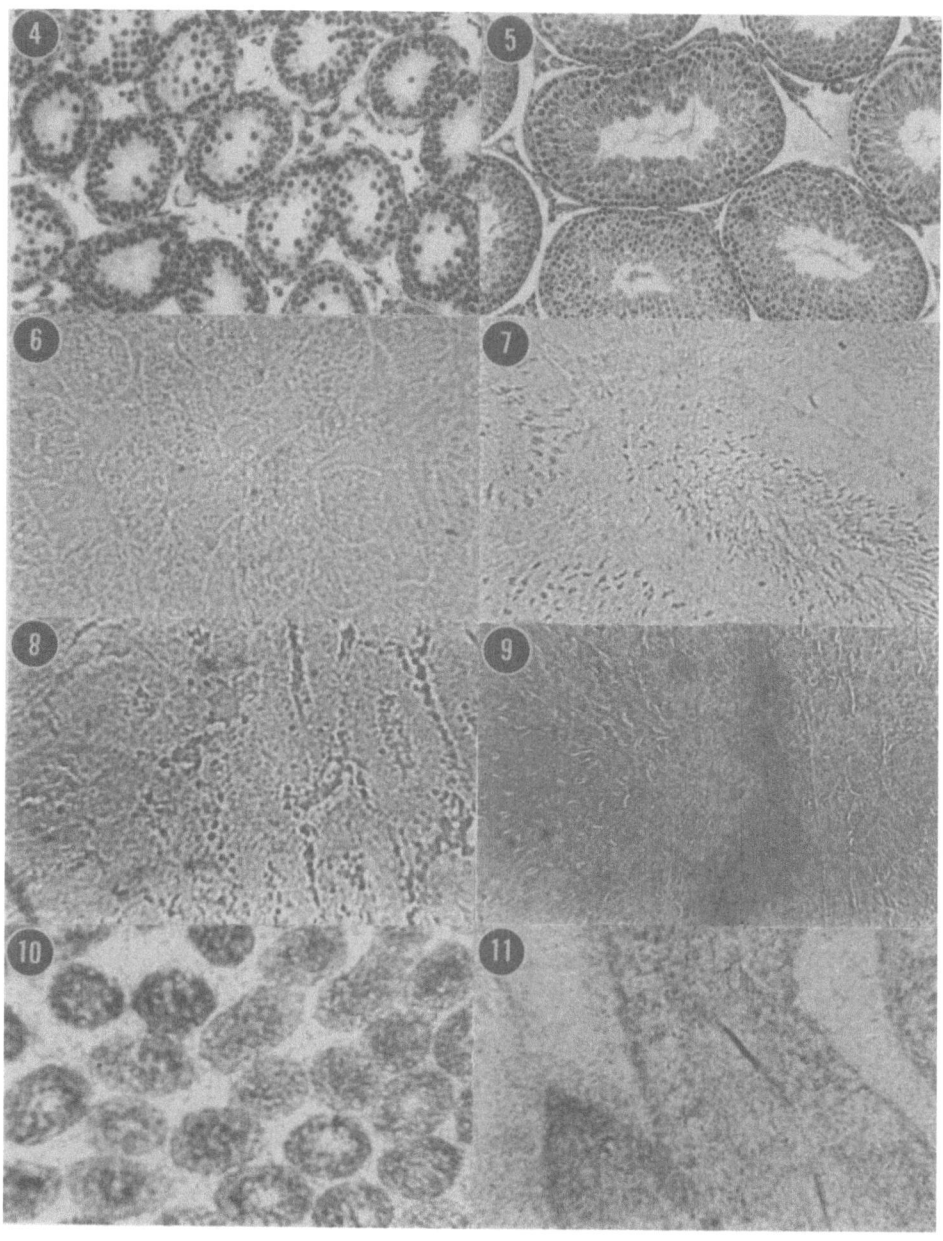

15 day old testes (compare Figs. 10,11). Although it was always
apparent that silver grains attributed to ^{125}I-rFSH were localized
in the intratubular regions of the testes of older rats, an appreciably greater proportion of these grains were found in the basal
rather than the apical portion of the seminiferous tubule (Fig. 11).
Treatment of ^{125}I-rFSH autoradiographs with a 1000-fold excess
of rLH or hCG failed to cause any apparent reduction in the number
of reduced silver grains localized over the seminiferous epithelium. However, sections that were incubated with ^{125}I-rFSH and
1000-fold excess of rFSH resembled control tissues (Figs. 6,7).

Discussion

The present results demonstrate, for the first time, the interaction of radioiodionated hCG and rFSH with testicular gonadotropin receptors at two different levels of cellular organization,
tissue slices and 1500X g sedimentable material prepared from
testicular homogenates. The evidence developed from both sets
of observations strongly indicates the interaction of these hormones with their respective binding sites was tissue and hormone
specific and that the binding of ^{125}I-hCG and ^{125}I-rFSH may be
attributed to receptor sites located, respectively, in the inter-
and intra-tubular compartments of the rat testis throughout
development.

A further significant feature of the present study pertains to
the qualitative and quantitative findings that ^{125}I-hCG and ^{125}I-
rFSH binding was influenced by the developmental status of cells
present in the interstitial and tubular regions of the testis. Thus,
^{125}I-rFSH binding increased 2.5-fold between 5 and 15 days of age
and remained relatively constant after this initial increase
throughout subsequent testicular development (12). The observation that ^{125}I-rFSH was localized within the seminiferous tubules
coupled with the finding that the early rise in ^{125}I-rFSH binding
coincided with increments in Sertoli cell numbers between 5 and
15 days prompts the speculation that this hormone was bound by
Sertoli cells or spermatogonia (all classes) since these cells were
the primary components of the seminiferous epithelium at 15 days
of age (16). It is also noteworthy that fresh-frozen sections of
testes from mature rats (i.e., 45 and 55 days of age) exhibited
intense ^{125}I-rFSH binding and that a high proportion of silver
grains attributed to ^{125}I-rFSH were found in the basal rather than
the apical portion of the seminiferous tubules since this region
tends to contain the greatest number of spermatogonia and Sertoli
cells. Evidence indicating that ^{125}I-rFSH was selectively localized by cells in the seminferous epithelium parallels earlier
reports showing that radiolabeled FSH was bound to preparations
of seminiferous tubules in vitro and that ferritin-labeled FSH pre-
ferentially accumulated in the tubular wall and cytoplasm of
Sertoli cells after this hormone was administered in vitro (4,8,

15, 19).

In contrast to ^{125}I-rFSH binding, ^{125}I-hCG binding increased over a prolonged time span ranging from 5 to 55 days and appeared to remain at adult-like levels beyond this point. Importantly, the temporal increases seen in ^{125}I-hCG binding were correlated directly with increments in Leydig cell numbers and the appearance of elevated concentrations of testosterone in blood plasma (16). In spite of the apparent conformity between ^{125}I-hCG binding and Leydig cell numbers, the increase in Leydig cell numbers appeared to precede the rise in plasma testosterone levels and ^{125}I-hCG binding by 5 to 10 days. These observations support the results of Knorr et al. (20) and suggest that Leydig cells may require more time to differentiate before maximal binding and secretion can occur.

Localization of ^{125}I-hCG and ^{125}I-rFSH within testes by topical autoradiography differs markedly from that of other autoradiographic investigations from two standpoints. Firstly, in previous autoradiographic studies it was not possible to distinguish between the localization of the intact labeled hormone or one of its labeled metabolites since labeled hormones were administered in vivo or incubated in vitro with interstitial tissue (5-8). The possibility that the present results may be explained on the basis of labeling artifacts was excluded because of the brief exposure of the radiolabeled hormone to tissue sections after freezing and thawing and the fact that the labeled hormone was displaced by excess unlabeled homologous but not heterologous hormone. Secondly, previous studies involving labeled gonadotropins were limited to investigating the localization of a single gonadotropic hormone within the testis. However, in the present study it was possible to assess the localization of both labeled gonadotropins within the same testis by simply using the adjacent sections. Under these conditions, the present results clearly indicate that ^{125}I-hCG and ^{125}I-rFSH were bound specifically in two different anatomical compartments with widely different physiological functions in the same testis. The possibility exists, however, that "low-affinity" receptors for both LH and FSH are distributed uniformly throughout the testis and that their detection went unnoticed because topical autoradiographic procedures are not sufficiently sensitive to reveal binding at these sites. This possibility may not be discounted (21, 22) even though others have indicated that radiolabeled hCG/LH and FSH bound only to interstitial tissue and seminiferous epithelial cells, respectively (2, 4).

Since the present observations were made at a time when knowledge about the effects of highly purified gonadotropic hormones on the testis is rapidly expanding it seems pertinent to speculate on the physiological significance of our results. Firstly, with regard to hCG, both present and previous studies indicate that this hormone and its phypsiological counterpart, LH, were bound and localized by similar receptors in the interstitial compartment of the testis (2, 5, 6). This evidence coupled with that pertaining to the physiological and biochemical response of the testis following exposure to hCG/LH supports the concept that these hormones primarily promote the synthesis and secretion of androgens by Leydig cells (23-26).

Secondly, the present indication that ^{125}I-rFSH binding was maximal in immature testes and that this hormone was consistently localized within seminiferous tubules at all stages of testicular development is consonant with other reports concerning FSH binding and the observation that FSH may play an activational role in the immature testis and/or promote spermatid development in testes of adult rats (4, 15, 19, 27, 28). Despite this and other evidence for the action of FSH on testes no consensus has been reached concerning the specific role this hormone may play on the process of spermatogenesis in adult mammals (28-29). However, in light of our results and those of others, we postulate that the interaction of FSH with the seminiferous epithelium may be related to a permissive role of this hormone in facilitating the binding, transfer or transformation of testosterone or other androgens within seminiferous tubules. Evidence supporting this speculation stems from the finding that FSH enhanced testosterone secretion by the perfused rabbit testis-epididymis and whole rat testes incubated in vitro beyond that seen in the presence of saturating levels of LH (30-31). Moreover, spermatogenesis was maintained quantitatively, in the absence of immunoreactive serum LH and FSH, in adult rats receiving subdermal testosterone-filled Silastic capsules designed to maintain the peripheral concentration of testosterone at levels slightly greater than that emanating from the spermatic venous effluent (32). While these results imply that testosterone (or one of its metabolites) may be the primary agent(s) needed to maintain sperm production, they are not at variance with the notion of FSH involvement in the completion of spermiogenesis (28). The nexus between these seemingly conflicting observations resides in the fact that the beneficial effects of FSH on spermatid formation have always been found in rats that received exogenous testosterone in doses that were insufficient to maintain peripheral levels of this hormone at concentrations mimicking that normally available to seminiferous tubules. Hence, if the concentration of testosterone in the intratubular compartment was low or below normal FSH could have promoted spermatid development by exerting a permissive effect by enhancing the binding, transfer, or transformation of this androgen in the seminiferous epithelium. This speculation conforms with the finding that FSH must be administered with LH to facilitate sperm production in hypophysectomized rats after testes were allowed to regress (33) and evidence indicating that greater increases in testis weight were obtained when immature hypophysectomized rats received combinations of FSH and LH rather than either hormone alone (34). Thus if FSH is to play a facilitatory or permissive role in the action of androgens on the seminifeorus epithelium one would expect that its secretion should not be easily suppressed by testosterone or other androgens. That this is indeed the case is seen from numerous studies documenting the preferential suppression of LH over FSH by testosterone or one of its esters in either acutely or chronically orchidectomized adult rats (35-37). Finally our postulate that FSH exerts a permissive influence on androgens in the seminiferous epithelium is consonant with observations indicating that testosterone may not be the chief factor regulating feedback to the hypothalamo-hypophyseal neuroendocrine axis since elevated serum FSH concentrations have been reported in males experiencing selective damage to seminiferous epithelium in the presence of normal LH and testosterone concentrations (38-40).

Obviously the validity of our speculation remains to be shown, but it is hoped that it may be viewed within the framework of providing added impetus to solve the enigmatic role of FSH action on the testis. From the standpoint of the present evidence and that reviewed here, it seems reasonable to conclude that hCG/LH exert their effects on the Leydig cells and that FSH acts on the seminiferous epithelium.

Summary

Rat testes were obtained between 5 and 90 days of age to prepare: 1) fresh-frozen sections for topical autoradiographic localization of ^{125}I-hCG and ^{125}I-rFSH, and 2) 1500X g sedimentable material for in vitro assessment of ^{125}I-hCG and ^{125}I-rFSH binding. Autoradiographic studies established that ^{125}I-hCG and ^{125}I-rFSH were localized respectively in the inter- and intra-tubular compartments of the testis at all stages of development. Similarly in vitro binding analyses demonstrated that ^{125}I-hCG and ^{125}I-rFSH were bound specifically to receptors prepared from testes of rats between 5 and 90 days of age. ^{125}I-rFSH binding increased 2.5-fold between 5 and 15 days and remained unchanged ($P > 0.25$) throughout testicular maturation. In contrast, ^{125}I-hCG binding increased slowly between 5 and 20 days and rose markedly thereafter, reaching a peak at 55 days resulting in a 25-fold increment during testicular development. It was concluded that rat testes contain at least two sets of "high-affinity" receptors for hCG/LH and FSH and that these receptors were associated with the interstitial elements and seminiferous epithelium, respectively. These conclusions support a working hypothesis in which hCG/LH exerts its effects on cells involved in the synthesis and secretion of androgens with FSH acting on cells present in the seminiferous tubule.

Acknowledgements

The authors express their appreciation to Joyce Duncan, Marjorie Hepburn and Shirley Wooten for their assistance with these experiments. This research was supported in part by U. S. Public Health Service Research Grants HD-05318 (A. R. M.), HD-07381 (C. D.) and HD-08228 (L. E. R.) from The National Institute of Child Health and Human Development. Other support was provided by a Predoctoral Fellowship to A. J. A., from The Ford Foundation and by a Career Development Award to A. R. M. from The National Institute of Child Health and Human Development.

References

1. Butcher, R. W., Robison, G. A., and Sutherland, E. W., In Biochemical Actions of Hormones, Litwack, G. (ed.), Academic Press, 1972, p. 21.

2. Catt, K. J., and Dufau, M. L., In Receptors for Reproductive Hormones, O'Malley, B. W., and Means, A. R. (eds.), Plenum Press, New York, 1973, p. 379.

3. Reichert, L. E., Jr., Leidenberger, F., and Trowbridge, C. G., Recent Progr. Hormone Res. 29 497, 1973.

4. Means, A. R., In Receptors for Reproductive Hormones, O'Malley, B. W., and Means, A. R. (eds.), Plenum Press, New York, 1973, p. 431.

5. deKretser, D. M., Catt, K. J., Burger, H. G. and Smith, G. C., J. Endocrinol. 43: 105, 1969.

6. deKretser, D. M., Catt, K. J., and Paulsen, C. A., Endocrinology 88: 332, 1971.

7. deKretser, D. M., Catt, K. J., Dufau, M. L. and Hudson, B., J. Reprod. Fertil. 24: 311, 1971.

8. Mancini, R. E., Castro, A., and Seigeur, A. C., J. Histochem. Cytochem. 15: 516, 1967.

9. Midgley, A. R., Jr., In Receptors for Reproductive Hormones, O'Malley, B. W., and Means, A. R. (eds.), Plenum Press, New York, 1973, p. 365.

10. Midgley, A. R., Jr., Zeleznik, A. J., Rajaniemi, H. J., and Richards, J., In Proceedings of the Symposium on Advances in Chemistry, Biology, Immunology of Gonadotropins, Moudgal, N. R. (ed.), in press.

11. Reichert, L. E., Jr., In Advances in Enzymology, O'Malley, B. W., and Hardman, J. G. (eds.), Academic Press, New York, 1974, in press.

12. Desjardins, C. A., Zeleznik, A. J., Midgley, Jr., A. R, and Reichert, Jr., L. E., unpublished observations.

13. Miyachi, Y., Vaitukaitis, J. L., Nieschlag, E., and Lipsett, M. B. L., J. Clin. Endocrinol. Metab. 34: 23, 1972.

14. Midgley, A. R., Jr., Niswender, G. D., Gay, V. L., and Reichert, L. E., Jr., Recent Progr. Hormone Research 27: 235, 1971.

15. Reichert, L. E., Jr., and Bhalla, V. K., Endocrinology 94: 483, 1974.

16. Desjardins, C. A., Zeleznik, A. J., Midgley, Jr., A. R., and Reichert, Jr., L. E., unpublished observations.

17. Rajaniemi, H. J., and Midgley, A. R., In Advances in Enzymology, O'Malley, B. W., and Hardman, J. G. (eds.), Academic Press, New York, 1974, in press.

18. Snedecor, G. W., and Cochran, W. G., Statistical Methods, 6th Ed., Iowa State University Press, Ames, Iowa, 1967, p. 273.

19. Bhalla, V. K., and Reichert, Jr., L. E., J. Biol. Chem. 249: 43, 1974.

20. Knorr, D. W., Vanha-Perttula, T., and Lipsett, M. B., Endocrinology 86: 1298, 1970.

21. Bahalla, V. K., and Reichert, Jr., L. E., This volume, pg. 196.

22. Kuehl, F. A., Jr., Patanelli, D. J., Tarhoff, Jr. and Humes, Biol. Reprod. 2: 154, 1970.

23. Christensen, A. K., and Gillim, S. W., In The Gonads, McKerns, K. W. (ed.), Appleton-Century-Crofts, New York, 1969, p. 415.

THE EFFECTS OF FSH ON CELL PREPARATIONS FROM

THE RAT TESTIS

J. H. Dorrington, N. F. Roller and I. B. Fritz

Banting and Best Department of Medical Research
University of Toronto
Toronto, Ontario, Canada M5G 1L6

Follicle stimulating hormone (FSH) and luteinizing hormone (LH) are required for the initiation of spermatogenesis in the immature rat (1), and for the restoration of spermatogenesis in the regressed hypophysectomized rat (2, 3).

We have previously reported that both gonadotropins increase cyclic AMP levels in whole testis preparations from the hypophysectomized rat (4). Evidence for an effect of LH, but not FSH on cyclic AMP production in isolated interstitial cell preparations has been presented. Isolated seminiferous tubules on the other hand responded to FSH but not to LH (5). Studies on tubule preparations from hypophysectomized rats, and cryptorchid and irradiated testes suggested that the Sertoli cells in the testis responded to FSH with an increase in cyclic AMP accumulation (5).

Recently, we have been primarily concerned with the isolation of the various cell types present in the seminiferous tubule in order to determine with minimal ambiguity which cells are under direct hormonal control.

Tubules from 26 day old rats were used to prepare spermatocyte-enriched suspensions, as described by Dorrington and Fritz (6). These suspensions consisted of approximately 86% spermatocytes at the leptotene stage of prophase or a more advanced stage, 6% were either spermatogonia or preleptotene spermatocytes, 6% were immature spermatids and 2% were Sertoli cells. Whereas the isolated tubules responded dramatically to FSH in the presence of theophylline (10 mM), the

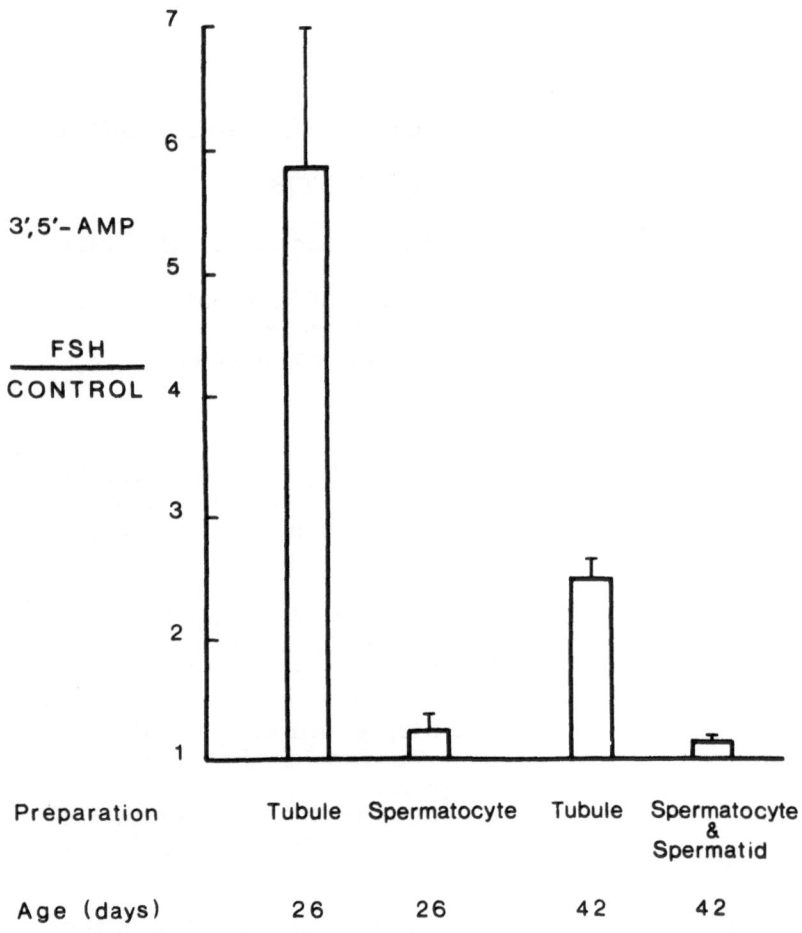

Figure 1. Ratios of the cyclic AMP level after the addition of
FSH (10 μg NIH-FSH-S9/ml) to that obtained in the absence
of exogenous FSH, in tubules (isolated from 26 and 42 day old
rats) and in cell suspensions. All incubations were carried out
in 1 ml Krebs-Ringer bicarbonate buffer pH 7.4, containing glucose (5 mM) and theophylline (10 mM) for 20 min at 32° C.

spermatocyte-enriched preparation failed to respond to FSH in
the presence or absence of theophylline (Fig. 1). The response
to FSH was reduced in tubules from more mature testes which
contained spermatids, compared with the response observed
in tubules from the 26 day old animal, indicating that spermatids were unresponsive. This was investigated further by preparing a cell suspension of spermatids and spermatocytes from

tubules of 42 day old rats (6). These cell suspensions consisted of approximately 65% spermatids, 28% spermatocytes at the leptotene stage of prophase or a more advanced stage, 5% spermatogonia or preleptolene spermatocytes and 2% Sertoli cells. FSH had no effect on the cyclic AMP level of these preparations in the presence or absence of theophylline (Fig. 1).

Sertoli cell preparations were obtained from testes of 20 day old rats by sequential treatment with trypsin and collagenase. Cell pellets were fixed in Bouin's solution, embedded in paraffin and 5 μ sections were stained with periodic acid-Schiff-hema toxylin. One thousand cells were counted in each of two preparations, and indicated that approximately 77% were Sertoli cells (in aggregates of up to 30 cells) 18% were spermatogonia and spermatocytes and 5% were unidentified or degenerating cells. FSH (10 μg/ml) stimulated cyclic AMP production by these cells when incubated in the presence of 10 mM theophylline for 20 mins at 32° C (Fig. 2) LH (10 μg/ml) had no effect on this preparation. The Sertoli cell preparation was

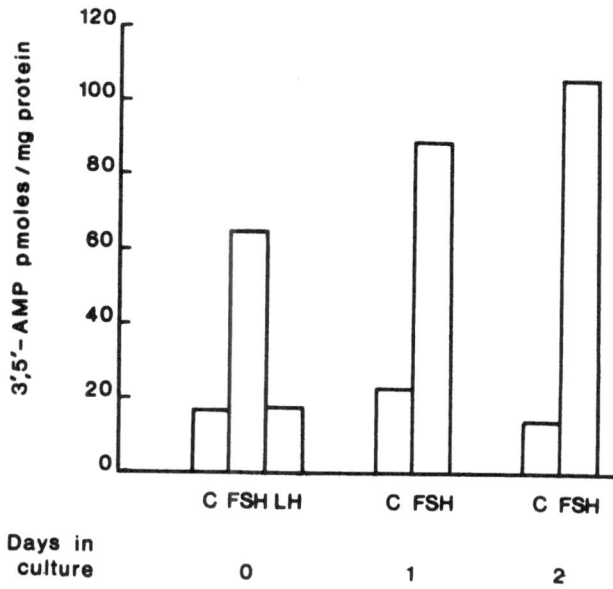

Figure 2. The effects of FSH (10 μg NIH-FSH-S9/ml) and LH (10 μg NIH-LH-S16/ml) on the cyclic AMP levels of Sertoli cell-enriched preparations (obtained from 20 day old rats), 1) immediately after preparation; 2) after 1 day in culture; 3) after 2 days in culture. All incubations were carried out in Krebs-Ringer bicarbonate containing glucose (5 mM) and theophylline (10 mM) for 20 min at 32° C.

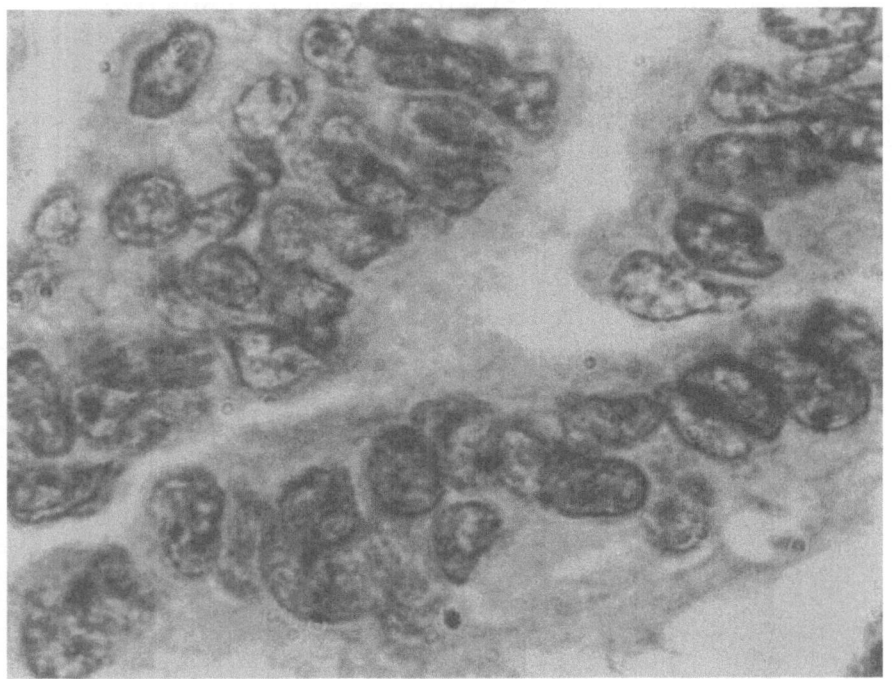

Figure 3. Microphotograph of a Sertoli cell preparation (from
20 day old rat testes) after 2 days in culture. The cells which
adhered to the culture flask were removed by trypsinization,
the cell pellet was fixed in Bouin's solution, embedded in paraffin and 5 μ sections were stained with periodic acid-Schiff-
hematoxylin.

placed in culture flasks in the medium described by Steinberger and Steinberger (7). After 1 and 2 days in culture the Sertoli cell aggregates were attached to the surface of the culture flask, whereas germinal cells were found freely suspended in the medium. After either 1 or 2 days in culture the medium was removed and the remaining cells were detached from the surface of the culture flask by treatment with 5 ml 0.25% trypsin solution. Soy-bean trypsin inhibitor was added and the cells were washed three times in Krebs-Ringer bicarbonate buffer. Cell pellets were fixed in Bouin's solution for the preparation of slides for light microscopy, or in 3% glutaraldehyde in 0.2 M phosphate buffer for electron microscopy. Cell counts indicated that after 1 day in culture the attached cells consisted of approximately 89% Sertoli cells, 5% spermatogonia or spermatocytes, and 6% unidentified cells, and after 2 days in culture the proportions were 95%, 2% and 3% respectively (Fig. 3). FSH (10 μg/ml) increased cyclic AMP levels in Sertoli cell preparations (removed from culture after 1 and 2 days) when the cells were incubated in the presence of theophylline (10 mM) for 20 mins at 32°C (Fig. 2).

The results suggest that FSH does not elicit an increase in adenylate cyclase activity of interstitial cells or germinal cells, but clearly demonstrate that Sertoli cells are FSH-responsive.

References

1. Steinberger, E., Physiol. Rev. 51, 1, 1971.

2. Lostroh, A. J., Acta Endocr. 43, 592, 1963.

3. Go, V. L. W., Vernon, R. G., and Fritz, I. B., Can. J. Biochem. 49, 768, 1971.

4. Dorrington, J. H., Vernon, R. G., and Fritz, I. B., Biochem. Biophys. Res. Commun. 46, 1523, 1972.

5. Dorrington, J. H., and Fritz, I. B., Endocrinology (in press).

6. Dorrington, J. H., and Fritz, I. B., Biochem. Biophys. Res. Commun. 54, 1425, 1973.

7. Steinberger, A., and Steinberger, E., Experimental Cell Research 44, 443, 1966.

EVIDENCE FOR MULTIPLE, CELL SPECIFIC, DISTINCTIVE

ADENYLATE CYCLASE SYSTEMS IN RAT TESTIS

T. Braun

Department of Physiology
Northwestern University Medical Center
Chicago, Illinois

Introduction

Considerable evidence has been accumulated during the last decade which indicates that a large group of hormones acts through the mediation of the adenylate cyclase system in the target cell plasma membrane (1). It has been established that adenylate cyclase systems in various cell types are hormone selective, and many exhibit specific metal and/or nucleotide requirement for 'optimal' catalytic activity and/or for hormonal activation (2, 3). Hormone selectivity of adenylate cyclase systems in various target cells depends upon distinctive receptors which 'recognize' and interact with the hormone in a specific binding reaction which leads to adenylate cyclase activation and cyclic AMP (cAMP) generation.

Recent investigations from several laboratories, including ours, suggest the possibility that the effects of LH and FSH in testis are likewise mediated via adenylate cyclase systems (4-9). We have thus investigated rat testicular adenylate cyclase systems in relation to the formation and differentiation of specific cell groups during spermatogenesis. The purpose of these studies was to identify the testis cell types associated with the hormone specific and/or distinctive adenylate cyclase systems, i.e., to utilize these distinctive cyclases as markers of specific cell groups. This review primarily summarizes investigations from this laboratory, which have established the general and distinctive properties of the rat testis adenylate cyclase systems from the early neonatal period to the time of maturity.

Table 1

Effect of FSH on ^{14}C-cAMP Accumulation in Isolated
Seminiferous Tubules in the Absence and Presence of MIX[1]

Age	MIX [1mM]	^{14}C-cAMP Basal	Accumulation[2] FSH
10	-	.0	.08
	+	.01	1.48
16	-	.0	.03
	+	.10	.78
50	-	.0	.01
	+	.02	.21
74-85	-	.0	.02
	+	.03	.19

[1] 1-methyl, 3-isobuthylxanthine

[2] % of total intracellular radioactivity converted into ^{14}C-cAMP.

Of the ^{14}C-adenine taken up by testis tissue 96% is converted into
adenine nucleotides (61% into ATP and 35% into ADP and AMP). The
uptake of labeled adenine is greatest in younger rats and decreases
with age (9). The % conversion of the precursor pool to cAMP has
been found to be relatively independent of pool size (25). We
prefer therefore to express the results as % conversion of intracellular radioactivity to ^{14}C-cAMP. For details concerning the
principals and evaluation of the prelabeling technique the reader
is referred to a comprehensive review on this topic by Daly (10).

Data from 10 and 50 days of age groups are from a single experiment, while data from 16 and 74-85 days are from 2 separate
experiments. Values are the mean of 2-7 determinations.

Materials and Methods

Sprague-Dawley descended rats obtained from Charles River Breeding Laboratories were used. Whole testis fragments were prepared by teasing apart testis with fine forceps (Dumont No. 5). Unless otherwise stated, seminiferous tubules were isolated by microdissection. These procedures have been described previously in detail (9). Isolated testis cells were prepared from whole testis tissue and isolated seminiferous tubules by treatment with crude collagenase (Worthington CLS 9KC). Broken-cell preparations of whole testis tissue and isolated seminiferous tubules were prepared by homogenization in glass Dounce homogenizers using 2-3 strokes. Cellular fractions from homogenates were prepared by differential centrifugation. Accumulation of ^{14}C-cAMP in tissue preparations and isolated cells was determined by the prelabeling technique using ^{14}C-adenine as precursor for the intracellular ATP pools (10). Adenylate cyclase activity in broken-cell preparations was determined by measuring the formation of ^{32}P-cAMP from α - ^{32}P-ATP. The prelabeling technique, the assay for adenylate cyclase activity and the separation of the formed radioactive cAMP from other radioactive material has been previously described (9,11). Guanylate cyclase activity was determined by measuring the formation of ^{32}P-cGMP from α-^{32}P-GTP. Guanylate cyclase activity was assayed and the formed ^{32}P-cGMP separated from other radioactive material by a modification (Nissenson, R. A. and Hechter, O. M., unpublished), of the White and Zenser (12) procedure.

Results and Discussion

1) FSH and LH effects upon rat testis adenylate cyclases

FSH and LH stimulates ^{14}C-cAMP accumulation in intact-cell preparations of rat testis (1-3). This stimulation is dose-dependent. The ED_{50} for FSH (ovine NIH-FSH-81) is $2.4 + 0.37 \mu g/ml$ (average + SE of 6 experiments), while the ED_{50} for LH (ovine-LH-S16) is $0.25 + 0.06 \mu g/ml$ (average of 4 experiments). Thus, LH is about ten times more potent than FSH in this system. These in vitro stimulatory effects of FSH and LH in intact-cell preparations of testis are obtained with hormone concentrations within the range of their levels measured in serum.

2) FSH stimulation of adenylate cyclase in the testis of maturing and adult rats: Revealed by effective inhibition of phosphodiesterase

FSH effects in rat testis have been previously demonstrated to be age-dependent (13). Stimulation of adenylate cyclase in testis has been observed only in immature (less than 21 days old), but not in older rats, unless hypophysectomized (7,8). Monn et al. (14) have

Table 2

Effect of FSH and LH Tested Individually and in Combination on ^{14}C-cAMP Accumulation in Rat Testis Preparations.

FSH (μg/ml)	LH	^{14}C-cAMP Accumulation[1]	Hormone Effect[2]
		Whole testis tissue fragments[3]:	
--	--	.020	--
20	--	1.170	58.5
--	3	.630	31.5
20	3	1.720	86.0
		Isolated seminiferous tubules[4]:	
--	--	.018	--
10	--	.120	6.8
--	10	.026	1.4
--	30	.048	2.7
--	60	.069	3.8
10	10	.147	8.2
10	30	.142	7.9
10	60	.142	7.8
		Testis cell suspension[3]:	
--	--	.03	--
20	--	.37	12.3
--	3	3.07	102.0
20	3	3.73	124.0

1 % of total intracellular radioactivity converted into ^{14}C-cAMP.
2 Ratio of hormone value to basal.
3 Tissue fragments and cells obtained from 10-day-old rats.
4 Seminiferous tubules obtained from 34-day-old rats.

Isolation of cells from testis is described in the legend to Table 3.
Testis cell suspension is identical to cells referred to in Table 3 as Fraction 1.
Each value is the mean of duplicate determinations. Part of the data listed in Table are reprinted from Braun, T. and Sepsenwol, S. (9).

shown that phosphodiesterase activity in rat testis gradually increases 5-fold from 20-50 days of age. Since intracellular accumulation of cAMP formed depends on the ratio of rates of its formation and degradation, we have considered the possibility that increased cAMP degradation would mask FSH effect on cAMP formation, and this would account for the apparent ineffectiveness of the hormone in maturing and adult rats. In the first series of our studies, we established that among the available phosphodiesterase inhibitors, the theophylline derivative, 1-methyl, 3-isobutylxanthine (MIX) was more potent and effective in enhancing FSH-evoked ^{14}C-cAMP accumulation in testis tissue preparations from immature rats than the more commonly used aminophylline or papaverine (9). Subsequently, we have compared the effectiveness of FSH in evoking ^{14}C-cAMP accumulation in testis from immature, maturing and adult rats in the presence of MIX. Table 1 shows that significant and reproducible FSH stimulation of C-cAMP accumulation in testis tissue from maturing and adult rats was detected only with MIX. In the absence of MIX and hormonal stimulation, there is no net ^{14}C-cAMP accumulation in testis tissue of either immature or adult rats. In the absence of MIX, FSH evokes a slight increase in ^{14}C-cAMP levels in immature rats. However, even in immature rats, the stimulatory effect of FSH in the absence of phosphodiesterase inhibition is only a small fraction (5-6%) of that obtained with FSH in the presence of MIX. [Hence, all determinations of ^{14}C-cAMP accumulation in intact cell preparations were carried out in the presence of MIX (1 mM)].

Thus, an FSH effect eliciting a biological response in testis from maturing and adult rats was demonstrated by effectively inhibiting phosphodiesterase activity (9). This finding is consistent with the observation of Means and Vaitukaitis (15), that ^{3}H-FSH specifically binds to testicular tissue preparations from sexually mature as well as immature rats.

3) Evidence for separate FSH and LH-responsive adenylate cyclases in testis

A) Additive effects of FSH and LH in intact cell preparations containing interstitial and seminiferous tubule cells

Since LH has been shown to act upon the interstitial Leydig cells, and FSH upon the cells of the seminiferous tubule, we would expect a priori that each of the hormones will interact with an anatomically separate adenylate cyclase, located in different cell types. Indeed, Dorrington et al. (8), and Braun and Sepsenwol (9), have shown that FSH stimulates an adenylate cyclase in the cell(s) of the seminiferous tubules, while LH stimulates a cyclase in the interstitium (8,9,16). In our studies, the specificity of these cyclases for either FSH or LH has been rigorously examined. Table 2 shows that in tissue fragments of whole testis, both FSH and LH stimulate ^{14}C-cAMP

Table 3

Effect of FSH and LH on ^{14}C-cAMP Accumulation
in Cell Fractions Isolated from Testis

^{14}C-cAMP Accumulation[1]

	Basal	FSH	LH
Cell Fraction 1	0.03	0.37	3.07
Cell Fraction 2	0.12	1.01	0.45

Relative Cell Composition (%)

	Interstitial cells	Tubular cells	Red Blood cells
Cell Fraction 1	65	15	20
Cell Fraction 2	33	59	8

1   % of total intracellular radioactivity converted into ^{14}C-cAMP.

Cell fractions were prepared by collagenase (1 mg/ml) treatment of testes (1 g of tissue pooled from 30 rats 10-day old) in 10 ml of Krebs-Ringer-phosphate buffer (pH 7.2) containing half the usual amount of Ca^{++} and 1% bovine serum albumin (9). After 5 min incubation the cells were separated from the undigested tubules by filtering through nylon mesh. This cell fraction is designated as Fraction 1. The washed tubules were resuspended in 10 ml of the buffer (without collagenase) and for 30 min incubated in a metabolic shaker at 60 cycles/min. The cells recovered in the medium after 30 min incubation are designated as Fraction 2. The cell composition of the suspension was assessed in sections (1 μ) of Epon plastic embedded testis cells stained with borate-buffered toludine blue. The cell types were classified on the basis of nuclear size and morphology, chromatin distribution, interchromatin density and cytoplasmic characteristics (18) by light and electron microscopy.

Cell Fraction 1 contains Leydig, endothelial capillary and myoid cells. The tubular cells in this fraction are germ and Sertoli cells and their proportion is about 1:1.

Cell Fraction 2 contains spermatogonia types A, Intermediate and B, pre- and leptotene spermatocytes and Sertoli cells. The proportion of germ to Sertoli cells in this fraction is about 30:1, and spermatocytes comprise about 14%.

accumulation. Their effects in combination at supramaximal doses are additive, i. e., equal to the sum of the effects obtained with the individual hormones. In seminiferous tubules isolated by micro-dissection, ^{14}C-cAMP accumulation is augmented significantly only by FSH. LH effects in seminiferous tubules are slight and are obtained only a high (10-60 μg/ml) concentrations, and are readily accounted for by its contamination with FSH. This conclusion is further supported by the fact that in the seminiferous tubules, FSH and LH, when tested in combination is not greater than the effect obtained with FSH alone. In cell aggregates, isolated from testis by collagenase which contain both interstitial and tubule cells, LH and FSH both stimulate ^{14}C-cAMP accumulation. Their effect when tested in combination is greater than that attained by the hormones individually (Table 2). In other experiments, (not shown here), we have found that the combined effects of FSH and LH tested in isolated cells are 27-30% greater than expected on the basis of simple addi-tivity. The significance of this latter finding remains to be estab-lished. It may reflect synergism in the action of FSH and LH in isolated testis cells; alternatively LH and/or FSH receptors coupled to adenylate cyclase inaccessible in intact tissue may become ex-posed. Our preliminary findings suggest that in isolated testis cells, receptors coupled to adenylate cyclase become accessible to LH. These cells originate in the seminiferous tubules (see also footnote 1).

In these studies of isolated testis cells, we have found that the magnitude of the FSH and LH responses depends on the proportion of interstitial and tubule cell types. Cellular fractions enriched with interstitial cells exhibit high LH- and low FSH-responsiveness. In contrast, cellular fractions which exhibit high FSH- and low LH-responsiveness contain greater number of tubules than interstitial cells. These cell fractions showing high FSH-responsiveness were found to contain an abundance of spermatogonial over Sertoli cells (Table 3).

B) Differential changes in the responsiveness of the FSH and LH specific adenylate cyclase system during initiation and development of spermatogenesis

The effect of FSH and LH upon adenylate cyclase was examined using intact- and broken-cell preparations of rat testis starting from the early neonatal period to the time when speramtogenesis is fully established. In intact-cell preparations of seminiferous tubules and whole tissue fragments FSH stimulation of adenylate cyclase can be demonstrated in rats of all ages, including newborns (Figure 1). There is a remarkable increase in the response to FSH at 4-12 days of age with a distinct peak at 11-12 days. The transient burst in the response to FSH is followed by an abrupt decline between 13-18 days. A more gradual decline occurs between 18-40 days of age, until it reaches stable levels

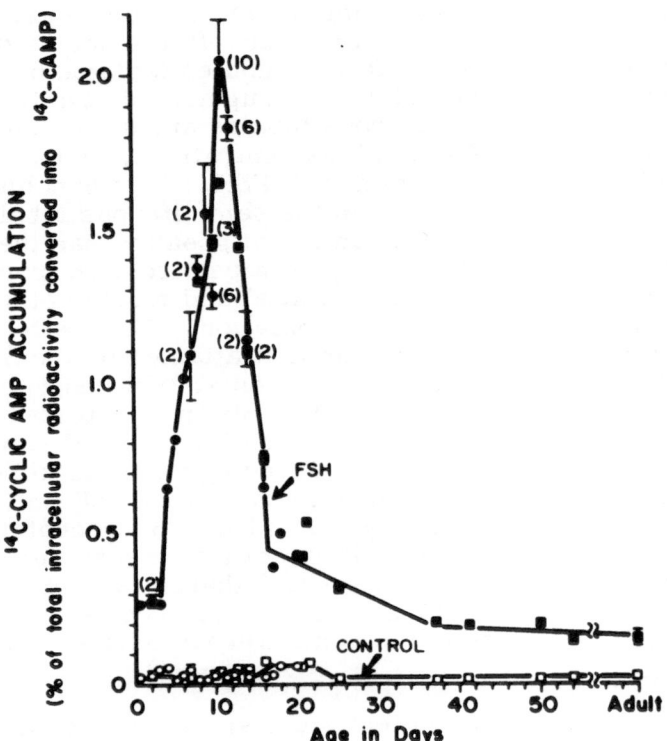

Figure 1. Accumulation of ^{14}C-cAMP in the absence (control) and the presence of FSH in whole tissue fragments (circles) and in isolated seminiferous tubules (squares) from rats of various age groups. The effect of 10-20 µg/ml of FSH (doses evoking a maximal response) is depicted in the Figure. However, in many experiments 5-6 different concentrations of the hormone were tested. Each point is the mean of 1-10 separate experiments assayed in duplicates. All assays were performed at 32° C. The numbers in brackets indicate the number of experiments and the vertical lines represent SEM. In each experiment testes from 4-10 rats were pooled for preparing the tissue preparations.

characteristic of adult rats.

This transient burst in the responsiveness to FSH was also observed in unfractionated homogenates from whole testis tissue and isolated seminiferous tubules (Figure 2). The fact that this phenomenon is observed also in homogenates of whole tissue and isolated seminiferous tubules indicates that the FSH-evoked ^{14}C-cAMP accumulation in intact cells is due to an increase of cAMP formation,

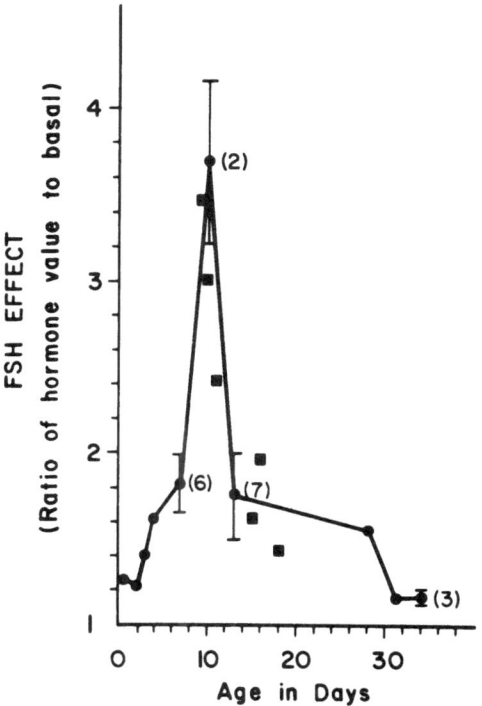

Figure 2. FSH-stimulated adenylate cyclase activity in unfractionated homogenates of whole testes tissue (circles) and in isolated
seminiferous tubules (squares) from rats of various age groups.
Adenylate cyclase activity was performed in a final volume of 50 μl
containing 40 mM Tris-HCl buffer (pH 8.0), 5 mM $MgCl_2$, 0.5 mM
unlabeled cAMP, 0.1% bovine serum albumin, 10 mM Creatine-phos-
phate, 0.1 mg/ml Creatine-kinase, 0.1 mM EDTA, 0.1 mM α- ^{32}P-
ATP and testis homogenate equivalent to 10-20 μg of protein.
Assayed at 32° C for 20 min. Each point is the mean of 1-7 separate
experiments assayed in duplicate. The numbers in brackets indicate
the number of experiments and the vertical lines represent SEM.

and indeed reflects the activity of the FSH-stimulated adenylate
cyclase system.

   Stimulation of adenylate cyclase by LH was found in intact cell
preparations of whole tissue fragments of newborn, as well as
immature and sexually mature rats (Figure 3). However, the pattern of changes in the activity of the LH-stimulated adenylate cyclase
during ontogeny is clearly different from that of the FSH-stimulated
cyclase. There appears to be a transient, moderate (50%) increase

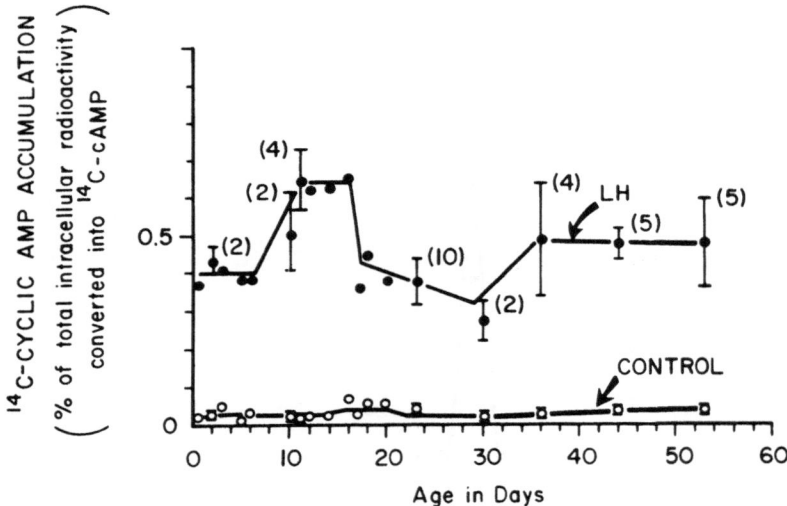

Figure 3. Accumulation of ^{14}C-cAMP in the absence (control) and presence of LH in whole tissue fragments from rats of various age groups. The effect of 2-3 μg/ml of LH (doses evoking maximal response) is depicted in the Figure. Other pertinent information is the same as described in the legend for Figure 1.

in the activity of the LH-stimulated adenylate cyclase at 11-16 days of age. However, the onset and decline of this relatively broad LH-peak does not parallel the sharp peak observed with FSH. Moreover, a second permanent increase in the LH-stimulated effect occurs at 30-50 days, at a time when the FSH effect has declined and levelled off.

4) <u>Spermatogonial cells as a possible target cell for FSH in seminiferous tubules</u>

One of the most striking findings in studying the ontogeny of the FSH-stimulated adenylate cyclase system in relation to the development of spermatogenesis is the transient burst of FSH-stimulated adenylate cyclase activity at 4-11 days of age (Figure 1). This burst could be due either to the appearance of a factor(s) augmenting the hormone effect or to an increase in the amount of the FSH-responsive adenylate cyclase system i.e., either receptors or the catalytic component. An increase in the amount of the FSH-sensitive adenylate cyclase could be due to an increased rate of <u>de novo</u> synthesis in existing cells, or result from the formation of the cyclase system in new cells which form during development. In consideration of this latter possibility, it is well established that multiple mitotic divisions of both Sertoli and spermatogonial cells take place in neonatal rats (17,18). Steinberger et al. (17) have shown that Sertoli cells divide most actively, and at a constant rate, during the first six days after birth. Accordingly, the total number of Sertoli cells increases already during the first three days. However, it should be emphasized that the activity of the FSH-responsive adenylate cyclase remains constant during this period. Spermatogonia first appear in testis at day 4 and spermatocytes at about 10-12 days postnatally; spermatogonia, after six successive mitotic divisions between 4-12 days, enter the spermatocyte pool. Considering the possibility that the cells in the seminiferous tubules responsive to FSH are solely Sertoli cells, we would expect that the appearance of a large number of spermatogonia should lead by dilution to a decline in the measurable activity of the FSH-sensitive cyclase. However, this is not the case. On the other hand, the burst of FSH-responsive adenylate cyclase in the seminiferous tubules appears to correlate with the appearance and onset of spermatogonial cell divisions.

Closer examination of the shape of the FSH-peak (Figure 1), reveals a non-linear ascending and a linear descending component. The non-linearity of the ascending limb of the peak can be explained by the fact that a certain number of spermatogonia (primarily type A_2 and A_3) degenerate; thus, the increase in the number of new spermatogonial cells is less than geometric. The profound steep decline in the activity of the FSH-sensitive cyclase at days 13-18, coincides with the appearance of a considerable number of spermatocytes. Moreover, at this developmental stage, extensive degeneration of spermatogonia is taking place. At this stage of development, Sertoli cells reach their total maximal number and cease to divide, while the number of spermatocytes is rapidly increasing. Apparently the spermatocytes do not possess FSH-responsive adenylate cyclase and are diluting the FSH-sensitive cell type(s) in the seminiferous tubules.

Dorrington and Fritz (19) on the basis of studies using tubule preparations from hypophysectomized, cryptorchid or irradiated rats suggested that Sertoli cells "may constitute the principle cell type within the seminiferous tubules which responds to FSH with an increase in cAMP levels". Our present findings suggest the possibility that in tubules from untreated rats, an FSH-sensitive adenylate cyclase may be associated with gonocytes (in newborn and 1-3 day-old rats) and spermatogonial cells (in rats older than 4 days). This possibility is supported by the finding that cell fractions containing an abundance of spermatogonial over Sertoli cells show the greatest FSH-responsiveness (Table 3).

Table 4

Distribution of Adenylate Cyclase Activity in Subcellular Fractions of Adult Rat Testis

Fraction	Specific Activity[1]		% of Total Activity[2]		Protein % of Total
	Mg++	Mn++	Mg++	Mn++	
Whole homogenate	2.5	10.9	100	100	100
600 x g x 10 min pellet	2.3	10.1	12.4	15.0	14.5
10,000 x g x 10 min pellet	2.7	7.5	13.1	9.8	12.8
105,000 x g x 60 min pellet	1.8	5.9	6.8	5.7	9.4
105,000 x g 60 min supernatant	.7	20.8	12.6	89.0	46.8
180,000 x g x 60 min pellet	.0	19.1	.0	4.2	2.6
180,000 x g x 60 min supernatant	.8	18.4	15.5	72.5	46.0

1 Picomoles cAMP/mg protein/min.

2 Total adenylate cyclase activity and protein content in the whole homogenate = 100.

Whole homogenate (20%) was prepared by homogenizing whole testis in hypotonic 5 mM Tris-HCl buffer (pH 7.2) containing 3 mM $MgCl_2$ and 1 mM EDTA. Subcellular fractions from filtered homogenates were prepared by differential centrifugation (using the Sorvall Model RC2-B centrifuge and Beckman Model 12-65B ultracentrifuge). The sedimented pellets were washed once and resuspended in the homogenizing buffer. The supernatant fraction from the 600 x g x 10 min centrifugation was successively recentrifuged at higher speeds as indicated.

Adenylate cyclase activity in each fraction was assayed in duplicate in the presence of either Mg++ or Mn++ (5 mM) in the assay medium. The details of the assay procedure are described in the legend of Figure 2. The values listed in the Table are the means from two separate experiments.

Table 5

Adenylate Cyclase Activity in Rat Testis Homogenate
and High-Speed Supernatant Subcellular Fraction

Tissue Preparation	picomoles Cyclic AMP/ mg protein/min
Total Homogenate	11.5 ± 0.54[a]
High-Speed Supernatant	18.5 ± 1.31[a]
105,000 x g x 60 min Supernatant	18.3
180,000 x g x 60 min Supernatant	19.8
300,000 x g x 5 hr Supernatant	21.7
180,000 x g x 24 hr Supernatant	22.2
180,000 x g x 60 min Supernatant	
1. Unfiltered (Rats 120 days of age)	23.9 ± 0.12[b]
2. Unfiltered, boild 10 min	0.0
3. Filtered through 0.22μ millipore filter	25.3 ± 1.54[b]
180,000 x g x 60 min Supernatant	
1. Unfiltered (Rats 22 days of age)	1.25
2. Filtered through 0.22μ millipore filter	0.96

[a]Mean $\pm$ SE from 6 individual preparations, each of which was assayed in duplicate.

[b]Mean $\pm$ SE of triplicate, all other values are the mean of duplicate determinations.

Preparation of total homogenates and subcellular fractions is described in the legend of Table 4.

5) <u>Development of a distinctive adneylate cyclase during spermio-</u>
<u>genesis in rat testis</u>

As corollary to the studies in intact cell preparations, we have
investigated the development of adenylate cyclase activity in testis
homogenate from neonatal, immature and sexually mature rats
(Figure 4). The adenylate cylase in the testis has a divalent cation
requirement (Mg^{++} or Mn^{++}) for catalytic activity. In newborn and

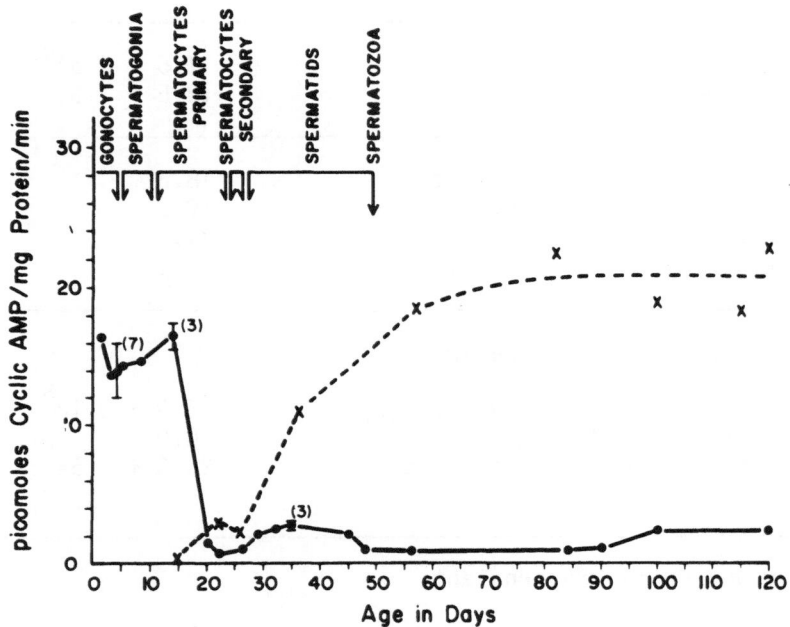

Figure 4. Adenylate cylcase activity in testis homogenates and
in 105,000 x g x 60 supernatant fraction from rats of various ages.
Adenylate cyclase activity was assayed in the homogenates in the
presence of 5 mM MgCl (●——●) and in the high-speed supernatant
in the presence of 5 mM MnCl (x--x). The concentration of
α-^{32}P-ATP was 0.2 mM; otherwise the composition of the incubation medium and other pertinent information is the same as described in the legend to Figure 2.

1-14 day-old rats, the adenylate cyclase activity in the presence of
Mn^{++} is 5-8 times higher than in older rats. This cyclase activity
declines abruptly between 14-20 days of age. Using Mg^{++} it is
stimulated by fluoride, FSH and LH[1]. This adenylate cyclase
activity corresponds to the cyclase systems described above in
intact cell preparations. The adenylate cyclase, at this early

Table 6

Distribution of Adenylate Cyclase Activity in Subcellular
Fractions of Rat Epididymal Spermatozoa

Fraction	Specific Activity[1]		% of Total Activity[2]		Protein % of Total
	Mg++	Mn++	Mg++	Mn++	
Whole homogenate	1.4	24.7	100	100	100
600 x g x 10 min pellet	.6	8.3	9.8	7.4	33.3
10,000 x g x 10 min pellet	1.9	71.2	20.0	42.0	21.8
105,000 x g x 60 min pellet	33.5	558.0	49.5	47.0	3.1
105,000 x g x 60 min supernatant	.0	28.7	.0	3.2	4.2
180,000 x g x 60 min pellet	.0	180.0	.0	3.6	2.6
180,000 x g x 60 min supernatant	.0	51.8	.0	1.6	.1

[1] Picomoles cAMP/mg protein/min.

[2] Total adenylate cyclase activity and protein content in the whole homogenate = 100.

Epididymal spermatozoa were collected from the caudal epididymis of adult rats in hypotonic Tris-HCl buffer (pH 7.2) containing 3 mM MgCl2 and 1 mM EDTA and sedimented by centrifugation at 600 x g x 5 min. Spermatozoa were washed once, resuspended and homogenized in the hypotonic buffer in a glass tight-fitting Dounce homogenizer using 20 strokes. The preparation of subcellular fractions is described in the legend of Table 4. Adenylate cyclase activity in each fraction was assayed in duplicate in the presence of either Mg++ or Mn++ (5 mM) in the assay medium. The details of the assay procedure are described in the legend of Figure 2. The results of a single experiment are shown. Data from Braun, T. and Dods, R. F. (in preparation).

stage, appears to be membrane bound, since by centrifugation of the homogenates at 600 and 10,000 x g x 10 min and 105,000 x g x 60 min, it is almost completely sedimented, and the activity is recovered in the sedimented pellets. However at about 22-26 days of age, a separate adenylate cyclase system developes in the rat testis, which is Mn^{++}-dependent, but Mg^{++}-insensitive. This cyclase is not influenced either by fluoride or by FSH and LH. The specific activity of this Mn^{++}-dependent cyclase at first is very low, but increases substantially at the age of 26-36 days and reaches maximum values in adult, sexually mature rats. When we examined the distribution of this Mn^{++}-dependent adenylate cyclase in the isolated interstitial cells and seminiferous tubules, it was found mainly in the tubules. The Mn^{++}-dependent cyclase sytem was almost completely recovered in the high-speed supernatant following centrifugation of testis homogenates (Table 4). It has been established that the Mn^{++}-dependent cyclase passes through a .22 Millipore filter and remains in solution even after centrifugation for 5 hours at 300,000 x g (Table 5). It seems that this soluble Mn^{++}-dependent cyclase system is located in the cell cytoplasm since neither detergents nor mechanical shearing force was required for its solubilization.

The Mn^{++}-sensitive adenylate cyclase has been distinguished from guanylate cyclase, which has been shown by previous studies to be both soluble and Mn^{++}-dependent. We have found both cyclases in the 180,000 g x 60 min supernatant. They differ with regard to nucleotide substrate specificity. Figure 5 shows the rate of activity of the two cyclases as a function of either ATP or GTP concentration, used as substrate. The simultaneous addition of α-^{32}P labelled ATP and unlabelled GTP has no effect on the rate of activity of the adenylate cyclase. In contrast, the addition of ATP inhibits the rate of activity of the guanylate cyclase.

In further studies, the soluble adenylate cyclase was partially purified by column chromatography on Sephadex G-150. By using a Sepharose B column calibrated with polymers of known molecular weight, the molecular weight of this soluble adenylate cyclase is estimated to be in the range of 80,000 of 160,000 (Figure 6).

6) Some of the properties of the rat epididymal sperm adenylate cyclase

In the rat epididymal sperm the adenylate cyclase has properties similar to the adenylate cyclase which develops in the spermatids with regard to its Mn^{++}-requirement and fluoride insensitivity. Moreover, in the rat epididymal sperm adenylate cyclase, as in the cyclase system of the spermatid stage, the stimulatory effect of Mn^{++} is potentiated by Ca^{++}. However, the adenylate cyclase in the epididymal sperm is membrane bound; in contrast to the soluble

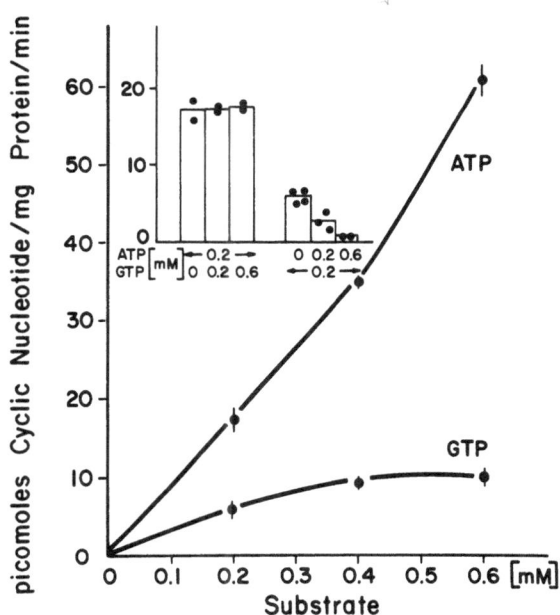

Figure 5. Adenylate and guanylate cyclase activity in the 180,000 x g x supernatant fraction as a function of ATP and GTP concentration. In the upper left corner, the results of an experiment are illustrated in which radioactive ATP and unlabeled GTP and vice versa were added simultaneously. Both cyclases were assayed in the presence of 5 mM $MnCl_2$. In guanylate cyclase assays 1-methyl, 3-isobutylxanthine was used as the phosphodiesterase inhibitor. In adenylate cyclase assays unlabelled cAMP was used to protect ('trap') the ^{32}P-cAMP formed (11).

cyclase of the spermatid stage, it is found associated mainly with the 10,000 x g x 10 min and 105,000 x g x 60 min particulate fractions (Table 6). These findings suggest that the spermatid stage adenylate cyclase is synthesized and remains soluble in the cytoplasm and only later in development becomes associated with the membrane in sperm. Whether the attachment of the sperm adenylate cyclase to membrane occurs in the testis, or during the subsequent stay of the sperm in the epididymis is presently uncertain.

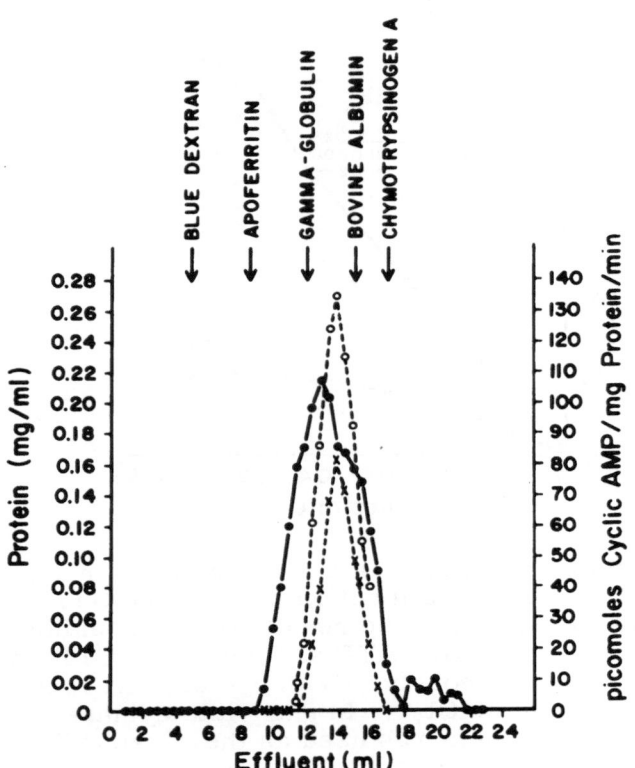

Figure 6. Gel filtration on a Sepharose B column (0.9 x 19 cm) of the 180,000 x g x 60 min supernatant fraction prepared from adult rat testis homogenates. The column was precalibrated with substances of known molecular weight (Calibration Kit, Pharmcia Fine Chemicals, Inc.). Eluted with 5 mM Tris-HCl buffer (pH 7.2) containing 3 mM $MgCl_2$ and 1 mM EDTA at a flow rate of 13 ml/60 min. Fractions (0.5 ml) were collected and albumin added to a final concentration of 0.1%. Adenylate cyclase activity in each fraction was assayed in duplicate in the presence of 5 mM (x---x), and 20 mM (o---o) of $MnCl_2$. The concentration of α- ^{32}P-ATP was 0.2 mM; otherwise, the composition of the incubation medium was the same as described in the legend to Figure 2. Protein elution pattern (•---•).

Concluding Remarks

Our present findings suggest that the FSH-sensitive adenylate cyclase in the seminiferous tubules might be associated with speramatogonia, the LH-sensitive cyclase with the interstitial Leydig cells. The transient burst of FSH-stimulated adenylate cyclase activity which occurs during the initiation of the first spermatogenic cycle begins at the time of the transformation of the gonocyte population into the least differentiated type A spermatogonia ('stem cells') and their proliferation to produce the first spermatogonial population. Others have suggested that in 'normal circumstances' there is an initial 'overproduction' of A_1 type spermatogonia, which subsequently degenerate as A_2 and A_3 (20) or A_4 and intermediate (21) type cells. In adult rats, this degeneration is extensive. In neonatal and in immature rats, when the first populations of spermatogonia differentiate the amount of degeneration is considerably less (20, S. Sepsenwol, unpublished observations). Our findings that there is a transient burst of the FSH-sensitive adenylate cyclase during the formation of the first population of spermatogonia is thus in line with the aforementioned observations.

Previous observations have demonstrated that FSH injected into immature rats increases the number of spermatogonial mitoses (13), and the number of spermatocytes per tubule (23). Recently, Huckins et al. (22), have indicated that FSH administered to 16 day-old rats decreases or prevents the degeneration of spermatogonial cells which normally occurs at this developmental stage. These findings can be interpreted to mean that the role of FSH is to control the size of the differentiating spermatogonial pool and, in this way, the number of cells which will enter the spermatocyte pool. The question arises hence, why extensive degeneration does not take place during the differentiation of the first spermatogonial population. Whether the first population of spermatogonia may be more sensitive to FSH, the hormone may be more readily accessible to the cells, merits further investigation.

The present study describes the development of the sperm adenylate cyclase system in the rat. Some of the properties of the rat sperm adenylate cyclase are similar to the properties of the gonadotropin-sensitive testis cyclase and cyclases from other mammalian tissues. The rat sperm adenylate cyclase exhibits certain striking properties which have been considered to be unique to guanylate cyclases (24). The sperm adenylate cyclase appears to be another form, distiguishable from most adenylate and guanylate cyclases of mammalian somatic cells. Spermatozoa are distinctive cell types formed by a complex, morphologically well characterized developmental process in which the original germ 'stem cell' undergoes profound structural and biochemical changes. The question arises whether this form of sperm cyclase is synthesized as such, or whether it is transformed from the more familiar adenylate or guanylate cyclase. Additionally, the molecular nature responsible for the distinctiveness of the sperm adenylate cyclase is presently not known, but its characterization is our aim in ongoing studies.

Acknowledgements

This project was supported by Rockefeller Foundation Grant RF 71075. I wish to thank my co-workers, Dr. S. Sepsenwol and Dr. R. F. Dods, for their contribution and participation in portions of this project, and Ms. B. Krohn and K. Cheney for excellent technical assistance. I am grateful to Dr. O. M. Hechter, Chairman of the Physiology Department, NUMC, for his continued interest and helpful discussions, and to NIADD (Bethesda, Md.) for the generous gift of FSH and LH, and to Searle Laboratories (Chicago, Il.), for the gift of 1-methyl, 3-isobutylxanthine.

Notes (p. 250, 252)

1. The LH-sensitive adenylate cyclase in the rat testis homogenates appears to originate in the seminiferous tubules. This conclusion is based on the following findings: When cell fractions enriched with interstitial Leydig cells are homogenized, the homogenates do not exhibit LH-responsiveness. Apparently, the LH-sensitive adenylate cyclase in the interstitium is labile and does not 'survive' homogenization. However, when homogenate is prepared either from whole testis tissue or isolated seminiferous tubules (free of interstitial cells), the adenylate cyclase in these homogenates does respond to LH. Thus, in the seminiferous tubules, LH-receptors coupled to adenylate cyclase exist which are unaccessible in intact tissue and become exposed after homogenization. Murad et al. (6) observed likewise LH-stimulation of adenylate cyclase in whole dog testis tissue homogenates. The physiological significance of these observations is not yet apparent.

2. Although some Mn^{++}-dependent adenylate cyclase activity was found in the interstitial cell fraction it is probably due to contamination of this cell fraction with cells originating in the seminiferous tubules. We have thus far been unable to prepare an interstitial cell fraction free of spermatids and testicular sperm from adult rats.

References

1. Robison, G. A., Butcher, R. W., and Sutherland, E. W., Cyclic AMP, Academic Press, New York, 1971.

2. Rodbell, M., Birnbaumer, L., Polh, S. L., and Krans, H. M. J., in Margoulies, M. and Greenwood, F. C. (eds.) Structure-Activity Relationship of Protein and Polypeptide Hormones, Excerpta Medica ICS, Amsterdam, 241: 211, 1971.

3. Hechter, O., and Braun, T., in Margoulies, M., and Greenwood, F. C. (eds.) Structure-Activity Relationships of Protein and Polypeptide Hormones, Excerpta Medica ICS, Amsterdam 241: 211 (1971).

4. Sandler, R., and Hall, P. F., Endocrinology 79: 647, 1966.

5. Dufau, M. L., Catt, K. J., and Tsuruhara, T., Endocrinology 20: 1032, 1972.

6. Murad, F., Strauch, S., and Vaughan, M., Biochim. Biophys. Acta 177: 591, 1969.

7. Kuehl, F. A., Panatelli, D. J., Tarnoff, J., and Humes, J. L., Biol. Reprod. 2: 154, 1970.

8. Dorrington, J. H., Vernon, R. G., and Fritz, I. B., Biochim. Biophys. Res. Comm. 46: 1523, 1972.

9. Braun, T., and Sepsenwol, S., Endocrinology 92: Suppl. A-98, 1973; ibid. 94, 1974 (in press).

10. Daly, J. W., in Chasin, M. (ed.) Methods in Cyclic Nucleotide Research, Dekker, Inc., New York, p. 255, 1972.

11. Bar, P., and Hechter, O., Anal. Biochem. 29: 476, 1969.

12. White, A. A., and Zenser, T. V., Anal. Biochem. 41: 372, 1971.

13. Means, A. R., Adv. Exp. Med. Biol. 36: 431, 1973.

14. Monn, E., DeSautel, M., and Christiansen, R. O., Endocrinology 91: 716, 1972.

15. Means, A. R., and Vaitukaitis, J., Endocrinology 90: 39, 1972.

16. Cooke, B. A., Van Beurden, W. M. O., Rommerts, F. F. G., and van der Molen, H. J., FEBS Letters 25: 83, 1972.

17. Steinberger, E., Steinberger, A., and Ficher, M., Recent Progr. Hormone Res. 26: 547, 1970.

18. Clermont, Y., and Perey, B., Am. J. Anat. 100: 241, 1959.

19. Dorrington, J. H., and Fritz, I. B., Endocrinology 94: 395, 1974.

20. Huckins, E., in Velardo, J. T. and Kasprow, B. A. (eds.) Biology of Reproduction, Basic and Clinical Studies, Pan American Association of Anatomy, New Orleans, p. 395, 1972.

21. Courot, M., Hochereau-de Rivers, M. T., and Ortavant, R., in Johnson, A. D., Gomes, W. R. and Vandermark, N. L. (eds.) The Testis, Vol. I., Academic Press, New York, p. 339, 1970.

22. Huckins, C., Mills, N., Besch, P., and Means, A. R., Endocrinology, Suppl. 92, A-94, 1973.

23. Greep, R. O., Fevold, H. L., and Hisaw, F. L., Anat. Rec. 65: Suppl. 261, 1936.

24. Hardman, J. G., Robison, G. A., and Sutherland, E. W., Ann. Rev. Physiol. 33: 311, 1971.

25. Shizimu, H., and Daly, J., Biochem. Biophys. Acta 222; 465, 1970.

ANDROGEN TRANSPORT AND RECEPTOR MECHANISMS IN

TESTIS AND EPIDIDYMIS

F. S. French, W. S. McLean, A. A. Smith, D. J. Tindall,
S. C. Weddington, P. Petrusz, M. Sar, W. E. Stumpf and
S. N. Nayfeh

Departments of Pediatrics, Biochemistry and The Laboratories
for Reproductive Biology, University of North Carolina
School of Medicine, Chapel Hill, North Carolina, U.S.A.

V. Hansson and O. Trygstad

Institutes of Pathology and Pediatric Research
Rikshospitalet, Oslo, Norway

and

E. M. Ritzén

Pediatric Endocrinology Unit, Clinical Reserch Laboratory
Karolinska sjukhuset, Stockholm, Sweden

Spermatogenesis is an androgen dependent process which can
be maintained in hypophysectomized rats by the administration
of either testosterone (1) or 5α-dihydrostestosterone (2).
Gonadotrophins may exert their effects on spermatogenesis
indirectly by way of androgens. The sole action of LH appears
to result from the stimulation of testosterone synthesis by the
interstitial cells of Leydig. FSH is necessary for the full maintenance of spermatogenesis, but its effects can be mimicked
by androgen and blocked by the anti-androgen, cyproterone,
indicating that its action is linked in series with androgen (1)
or that androgen is the mediator of FSH action.

Androgen is also essential for normal maturation of the
spermatozoa within the epididymis (3, 4). In order to influence
spermatogenesis as well as sperm maturation, androgen must
be transported from its site of synthesis in the Leydig cells to
its sites of action in target cells of the germinal epithelium and

epidiymis. The present article describes both extracellular
transport and intracellular receptor mechanisms for androgen
in testis and epididymis.

Rat Testis Produces an Androgen Binding Protein (ABP) Which is Secreted Into the Testicular Fluid

An androgen binding protein (ABP) with high affinity for $5 - \alpha$
dihydrotestosterone (DHT) ($K_a = 1.25 \times 10^9 M^{-1}$) and testosterone
($K_a = 0.5 \times 10^9 M^{-1}$) has been demonstrated in 105,000 x g supernatants of rat testis and epididymis (5-10). ABP is produced in
the testis, secreted into testicular fluid and carried to the epididymis by way of the efferent ducts (9,10). The concentration
of ABP in efferent duct fluid ($4-8 \times 10^{-8} M$) is sufficient to bind
testosterone and/or DHT in a concentration of 13-26 ng/ml,
assuming one binding site/molecule ABP (10). Ligation of efferent ducts causes ABP to disappear completely from caput epididymis supernatant within three days, indicating that the testis
is the only source of ABP in the epididymis (9). ABP must be
produced within the seminiferous tubules, since it is present in
efferent duct fluid (EDF) and is absent from testicular lymph.
Furthermore, the presence of undiminished amounts of ABP in
testis supernatant following complete destruction of the germ
cells by gamma-radiation or chemicals, like nitrofurazon,
suggests that ABP is formed by Sertoli cells. It appears that
ABP might have an important role in the transport of testicular
androgen to the germinal epithelium as well as to androgen dependent epithelial cells in the epididymis.

ABP Concentrations in Efferent Duct Fluid (EDF) and Super- natants of Testis and Epididymis

Concentrations of ABP were measured in testis, EDF, and
segments of epididymis from adult rats. Testis and segments
of epididymis were homogenized separately at 4° in 3 volumes
of 50 mM Tris-HCL, pH 7.4, containing 1.5 nM EDTA, 0.5 nM
2-mercaptoethanol, and 10% glycerol. Homogenates were centrifuged at 105,000 g for 60 min. To remove endogenous steroids,
supernatants and EDF were extracted with charcoal (1 mg/mg
protein) overnight at 0°, and the charcoal removed by centrifugation. Total protein was measured in each sample by the
method of Lowry et al. (11).

Binding capacity of ABP was measured by "steady state" polyacrylamide gel electrophoresis (SS-PAGE) (Fig. 1). By this
method, $[1,2-^3H]5_\alpha$-dihydrotestosterone (^3H-DHT) is dissolved in
the acrylamide solution before it polymerizes. ^3H-DHT is distributed uniformly in the polymerized gel and remains stationary
in the electrophoretic field until it is bound by protein moving
through the gel. Following electrophoresis, the gels are sliced

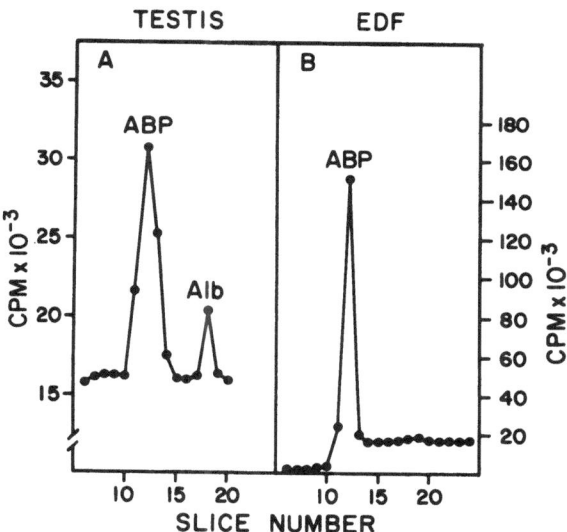

Figure 1. Steady state polyacrylamide gel electrophoresis (SS-PAGE). Samples were absorbed overnight with dextran coated charcoal at 0° C (1 mg Norit A/mg of protein). Charcoal was removed by centrifugation twice at 10,000 x g in a Beckman microfuge, and samples of 500 μl were layered onto 6 1/2% acrylamide gels (10 x 70 mm) containing 10% glycerol, to which 2 nM ^{3}H-DHT had been added before polymerization. Electrophoresis was run at 0° C for 5 hrs, and 5 mAmp/tube was applied. Following electrophoresis, the gels were transversely sliced into 2.3 mm segments which are placed directly into counting vials with toluene scintillation fluid. After standing overnight at room temperature, more than 98% of the radioactivity was extracted into the toluene. Steady state between bound and free ^{3}H-DHT is obtained when the level of radioactivity in front of the ABP peak is identical to that behind the peak. At steady state the amount of ^{3}H-DHT in the peak is a linear function of the total amount of binding protein (ABP) present in the sample:

$$\text{Total ABP} \quad \text{Peak ABP}\left(\frac{KD}{[H]} + 1\right)$$ where K is the equilibrium constant of dissociation and [H] is the concentration of the H-DHT in the gel.

 A: Testis cytosol fraction (0.4 ml = 2.2 mg protein); binding to ABP at steady state

 B: Efferent duct fluid (20 μl = 50 μg protein); binding to ABP not at steady state.

and the radioactivity measured in each slice. A steady state between bound and free radioactivity is reached when the level of free radioactivity behind the peak of bound steroid equals the level in front (Fig. 1A). At steady state the law of mass action can be used to determine the concentration of binding protein, assuming one binding site per protein molecule, and that the amount of ^{3}H-DHT bound to ABP is a linear function of the total number of binding sites present (12).

The concentration of ABP in EDF expressed as ^{3}H-DHT binding capacity at saturation (pmoles/mg protein) was much higher than in testicular and epididymal supernatants (Fig. 2). There was sufficient ABP in EDF to account for all the ABP measured in supernatants of testis and epididymis. Since the primary fluid of the seminiferous tubules becomes diluted before reaching the rete testis (13), the concentration of ABP surrounding the germinal epithelium might be even higher than in EDF. The relatively large amount of ABP in caput epididymis supernatant, as compared with testis supernatant, probably results from absorption of water as the testicular fluid passes through the efferent ducts and the first segment of caput (14), and may also reflect a larger proportion of luminal fluid per unit of tissue weight. ABP concentration in epididymis supernatant decreases from segment I to V (Fig. 2). Furthermore, the amount of ABP leaving the epididymis through vas deferens is much less than the amount that enters into the caput, suggesting that the ^{3}H-DHT binding activity of ABP is destroyed during passage through the epididymis. Although the exact role of ABP in the caput epididymis is not yet known, it very likely serves to concentrate large

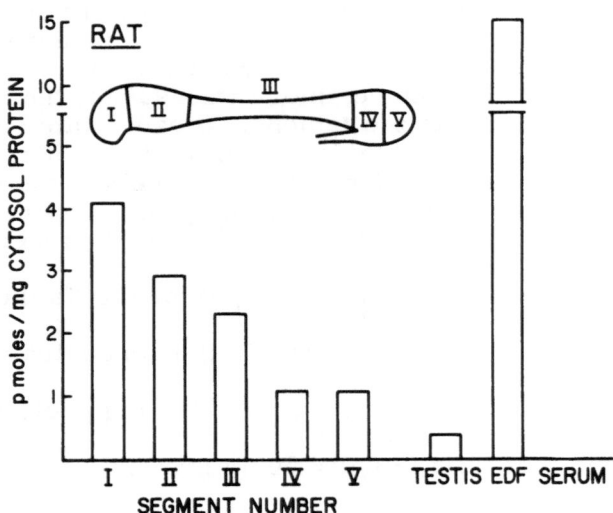

Figure 2. Concentration of ABP in 105,000 g supernatants prepared from segments of rat epididymis in comparison with rat testis, efferent duct fluid (EDF) and serum. ABP was measured as described in the legend to Figure 1.

amounts of androgen in the lumen in close proximity to the spermatozoa and surrounding epithelial cells (Fig. 3A). Indeed, the concentration of endogenous DHT in the caput epididymis of the rat (40-60 ng/g tissue) (16) is higher than in any other tissue of the body so far examined, and is very similar to the concentration of ABP, if one assumes one binding site per molecule of ABP.

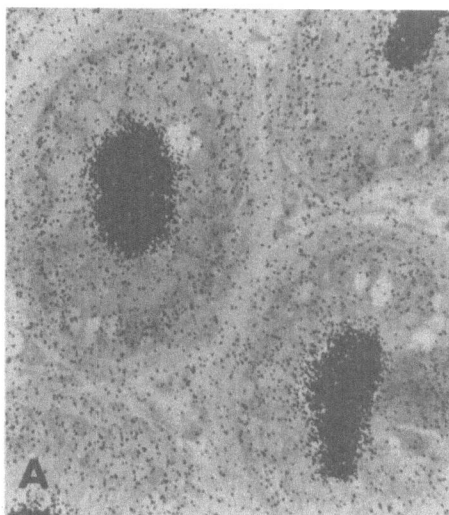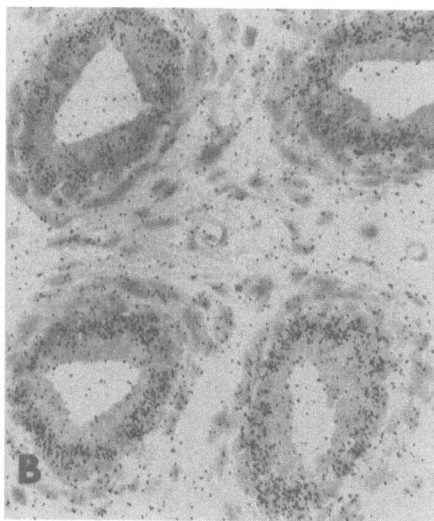

Figure 3. Autoradiograms of caput epididymis, prepared by the dry-mount technique, as described previously (15), 3 hrs after the injection of 1,2,6,7-^{3}H-testosterone into male 35-day Sprague-Dawley rats, intact (A) and ten days after hypophysectomy (B). Intraluminal localization of labeled androgen in caput epididymidis of the intact rat is shown in 3A. Concentration of label within the lumen occurred in the presence of ABP but was not seen in the hypophysectomized rat after ABP had disappeared from the lumen (3B). In the intact animal, intracellular receptors were saturated with endogenous androgen and there was very little intranuclear localization of labeled androgen. After hypophysectomy, however, nuclear localization of label was distinct and quite uniform throughout the epithelium.

ABP Production Stimulated by FSH, Not by LH or Androgens

To establish the relationship between the production of ABP and maturational changes in the testis, ABP was measured in rats of various ages. At 1 and 2 weeks of age, ABP was not detected in testis or epididymis. By 3-4 weeks of age however,

ABP could be measured in supernatants of testis and caput epididymis. After 4 weeks, ABP increased rapidly in the caput, reaching a peak during puberty (8 weeks) and decreasing in the adult rat to about 50% of the pubertal level (17). Since the appearance of ABP corresponded with the onset of gonadotrophin secretion in the immature rat (18), the effect of hypophysectomy on ABP was examined in rats 5 weeks of age. Three days after hypophysectomy, the concentration of ABP in caput epididymidis supernatants was only about 40% of the levels in intact littermates, and by the 10th day after hypophysectomy ABP had completely disappeared from both testis and epididymis. Evidence that this action of the pituitary is mediated through gonadotrophins, and not some other pituitary factor was obtained by treatment of adult hypophysectomized animals with human gonadotrophin containing both FSH and LH. As seen in Figure 4, FSH-LH administration for 5 days caused ABP to increase markedly in testis supernatant. The ABP concentration in treated rats was more than 10 times higher than in hypophysectomized controls and almost twice as high as in intact littermates. These findings indicated that ABP production is under pituitary control both in immature and adult rats.

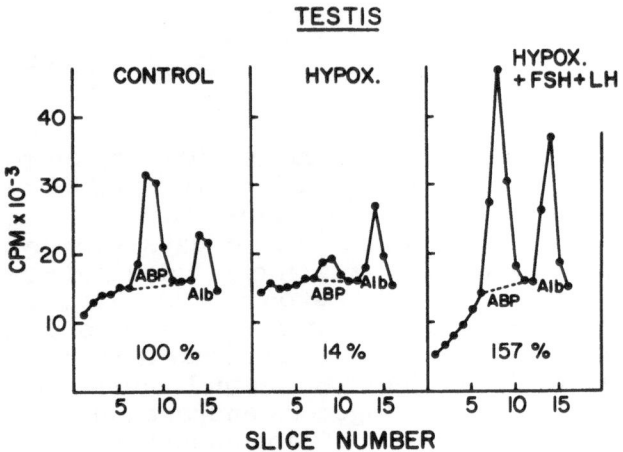

Figure 4. Effect of FSH + LH treatment on ABP levels in rat testis. Adult rats in groups of 4 were hypophysectomized for 19 days. From day 20 after hypophysectomy, each animal was injected daily with 75 IU FSH + 25 IU LH or saline only. After treatment for 5 days the testes were examined for ABP as described in the legend to Figure 1. Percentages indicate relative binding to ABP. Control: Sham operated; Hypox: Hypophysectomy for 19 days and saline for 5 days; Hypox + FSH + LH: Hypophysectomy for 19 days and FSH + LH treatment for 5 days.

Highly purified preparations of human FSH and LH were next used to examine their separate effects on ABP production. In 5 week old intact rats, FSH injected subcutaneously for 10 days markedly increased the concentration of ABP both in the testis and the caput epididymis, while LH treatment had no significant effect (17) (Fig. 5). Similar results were obtained when rats were hypophysectomized at 5 weeks of age and started on daily injections of FSH 10 days later. After 10 days of treatment, FSH restored ABP levels in testis and epididymis supernatants (17). When increasing doses of highly purified FSH were injected intramuscularly to immature rats there was a linear increase in ABP

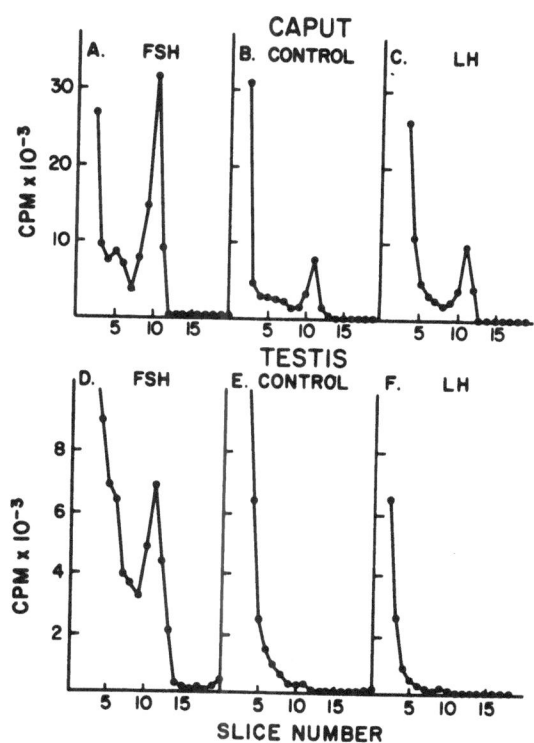

Figure 5. Effect of FSH (20 µg/day) and LH (20 µg/day) on 3H-DHT binding capacity of ABP in charcoal absorbed supernatants of caput epididymis and testis. Equal amounts of supernatant protein (caput 200 µg/100 µl and testis 800 µg/100 µl) were equilibrated with saturating amounts (88 nM) of ^{3}H-DHT and layered onto nonlabeled 7% acrylamide gels (5 mm x 60 mm) and electrophoresis run for 2 h at 0° C and 1.7 mAmp/tube.
From Hansson et al. (17)

concentration in caput epididymis at doses between 2-10 µg of FSH (Fig. 6). Furthermore, administration of testosterone

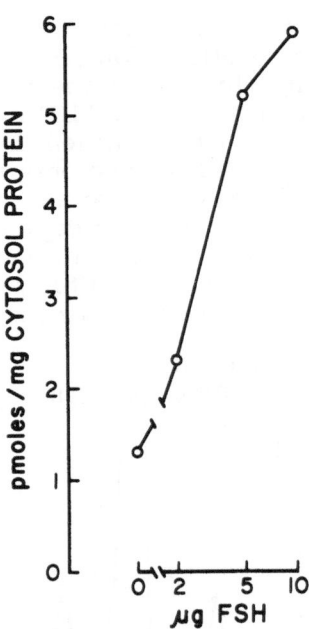

Figure 6. Effect of increasing doses of FSH on ABP levels in supernatants of caput epdidymis. Highly purified human pituitary FSH and LH were prepared from frozen pituitary glands according to the method of Roos (19) with some modifications (Trygstad, to be published). Purified FSH was assayed by the rat ovarian augmentation test (20) and had a biological activity of 15,000 IU/mg (680 NIH units/mg). LH was assayed by the seminal vesicle test (21) and contained 10,000 IU/mg (1600 HCG units/mg). Contamination of the preparations as determined by radioimmunoassay was negligible; FSH contained only 247 IU LH/mg and LH contained 142 IU FSH/mg. Thirty-five-day-old Wistar rats in groups of 4 were injected i.m. with FSH for 10 days, and ABP measured as described in the legend to Figure 1.

propionate in increasing doses (10-100 μg/90 g body weight) to intact 50 day old ("pubertal") rats caused a dose dependent decrease in ABP concentrations both in testis and epididymis indicating that stimulation of ABP is abolished by feedback suppression of pituitary gonadotrophins (22).

FSH stimulation of ABP both in intact and hypophysectomized animals is specific since no increase in ABP could be obtained using other pituitary hormones or sex steroids (Fig. 7). In hypophysectomized rats the sensitivity of the ABP response to FSH treatment for 3 days was similar to the ovarian augmentation test (20) as well as the ovarian weight response to FSH in the hypophysectomized rat (23). Significant stimulation of total

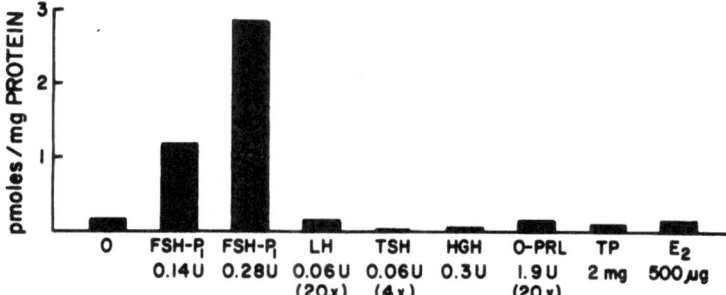

Figure 7. Specific stimulation of ABP by FSH. Rats in groups of 4 were hypophysectomized 28 days of age and injected with 0.14 or 0.28 NIH units FSH-P_1 (total dose). The injections were started on day 30. Parallel groups of animals were injected with high doses of LH, thyroid-stimulating hormone (TSH), ovine-prolactin (O-PRL), human growth hormone (HGH), testosterone propionate (TP) and estradiol-17ß (E_2).
    (20x) = twenty times the maximum contamination of LH or O-PRL in 0.28 unit FSH-P_1.
    (4x) = four times the maximum contamination of TSH in 0.28 unit FSH-P_1.

ABP in caput epididymis was obtained with as little as 2 IU FSH (equivalent to about 0.08 NIH units). The ABP response diminished with time after hypophysectomy but was restored by pretreatment with testosterone. Similar augmentation of the ABP response to FSH was obtained by pretreatment with LH. In either case the augmentation was associated with an increase in weight of the epididymis and was presumably an androgen effect. The enhanced response to FSH following androgen priming is reflected in increased concentrations of ABP both in testicular and epididymal supernatants, however it remains to be determined whether the priming increases Sertoli cell production of ABP or decreases the rate of ABP degradation.

Androgen Receptors in Epididymal Epithelium

After testosterone is taken up by epithelial cells of epididymis, it is rapidly converted to several metabolites with DHT and 5α-androstane-3α, 17ß-diol as major products (24, 25). Nuclear concentration in target cells is characteristic for androgens as well as other sex hormones (26, 27). (Fig. 3B). DHT is bound to intracellular androgen receptors in the cytoplasm (28, 29), subsequently transported into the nucleus and bound to nuclear chromatin. DHT-receptor complexes can be extracted from nuclei in 0.4 M KCl and have a sedimentation of 3-3.5 S (24, 27, 30).

Epididymal cytoplasmic receptor (CR) has physical properties
and steroid specificity very similar to the ventral prostate receptor (28, 29, 31). Both receptors are highly specific for DHT.
Furthermore, they have similar electrophoretic mobilities by
PAGE (R_x=0.4), similar sedimentation rates by sucrose gradient
centrifugation (8S and 4S) and similar elution volumes by Sephadex
G-200 gel filtration (28-31). Both are destroyed by heating at
50° C for 30 min and lose binding activity after treatment with sulfhydryl blocking agents, such as PCMPS (1mM) (28, 29). A characteristic feature of ^{3}H-DHT-CR complexes of epididymis and
prostate is the very slow rate of dissociation at 0° C (t 1/2 0° 4
days) (29, 31). This property clearly distinguishes ^{3}H-DHT-CR
from ^{3}H-DHT-ABP which dissociates much more rapidly (t 1/2 0° =
6 min) (29). The slow rate of dissociation of ^{3}H-DHT-CR is
consistent with a receptor function of CR. During the process of
translocation from cytoplasm to nucleus, androgen is firmly
bound to the receptor and cannot be exchanged by excess of free
DHT (30, 32). The rapid dissociation of DHT from ABP, on the
other hand, suggests that ABP functions as a carrier protein
capable of releasing its androgen to surrounding epithelial cells.
A striking difference between ABP and CR was also found in
their affinity for cyproterone (29). Cyproterone acetate inhibited
the binding of ^{3}H-DHT to epididymal CR to the same extent as
it reduced uptake and binding by epididymal nuclei (29). On the
other hand, binding of ^{3}H-DHT to ABP was not affected by this
treatment. These studies indicated that nuclear uptake and
binding of DHT are dependent on CR and independent of ABP.

Androgen Receptors in the Seminiferous Tubules

The accumulation of evidence for androgen action on spermatogenesis prompted a search for androgen receptors in rat seminiferous tubules. Studies were carried out in immature Sprague-
Dawley rats hypophysectomized at 25 or 35 days of age. Three
to twenty-four days following hypophysectomy, animals in groups
of 10 or 20 were eviscerated, functionally hepatectomized (24)
and injected intravenously with ^{3}H-testosterone. Whole testis
or washed seminiferous tubules were homogenized in 3 volumes
20 mM Tris-HCl buffer, pH 7.4, containing 0.32 M sucrose and
3 mM $MgCl_2$ (TSM buffer); and 105,000 g supernatant was prepared. Supernatants were made similarly from epididymis and
prostate. Binding was examined by polyacrylamide gel electrophoresis (6,8), Sephadex G-200 gel filtration (6,28), and sucrose
gradient centrifugation (6,24).

As seen in Figure 8, testicular supernatants contained an
androgen-protein complex (CR) moving as a symmetrical peak
of protein bound radioactivity with an R_f of 0.4. The mobility
of this androgen protein complex was clearly different from ABP

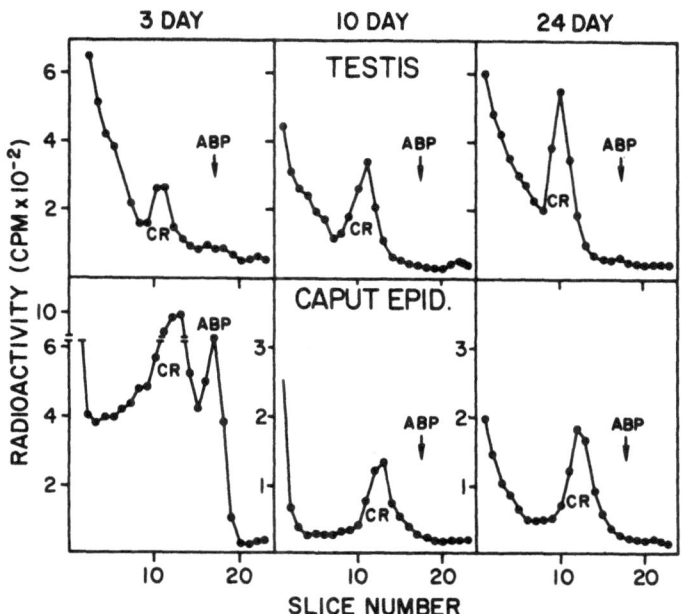

Figure 8. Cytoplasmic receptors (CR) in testis and epididymis different from testicular androgen binding protein (ABP). Sprague-Dawley rats were hypophysectomized at 35 days of age. At different intervals after hypophysectomy (3, 10 and 24 days), animals in groups of 10 or 20 were eviscerated and functionally hepatectomized (24). Five ml of 5% glucose in water and 200 μg cortisol were given subcutaneously 1 hr before the operation. ^{3}H-testosterone (91 Ci/mMole, 50 μCi) was then injected into the femoral vein, and the animals were killed after 3 hours. Testis and epididymis 105,000 x g supernatants (100 μl) were layered over 3 1/2% acrylamide gels (5 x 60 mm) containing 0.5% agarose (29). Electrophoresis was run for 2 hrs at 0° C and 1.5 mAmp/ tube. After electrophoresis the gels were sliced and counted as described in the legend to Figure 1.

(R_f =0.71), but very similar to the cytoplasmic receptors (CR) of the epdidymis and ventral prostate, which were run simultaneously for comparison. When the seminiferous tubules were separated from interstitial tissue, CR was present in the seminiferous tubule fraction. No binding of androgen was detected in supernatants of the interstitial tissue. Radioactivity bound to CR was eluted from the gel, and the isolated metabolites were identified by thin layer chromatography and crystallization to constant specific activity. Only testosterone (50%) and DHT (50%) were bound to testicular CR, even though these androgens were

relatively minor fractions of the total labeled metabolites. Most of
the radioactivity in testis supernatant chromatographed with 5α -
androstane-3 α, 17ß-diol and more polar metabolites. In the
same animals the radioactivity bound to the epididymal and prostate receptors was more than 90% ^{3}H-DHT.

Gel filtration chromatography of in vivo labeled testicular
supernatant yielded one peak of bound radioactivity in or close
to the void volume of the Sephadex G-200 column. The elution
position of the steroid-receptor complex was very similar to that
of the receptors in epididymis and prostate supernatants (28, 31),

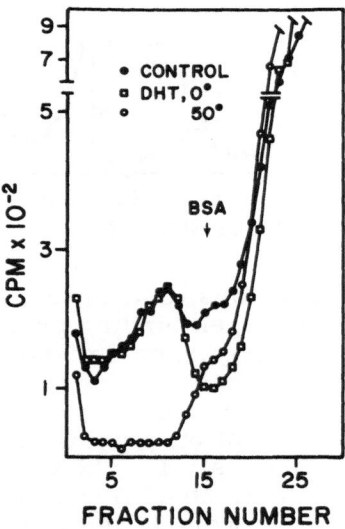

Figure 9. Sucrose density gradient centrifugation of testis
cytosol labeled with radioactive androgen in vivo. Thirty-five
day old rats, hypophysectomized for 10 days, were eviscerated,
functionally hepatectomized and injected intravenously with 50
μCi of 1, 2, 6, 7-^{3}H-testosterone. The animals were sacrificed
after 3 hours, the testis removed, and homogenized in 3 volumes
of 20 mM Tris-HCl containing 3 mM $MgCl_2$ and 0. 32 M sucrose.
The cytosol fraction was obtained by centrifugation at 105, 000
x g for 1 hour. An aliquot of the cytosol was layered directly
on 5-20% (w/v) linear sucrose gradients (20 mM Tris-HCl, 3 mM
$MgCl_2$, 10% glycerol). A second aliquot was incubated with 100
fold excess unlabeled DHT for 1 hour at 0° C, and a third aliquot
was incubated for 1 hour at 50° C prior to layering on the gradient. Tubes were centrifuged at 48, 000 rpm for 22 hours in an SW
50. 1 rotor. Gradients were fractionated from the bottom of the
tube in 10 drop fractions and counted in toluene counting solution.
Bovine serum albumin (4. 6 S$_{20,W}$) was used as a marker.

but different from the ^{3}H-DHT-ABP complex which has a Stokes radius of 47 A (6, 7, 28). The bound radioactivity was extracted and again identified by thin layer chromatography and crystallization as testosterone (55%) and DHT (45%). Centrifugation of supernatants through 5-20% linear sucrose gradients (sucrose solution prepared in 50 mM Tris-HCl, pH 7.4, containing 1 mM EDTA, 0.5 mM 2-mercaptoethanol and 10% glycerol) yielded one 6-8 S peak of bound radioactivity which was not displaced by incubation with excess unlabeled DHT at 0° but was destroyed by heating at 50° C (Fig. 9).

To establish further the receptor identity of CR in testis supernatant, the temperature stability and the dissociation of the androgen-protein complex were compared with cytoplasmic receptor in epididymis. Twenty rats, 25 days of age, were hypophysectomized and injected with ^{3}H-testosterone 3 days later. Testicular and epididymal 105,000 g supernatants were heated at either 25° or 50° C for 30 min, and binding was analyzed by PAGE (Fig. 10). Androgen-CR complexes in both testis and epididymis were stable after heating at 25° C, but were destroyed by heating at 50° C. Similar heating stability was found for the

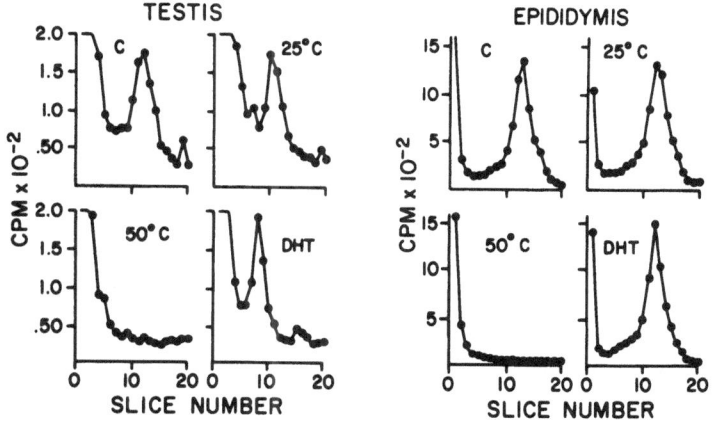

Figure 10. Effect of temperature and unlabeled dihydrotestosterone (DHT) on binding of radioactive androgens to cytoplasmic receptors in testicular and epididymal supernatants. Rats were hypophysectomized at 25 days of age. Three days later, the animals were injected with ^{3}H-testosterone, 105,000 x g supernatants prepared and binding examined by polyacrylamide electrophoresis as described in the legend to Figure 9. C: Control; 25° C: Supernatants labeled in vivo heated 30 min at 25° C; 50° C: Heated at 50° C for 30 min; Cold DHT: Excess of unlabeled DHT (10 μg) was added to 0.5 ml supernatants labeled in vivo 2 hrs before electrophoresis.

From Hansson et al. (33)

androgen-protein complex excluded from Sephadex G-200 and the
6-8 S complex obtained by sucrose gradient centrifugation.   This
heat sensitivity was identical to that of the prostate cytoplasmic
receptor (28-30), but different from ABP which was stable at
50° C (6-8, 28, 29).   Dissociation of labeled androgen-CR complexes was examined by PAGE after incubation of in vivo labeled
supernatant with a large excess (10 μg) of unlabeled DHT for 2
hours at 0° C.   Dissociation of the androgen-CR complex in testis
was negligible as was the dissociation of the androgen-receptor

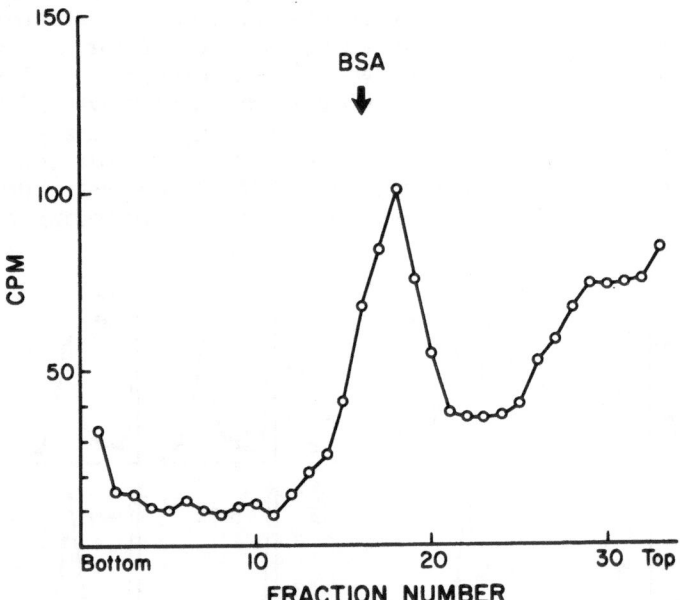

Figure 11.   Androgen receptors in purified nuclei from rat
testis.   Animals were injected with ^{3}H-testosterone in vivo
(see legend, Figure 9) and testicular nuclei were purified from
600 x g pellet of homogenized seminiferous tubules.   The 600 x g
pellet was carefully rehomogenized in 20 ml 2.0 M sucrose in
50 mM Tris-HCl containing 3 mM $MgCl_2$.   After centrifugation at
25, 000 x g for 30 min, the pellet was washed twice in 5 volumes
of 0.32 M sucrose, 50 mM Tris-HCl containing 3 mM $MgCl_2$
(TSM).   Nuclei were washed once in TSM containing 0.25% Triton
X-100 and again in 5 volumes of TSM.   After centrifugation at 600
x g for 10 min, the nuclear pellet was extracted for 1 hr with 1 M
KCl in 50 mM Tris-HCl, pH 7.4 containing 1 mM EDTA.   One ml
of the KCl was analyzed on a 5-20% sucrose gradient (48, 000 rpm,
24 hrs, SW 50.1 rotor, 0-2° C) containing 10% glycerol and 1 M
KCl.   Fractions of ten drops each were collected.

complex in epididymis. This extremely tight binding of androgen by the testis CR at 0° C (t 1/2 0° = 35 hrs) is similar to the binding by androgenic receptors in prostate as well as epididymis, giving further support to a receptor function of testicular CR.

Evidence for translocation of cytoplasmic androgen receptor complexes into testis nuclei was obtained from the demonstration of androgen binding macromolecules in purified nuclei with steroid specificity identical to CR. These androgen protein complexes could be extracted with 0.4-1 M KCl following injection of ^{3}H-testosterone and had a sedimentation constant of 3-4 S (Fig. 11).

These results support the view that the germinal epithelium of rat testis is an androgen dependent target tissue. The intracellular receptors for androgen demonstrated here very likely mediate the androgenic stimulus to spermatogenesis. It is not clear which cells within the seminiferous tubules contain CR. Recent studies by Dorrington and Fritz have demonstrated that the spermatocytes show typical "target tissue" metabolism of ^{14}C-testosterone to DHT and 5 α-androstane-3α-17ß-diol (34). Furthermore, the formation of these metabolites by the rabbit testis is greatly reduced after selective destruction of the germ cells by heat (35). The persistence of CR for as long as 24 days after hypophysectomy, however, indicates that CR is present in either Sertoli cells, spermatogonia or primary spermatocytes, since these were the only cell types remaining. Further studies on the localization of androgen receptors to specific types of cells within the seminiferous tubular epithelium are necessary to determine whether androgen acts directly on proliferating germ cells or stimulates spermatogenesis indirectly via the Sertoli cells.

Conclusion

The demonstration of androgen-receptor complexes in cytoplasmic and nuclear fractions of seminiferous tubules supports the concept that spermatogenesis is an androgen dependent process. LH stimulates spermatogenesis by increasing androgen production by the Leydig cells. FSH stimulates production of ABP presumably the Sertoli cells, thereby increasing the binding and accumulation of androgen within the seminiferous tubules in close proximity to androgen dependent cells of the seminiferous tubular epithelium. Thus, ABP might serve as an essential androgen concentrating factor under control of FSH. In addition, FSH stimulation of ABP secretion into testicular fluid increases the amount of ABP (and androgen) transported to the caput epididymis by way of the efferent ducts. Testosterone, which is taken up by epididymal cells both from the

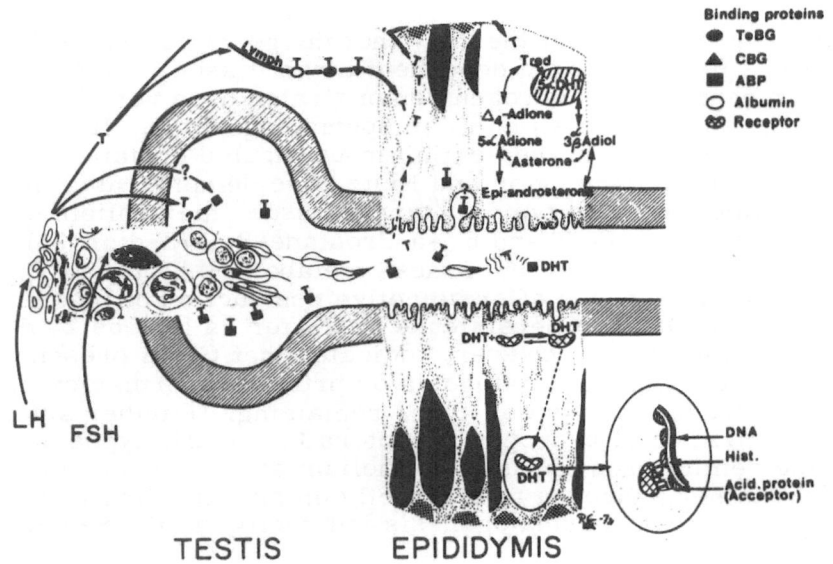

Figure 12.   Schematic drawing of androgen transport and receptor mechanisms in the testis and epididymis.

From Hansson et al. (18)

lumen and the circulating blood is "activated" by 5α-reduction to form DHT. DHT bound to cytoplasmic receptors is transported into the cell nuclei where the androgen complex binds to chromatin and initiates metabolic processes which are necessary for sperm maturation. After releasing its bound testosterone to epithelial cells ABP is free to bind testosterone or DHT which diffuses into the lumen from the blood or epithelium. Thus it could also serve to maintain a very high concentration of androgen in close proximity to epididymal epithelial cells and spermatozoa (Fig. 12).

Acknowledgements

Financial support was given by National Institutes of Health, US.A. (research grant HD04466 and training grant AM05330), The Rockefeller Foundation, World Health Organization (grant H9/181/83), Swedish Medical Research Council grant 3168), the Norwegian Research Council for Sciences and Humanities.

References

1. Steinberger, E., Steinberger, A., and Ficher, M., Rec. Prog. Horm. Res. 26: 547, 1970.

2. Ahmad, N., Haltmeyer, G. C., and Eik-Nes, K., Biol. Reprod. 8: 411, 1973.

3. Blaquier, J. A., Cameo, M. S., and Burgos, M. H. Endocrinology 90: 839, 1972.

4. Dyson, A. L. M. B., and Orgebin-Crist, M. C., Endocrinology 93: 391, 1973.

5. Ritzen, E. M., Dobbins, M. C., French, F. S., and Nayfeh, S. N., Excerpta Medica Int. Congress Series, No. 256: 79, 1972, Abstract 200.

6. Hansson, V., Steroids 20, 575, 1972.

7. Hansson, V., Djoseland, O., Reusch, E., Attramadal, A., and Torgersen, O., Steroids 21: 457, 1973.

8. Ritzen, E. M., Dobbins, M. C., Tindall, D. J., French, F. S., and Nayfeh, S. N., Steroids 21: 593, 1973.

9. French, F. S., and Ritzen, E. M., Endocrinology 93: 88, 1973.

10. French, F. S., and Ritzen, E. M., J. Reprod. Fertil. 32: 479, 1973.

11. Lowry, O. H., Rosenbrough, N. J., Farr, A. L., and Randall, R. J., J. Biol. Chem. 193: 265, 1951.

12. Ritzen, E. M., French, F. S., Weddington, S. C., Nayfeh, S. N., and Hansson, V., J. Biol. Chem., in press.

13. Tuck, R. R., Stechell, B. P., G. M. H., and Young, J. A., Pflügers Arch. ges. Physiol. 318: 225, 1970.

14. Crabo, F., Acta Vet. Scand. 6, suppl. 5, 1965.

15. Stumpf, W. E., J. Histochem. Cytochem. 18: 21, 1970.

16. Aafjes, J. H., and Vreeburg, T. M., J. Endocr. 53: 85, 1972.

17. Hansson, V., Reusch, E., Ritzen, E. M., French, F. S., Trygstad, O., and Torgersen, O., Nature New Biology 246: 56, 1973.

18. Swerdloff, R. S., Walsh, P. C., Jacobs, H. S., and Odell, W. D., Endocrinology 88: 120, 1971.

19. Roos, P., Thesis: "Human Follicle Stimulating Hormone" (Almquist and Wiksells, Uppsala, 1967).

20. Steelman, S. L., and Pohley, F. M., Endocrinology 53: 604, 1953.

21. Van Hell, H., Matthysen, R., and Overbeek, G. A., Acta Endocrinol. (Kbh.) 47: 409, 1964.

22. Hansson, V., Ritzen, E. M., and French, F. S., Proceedings of the IX Acta Endocrinologica Congress, Oslo, June 1973, in press.

23. Petrusz, P., Robyn, C., and Diczfalusy, E., Acta Endocr. (Kbh.) 63: 454, 1970.

24. Tindall, D. J., French, F. S., and Nayfeh, S. N., Biochem. Biophys. Res. Comm. 49: 1391, 1972.

25. Djoseland, O., Hansson, V., and Haugen, H., Steroids 21: 773, 1973.

26. Sar, M., Liao, S., Stumpf, W. E., Endocrinology 86: 1008 (1970).

27. Tindall, D. J., Hansson, V., Sar, M., Stumpf, W. E., French, F. S., and Nayfeh, S. N., Endocrinology, in press.

28. Hansson, V., Djoseland, O., Reusch, E., Attramadal, A., and Torgersen, O., Steroids 22: 19, 1973.

29. Tindall, D. J., Hansson, V., McLean, W. S., Nayfeh, S. N., and French, F. S., J. Biol. Chem., in press.

30. Blaquier, J. A., and Calandra, R. S., Endocrinology 93: 51, 1973.

31. Fang, S., and Liao, S., J. Biol. Chem. 246: 16, 1971.

32. Rennie, P., and Bruchovsky, N., J. Biol. Chem. 248: 328, 1973.

33. Hansson, V., McLean, W. S., Smith, A. A., Tindall, D. J., Nayfeh, S. N., French, F. S., and Ritzen, E. M., IRCS Medical Science (73-11) 3-10-34, 1973.

34. Dorrington, J. H., and Fritz, I. B., Biochem. Biophys. Res. Comm. 54: 1425, 1973.

35. Ewing, L., and Brown, B., Biology of Reproduction 9: 92, 1973.

ADDENDUM

Purification of Rabbit ABP

ABP was purified from caput epididymides of 100 adult rabbits using the following steps in series: homogenization in 50 mM Tris-HCl pH 7.4 containing 1 mM EDTA, ultracentrifugation 105,000 x g for 1 hr, precipitation of supernatant proteins with 40% (NH_4) SO_4 at 0° C, Sephadex G-200 chromatography of the resuspended precipitate, ion exchange chromatography on Whatman DE-52 cellulose, Sephadex G-25 chromatography to remove salt, preparative polyacrylamide gel electrophoresis in 6 1/2% gel.

As illustrated in Table 1, this procedure gave a recovery of ABP binding activity of about 3.5%, whereas the recovery of total protein was estimated to be about 0.05%. The increase in specific binding activity from the resuspended $(NH_4)_2SO_4$ precipitate to the final product was approximately 300-fold.

Table 1
Purification of Rabbit ABP

	Protein mg/ml	Protein Total mg.	ABP p moles/mg protein	p moles ABP total	% Protein	%ABP
1. Cytosol	8.8	660	4.0	2647.	100	100
2. $(NH_4)_2SO_4$ sup.	6.9	552	1.0	580	84	22
3. $(NH_4)_2SO_4$ sed.	28	266	1.4	385	40	15
4. Pooled Sephadex G-200 (Fractions 42-56)	1.81	48.9	8.0	390	7.4	15
5. Whatmann DE-52	-	-	-	-	-	-
6. Sephadex G-25 pooled peak	.31	3.9	52.4	203	.5	7.6
7. Fractophoresis in 6 1/2% gel	.08	.340	270	91.5	.05	3.5

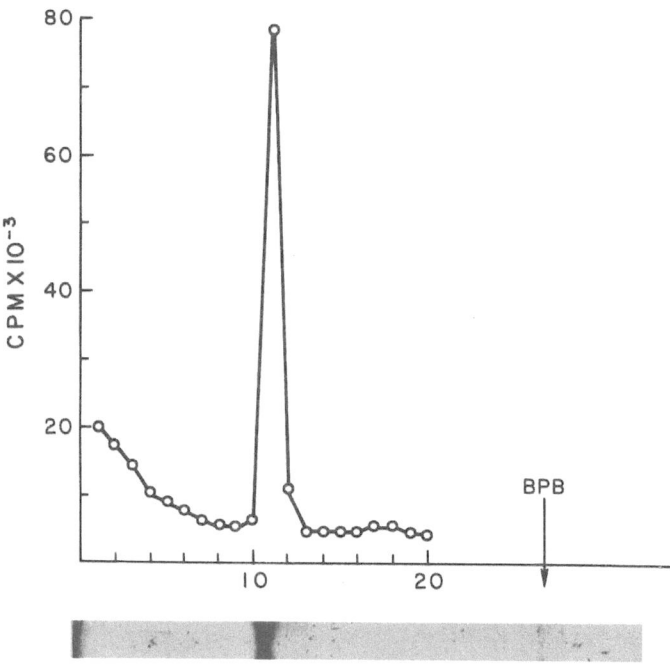

SLICE NUMBER

Figure 1. Polyacrylamide gel electrophoresis of 16 μg purified
ABP in 6 1/2% gels (5 x 70 mm) containing 2 nM ^{3}H-DHT.
Sample was equilibrated with 10 nM   H-DHT prior to layering
on the gel. Electrophoresis was run at 0° C for 2 1/2 hours,
100-150 V and 1.5 mAmp/tube. After electrophoresis, one
gel was sliced into 2.3 mm segments and the radioactivity
measured in each segment. One parallel gel was stained in
0.05% Coomassie Blue in 12.5% TCA. Arrow shows the position of Bromphenol Blue.

   Purified ABP migrated as a single band by gel electrophoresis
(Fig. 1) and preliminary studies of its physicochemical properties
(sedimentation rate, molecular radius, steroid binding) showed
that it was identical to the ABP in crude 105,000 g supernatants.
In the present experiment, we obtained about 300 μg of a highly
purified ABP, with a binding of about 300 pmoles/mg of total
protein. The yield of pure ABP from this type of procedure
should make it possible to raise specific ABP antibody and to
develop a radioimmunoassay for ABP.

FSH STIMULATION OF TESTICULAR ANDROGEN BINDING PROTEIN (ABP)
Androgen "priming" increases the response to FSH

Vidar Hansson

Institute for Pathology, Rikshospitalet, Oslo, Norway

Frank S. French, Samuel C. Weddington, and Shihadeh N. Nayfeh

Depts. of Pediatrics, Biochemistry and The Laboratories for
Reproductive Biology, School of Medicine, University of North
Carolina at Chapel Hill 27514, U.S.A.

E. Martin Ritzen

Pediatric Endocrinology Unit, Clinical Research Lab.
Karolinska sjukhuset, Stockholm, Sweden

Testicular androgen binding protein (ABP) is produced by the testis (1-3), presumably by the Sertoli cells, secreted into the testicular fluid and carried to the epididymis by way of the efferent ducts. ABP is completely dependent on FSH stimulation; it disappears rapidly after hypophysectomy and is dramatically stimulated by FSH (4), but not by LH or androgen alone. In the hypophysectomized rat, the accumulation of ABP in response to FSH is greatly enhanced by treatment with androgen.

As illustrated in Figure 1, FSH treatment caused a dose dependent increase in ABP in caput epididymidis of immature rats hypophysectomized two days prior to the injection of FSH. There was nearly a linear increase in ABP binding activity (plotted as log dose response) up to about 250 ug of FSH (NIH-P$_1$) daily, whereas further increase in FSH did not cause a proportionate increase in ABP. The sensitivity of the testis to FSH, as measured by the ABP response, decreased with time after hypophysectomy. When rats were hypophysectomized at 28 days of age and injected with 250 ug of FSH (NIH-P$_1$) for 3 days from day 7, 20 or 33 after hypophysectomy, the amounts of ABP in caput were much lower. There was a much larger ABP response to the same dose of FSH, if the hypophysectomized rats were treated with

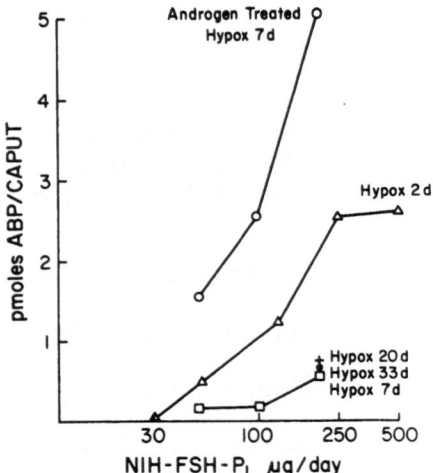

Figure 1. Effect of hypophysectomy and testosterone treatment on the FSH induced increase in ABP binding activity in caput epididymidis. Rats in groups of 4 were hypophysectomized at 28 days of age, and FSH treatment was started 2, 7, 20 or 23 days later. One of the groups was treated with 2 mg testosterone propionate i.m. daily from the day after hypophysectomy to the day of sacrifice. NIH-FSH-P_1 was administered to all groups twice daily the three last days before sacrifice. ABP was measured by steady state polyacrylamide gel electrophoresis (4,7).

testosterone propionate prior to and during FSH treatment (Fig. 1). This larger accumulation of ABP in caput must have resulted from an increased output of ABP in the testicular efferent duct fluid since augmentation of the ABP response to FSH could also be measured in testis supernatants (Fig. 2).

The mechanism by which TP increases the sensitivity of the testis for FSH is not known, however several possibilities might be considered. TP might prevent degradation of ABP by inactivating proteolytic enzymes or specific inhibitors for ABP in the testis and possibly within the epididymis as well. On the other hand TP could possibly enhance the action of FSH by increasing blood flow through peritubular capillaries thereby allowing more FSH to reach its target sites in the seminiferous tubules. TP might also diminish the degradation of FSH in liver, kidney, or within the testis itself. A further possibility is that TP stimulates the formation of FSH receptors on Sertoli cell membranes. Recently, the estradiol-17ß has been shown to increase dramatically the membrane binding capacity of prolactin and growth hormone in the liver (5). Demonstration of a direct effect of TP on

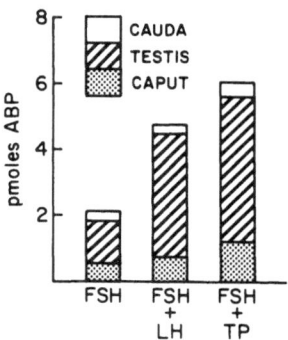

Figure 2. Effect of testosterone on ABP response to FSH. Augmentation of ABP response to FSH by LH and testosterone. Sprague-Dawley rats were hypophysectomized at 28 days of age. NIH-FSH-P_1 (0.76 U/mg) 150 μg/day was given to rats in groups of 4, alone or in combination with NIH-LH-S_{17} (1.01 U/mg) 33 μg/d or testosterone propionate 2.0 mg/day. Injections were started 2 days after hypophysectomy and given twice daily for 3 days. ABP was measured in 105,000 g supernatants of testis, caput and cauda by steady state polyacrylamide gel electrophoresis (7).

the Sertoli cells would indicate that the ABP producing cells (Sertoli cells) are androgen responsive. Most androgen target cells so far examined are equipped with an intracellular receptor system that is believed to mediate the androgenic stimulus to these cells. We have recently demonstrated such intracellular receptors for testosterone and DHT in cells within the seminiferous tubules (6). However, further studies are necessary in order to determine if these receptors are localized in germ cells or in Sertoli cells.

REFERENCES

1. French, F. S., and Ritzen, E. M., J. Reprod. Fert. 32: 479, 1973.

2. French, F. S., and Ritzen, E. M., Endocrinology 93: 88, 1973.

3. Hansson, V., Djoseland, O., Reusch, E., Attramadal, A., and Torgersen, O., Steroids 21: 457, 1973.

4. Hansson, V., Reusch, E., Trygstad, O., Torgersen, O., French, F. S., and Ritzen, E. M, Nature New Biol. <u>246</u>: 56, 1973.

5. Tsuhima, T., Posner, B. and Friesen, H., Presented at the Human Growth Hormone Symposium, Baltimore, Oct. 9-12, 1973.

6. Hansson, V., McLean, W. S., Smith, A. A., Tindall, D. J., Nayfeh, S. N., French, F. S., and Ritzen, E. M., IRCS Medical Science (73-11) 3-10-74.

7. Ritzen, E. M., French, F. S., Weddington, S. C., Nayfeh, S. N., and Hansson, V., This volume, p. 279 . (see description of method).

PROPERTIES OF RAT TESTICULAR ANDROGEN

BINDING PROTEINS

Barbara M. Sanborn, John S. H. Elkington and Emil Steinberger

Program in Reproductive Biology and Endocrinology
University of Texas Medical School at Houston
Houston, Texas

Introduction

The rat testis is highly dependent on gonadotropins for its function (1). Specifically, LH has been shown to be responsible for the stimulus to produce testosterone (2, 3, 4), presumably in Leydig cells, while FSH has been implicated in the maintenance of the germinal epithelium and in the later stages of spermio-genesis (1). In addition, testosterone (or a metabolite thereof) appears to have a direct role in spermatogenesis (1).

The biochemical effects of FSH and testosterone have not as yet been directly linked with their physiological influences on testicular function. The testis has been shown to possess specific FSH receptors (5). By analogy to the situation in most steroid target tissues, it seemed probable that androgen action might in-volve testicular androgen receptor proteins (6, 7).

We have found an androgen binding protein in rat testis and have studied a number of its physical and kinetic characteristics. In addition we have looked at the effect of hypophysectomy and FSH supplementation on the testicular level of this binding activity.

While this work was being carried out, a series of papers have appeared reporting the presence of such a binding protein in testis and epididymis (8, 9), its presence in tubular fluid (10, 11) and possible hormonal influences on its concentration (12).

Materials and Methods

Preparation of Cytosol

Animals (Sprague-Dawley or Long-Evans strain rats, >60 d of age) were killed by cervical dislocation or ether anesthesia. The testes were rapidly removed and perfused with 0.01 M Tris Cl pH 7.4 via the testicular artery.

Testes and epididymides were minced and homogenized in 2.5 and 3.0 volumes respectively of 0.01 M Tris Cl pH 7.4 at 0°. High speed cytosols were prepared by centrifugation at 10,000 x g (15 min) and then at 142,000 xg (90 min). After the addition of 10% glycerol, the cytosols were rapidly frozen in small aliquots and stored in liquid nitrogen or in a -80° freezer.

Prior to assay the cytosols were agitated in the presence of carbon (Norite A, Fisher 1 mg carbon/mg protein, 16 hr, 40°). The carbon was removed by centrifugation (10 min, 10,000 xg and 30 min, 142,000 xg) and the cytosols filtered through methanol washed glass wool prior to use.

Binding Data

Aliquots (0.150 ml) of cytosol were incubated in a total volume of 0.275 ml with 0.8-10 nM ^{3}H-testosterone (1$^\alpha$, 2$^\alpha$- ^{3}H-testosterone, 50 Ci/mmole, New England Nuclear) in 0.01 Tris Cl, 30% glycerol, pH 7.4 buffer for 16 hr at 0°. The contribution of low affinity binding components was assessed separately by including 400 ng unlabeled testosterone in the incubation medium. Unbound hormone was removed by addition of 0.7 ml of a carbon/dextran suspension (0.33%/0.033%) in 0.01 M Tris Cl buffer to 4 tubes at a time, shaking for 15 sec, and spinning for 2 min at 2600 rpm at 2°. All data represents high affinity binding unless otherwise indicated.

Samples were counted in Rpi-toluene/Triton-X-100:2/1 at 35% efficiency (Research Products International). Scatchard plots were analyzed by the method of least squares. Protein was determined as described by Layne (13).

Results and Discussion

Characteristics of Androgen Binding

Separation of Bound from Free Hormone

Using dextran-coated carbon to separate bound from free hormone, it was found that the proportion of low affinity binding increased with incubation time in the presence of carbon due to the rapid dissociation of the high affinity binding component. For example, low affinity binding comprised 33% of the total binding activity after 2 min exposure to dextran-coated charcoal and 81% of the activity after 30 min exposure. The dissociation reaction for the high affinity component was found to have a $t_{1/2}$ of 3 min at 0° in the presence of 30% glycerol (Figure 1). Therefore, to obtain a measure of the high affinity component, the carbon suspension was added rapidly and the tubes shaken (>15 sec) prior to centrifugation. This procedure, while admittedly approximate,

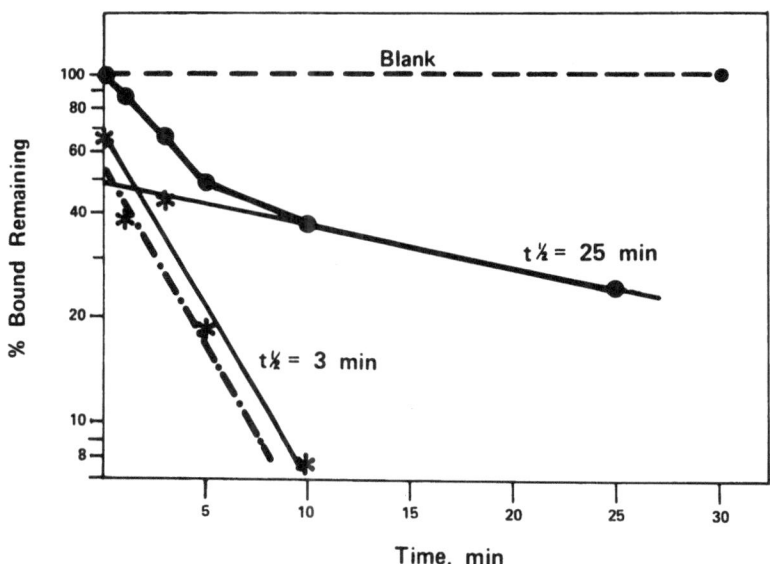

Figure 1. The dissociation of ^{3}H-testosterone from the androgen binding protein complex. Tubes containing 2.3 nM ^{3}H-testosterone (with or without 10 ng unlabeled testosterone) and 0.15 ml cytosol were incubated (16 hr, 0° C in 0.01 M Tris HCl, 30% glycerol, 1 mM EDTA, 1 mM ß-mercaptoethanol, pH 7.4) in a final volume of 0.275 ml. The dissociation reaction was initiated by the addition of 10 ng of unlabeled testosterone to all tubes. Free hormone was removed as described in the methods. The "Blank" line (--- no unlabeled hormone added), shows the stability of the complex over the time course. The dissociation of total bound counts (●) was resolved into slow ($t_{1/2}$ = 25 min and fast (·-·) components (23). The dissociation of high affinity binding (✳) showed the same $t_{1/2}$ as the fast component.

was quite reproducible with coefficients of variation of 0.35 - 2.5% between triplicates. Theoretically, it should measure more than 90% of the high affinity binding.

Influence of Endogenous Hormone on K_a and n:

Since the dissociation rate constant for the high affinity complex is so rapid, endogenous hormone should exchange with labeled hormone during the incubation period employed (12-18 hr, 0°). Under these conditions, the binding expression as arranged by Scatchard (14) becomes:

$$\frac{\bar{v}}{[H*]} = nK_a \left[\frac{1}{1 + K_a [H]} \right] - \bar{v} K_a \left[\frac{1}{1 + K_a [H]} \right] \qquad (1)$$

where $\bar{v}$ is expressed in units of mmoles labeled hormone bound per mg protein, $[H^*]$ is the concentration of free labeled hormone, K_a is the association constant, $[H]$ is the concentration of free endogenous hormone and n is the number of binding sites per mg protein. $[H]$ is essentially constant when the ratio of bound to free endogenous hormone is sufficiently small so that addition of increments of H^* does not displace enough bound H to significantly change the concentration of free H. Under these conditions, the slope of the Scatchard plot, or the apparent K_a, becomes

$$\frac{K_a}{1 + K_a [H]}$$

but the x-intercept or n is unchanged (15, 16).

To show that this was indeed the case experimentally, testicular cytosol was preincubated with unlabeled testosterone and then incubated further with ^3H-testosterone. As can be seen in Figure 2, the x-intercept remained unchanged in the presence of unlabeled hormone but the slope of the Scatchard plot decreased. The change in slope closely approximated the predicted value when the concentration of endogenous testosterone in the original extract was taken into account. Hence, the n measured in this system is the total number of binding sites as contrasted with available sites.

An important implication of this finding is that theoretically one should be able to measure the total number of binding sites in the cytosol from adult, intact rats despite the presence of testosterone in the cytosol of these animals. However, the high concentration of testosterone in the testicular cytosols from

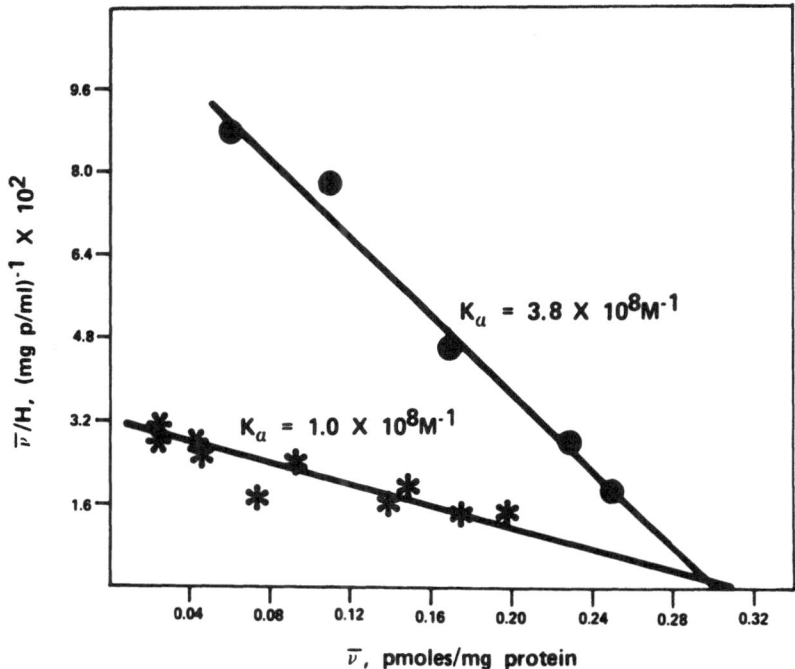

Figure 2. The effect of endogenous testosterone on the Scatchard plot. Cytosol (0.15 ml) was preincubated with (*) or without (●) 4.5 nM unlabeled testosterone (2 hr, 0°) and then incubated further with ^{3}H-testosterone (16 hr, 0°) prior to assay. A $\bar{v}$/H value of 0.09 corresponds to a bound/free ratio of 0.34.

normal rats (25 - 40 nM, (17)) decreased the slope so markedly that measurements were grossly inaccurate. Carbon extraction of the high speed cytosol consistently reduced the endogenous testosterone to 2-4 nM, a level where use of equation 1 was practical.

The use of dextran-coated carbon to separate bound from free hormone can be justified, although it is not an equilibrium method, in studies where the large amount of cytosol necessary for Sephadex gel equilibration is not available. In situations where a small concentration of binding protein is expected (see below) the Scatchard plot is preferable to analysis of peak area by polyacrylamide gel electrophoresis performed under saturating conditions (see below).

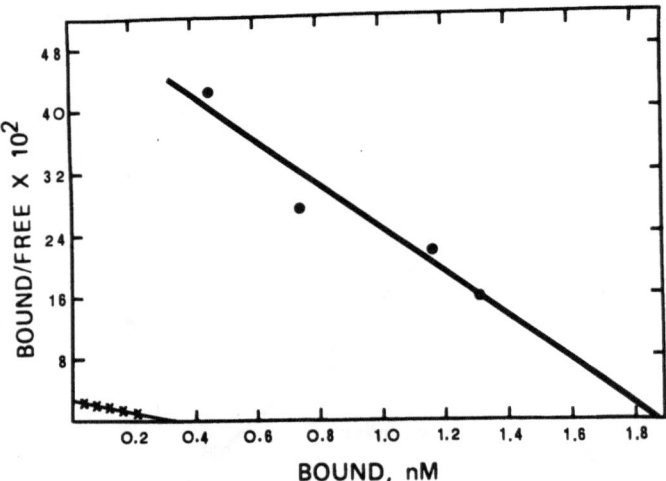

Figure 3. The binding affinity of a testicular cytosol preparation using two different exposure times to a carbon-dextran suspension for the separation of bound from free hormones. Carbon-
extracted cytosol from adult rats was incubated with ^{3}H-testos-
terone as described in Methods. The incubation mixtures were
exposed to the standard carbon-dextran suspension for 15 sec (●)
or 25 min (X) at 0° and centrifuged for 2 or 5 min at 2600 rpm
respectively. K_a for binding after 15 sec exposure was 2.9 x
$10^8 M^{-1}$ and after 25 min exposure was 0.80 x $10^8 M^{-1}$.

Binding Parameters and Specificity

     Multiple determinations on a single preparation produced K
of 4.3 + 0.45 x 10^8 M^{-1} and n of 0.19 + 0.014 pmoles/mg protein
for testosterone. K_a for 5 separate preparations from adult rats
gave a K_a of 5.5 + 0.83 x 10^8 M^{-1} and n of 0.32 + 0.019 pmoles/
mg protein. Figure 3 shows Scatchard plots of data for both the
fast-dissociating (15 sec carbon-dextran treatment) and slow-
dissociating (25 min carbon-dextran treatment) high affinity binding. The component remaining after extended carbon-dextran
incubation comprises about 16% of the binding activity or 2-3
pmoles/testis. Its binding affinity is of the same order of magnitude as the fast-dissociating activity.

     Binding activity was stable for several weeks at -80° or -190°
but gradually declined upon longer storage. It was also stable to
heating for 30 min at 0°, 37°, 45° and 50°.

Table I

Binding Parameters for Testosterone (T) and Dihydrotestosterone (DHT)

	$K_{assoc,} 10^8 M^{-1}$		n, pmoles/mg protein	
Cytosol	DHT	T	DHT	T
A (6 d hypox)	2.2	2.7	0.066	0.13
B (93 d)[a]	4.4	2.6	0.80	0.68
C (>100 d)[a]	2.1	3.8	0.67	0.31
(>100 d)[a,b]	1.3	4.3	0.82	0.28
D (100-190 d)[c]	1.5 $\pm$ 0.58*	4.2 $\pm$ 0.79	0.54 $\pm$ 0.083*	0.17 $\pm$ 0.015

[a]Carbon-extracted, all K_a are uncorrected for endogenous hormone (1-5nM).

[b]Binding data obtained on preparation C using a fixed amount of labeled hormone and increasing amounts of unlabeled hormone.

[c]Carbon-extracted, 5 groups with 3-4 rats/group, all of the same age on day of sacrifice. * <0.05 for the comparison of DHT and T by a paired "t" test.

The binding parameters of testosterone and dihydrotestosterone determined on several different preparations are shown in Table I. The endogenous testosterone concentrations in all cases were 1-3 nM. Binding data for one specific preparation (Preparation C) were constructed using increasing unlabeled hormone and, alternatively, a fixed amount of label and increasing unlabeled hormone. Results obtained by the two methods were comparable. It is apparent from Table I that by the method of analysis employed here, dihydrotestosterone binding in general exhibits a greater number of binding sites and a lower affinity for those sites than testosterone binding in the same cytosol. A statistical analysis of the data obtained from five such cytosols shows these differences to be significant ($p > 0.05$).

Regardless of the details of their relative binding affinities, these two steroids had a much greater ability to compete with labeled testosterone for binding than a variety of other steroids (Table II). The strongest competitors, androstanediol and estradiol, were only 10% as effective on a molar basis.

Table II

Relative Affinity Constants (RAC) of Steroids for Testosterone Binding Sites

Steroids (Steraloids, Schering Corp.) were dissolved in ethanol, added to the incubation tubes, and the solvent was evaporated. The steroids were redissoved in 2.5 µl ethanol followed by 0.10 ml of 0.01 M Tris Cl, 30% glycerol buffer pH 7.4, 0.31 pmole ^{3}H-testosterone, and 0.15 ml cytosol. Tubes were incubated (16 hr, 0°) and processed as described in Methods. At least 4 steroid concentrations were used for each determination. Free/bound hormone at 50% competition was 3.39. The relative affinity constant (RAC) was calculated as described by Korenman (25).

Steroids	RAC
Testosterone	1.0
Dihydrotestosterone	0.73
Androstane-3α, 17β-diol	0.13
Estradiol-17β	0.088
Progesterone	0.027
17α-Hydroxyprogesterone	0.015
Cyproterone acetate	0.0087
Cortisol	0.0030
17α-Hydroxypregnenolone	<0.0087
Δ^4-Androstenedione	<0.0087
Androsterone	<0.0087

Physical Properties

In the ultracentrifuge the androgen binding activity in both testis and epididymis sedimented at 3.5 - 4.2 S. The relative affinities of steroids for the testicular binding protein as judged by this technique were similar to those found using the carbon-dextran method.

Androgen binding activity migrated with an Rf of 0.54 relative to bromophenol blue when subjected to polyacrylamide gel electrophoresis. Since the hormone-binding protein complex dissociated rapidly, it was necessary to include steroid in the gel as well as in the incubation mixture to assure equilibrium. Under these conditions, the binding of steroid to the Rf 0.54 material was saturable (Figure 4). Under conditions where the binding sites were saturated, the binding of steroid was linear in the range of 0.41 to 3.2 mg protein added. A second peak (Rf 0.65) migrated in the position of albumin and bound an amount of dihydrotestosterone proportional to that added in this concentration range (Figure 4b).

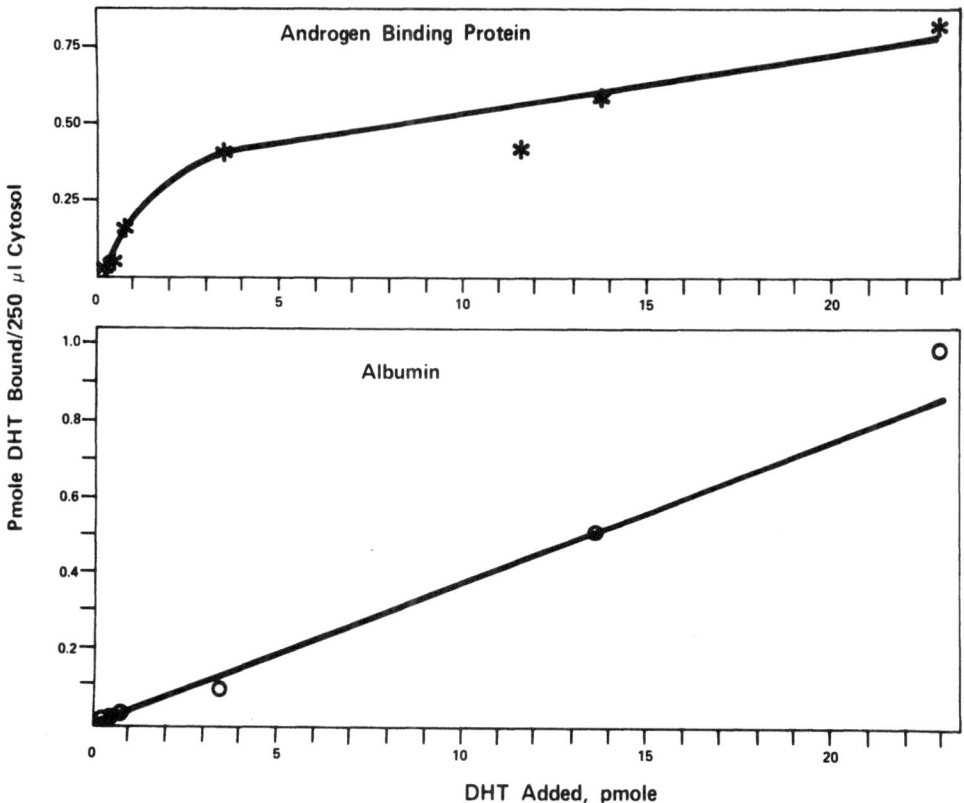

Figure 4.   The effect of increasing concentrations of ³H-dihydrotestosterone (DHT) in the incubation medium on the amount of DHT
bound to testicular androgen binding protein (Rf 0.54) and albumin
(Rf 0.65) measured by polyacrylamide gel electrophoresis (18,24).
Aliquots of cytosol (0.25 ml) were incubated with ³H-dihydrotestosterone (12 hr, 0°) prior to electrophoresis using 7.5% gels
prelabeled with 0.15 as much ³H-dihydrotestosterone (5 mAMP/
gel, 3 hr, 4°, pH 8.4).   The radioactivity in 2 mm slices of gel
was counted by liquid scintillation counting (toluene-Rpi-Triton X-
100:2/1) and the areas under regions of peak activity were estimated by weighing.

The addition of nM concentrations of unlabeled hormone to both the
incubation mixture and the gel diminished the Rf 0.54 peak area
significantly without greatly affecting the binding at Rf 0.65 (Figure 5).

Table III. Comparison of Binding Parameters by Different Methods[a]

Cytosol	Method	3H-Hormone	K_a, 10^9 M^{-1}	n	References
Testis, adult carbon extracted	SGE	DHT	0.12	3 nM	9
	SGE	DHT	-	200 pmoles/tesis	10
	PAGE	DHT	-	0.5 pmoles/mg protein (2 - 36 wks of age)	12
	C/D	T	0.5	0.2 pmoles/mg P(2 d hypox)	26
	C/D	T	0.55 ± 0.08	0.32 ± 0.02 pmoles/mg P	these authors
	C/D	T	0.42 ± 0.08	0.17 ± 0.02 pmoles/mg P[b]	"
	C/D	DHT	0.15 ± 0.06	0.54 ± 0.08 pmoles/mg P[b]	"
	C/D	T	0.44	0.27 pmoles/mg P[c]	"
	PAGE[d]	T	0.099	0.23 pmoles/mg P[c]	"
Epididymis, adult carbon extracted	SGE	DHT	0.4 (caput)	6 nM	10
				7 pmole/mg P (rabbit)	27
			0.4 (Cauda)	3.5 nM	10
	SGE	DHT	-	12 nM	9
	PAGE	DHT	0.13	2-3 pmoles/mg P	12
Epididymis, adult 2 d castrate	C/D	DHT	0.17	29 nM, 7.6 pmole/100 mg	18
	UC	DHT	0.18	22 nM	18
	SGE	DHT	0.11	22 nM	18
	Dialysis	DHT	0.18	12 pmole/100 mg	28
	C/D	DHT	0.20	3.3 pmoles/mg P, 10 pmoles/100 mg	these authors
Efferent Duct Fluid adult, 3 d ligation, carbon extracted	SGE	DHT	1.25	2.3 nM	11
		T	0.51	2.0 nM	11

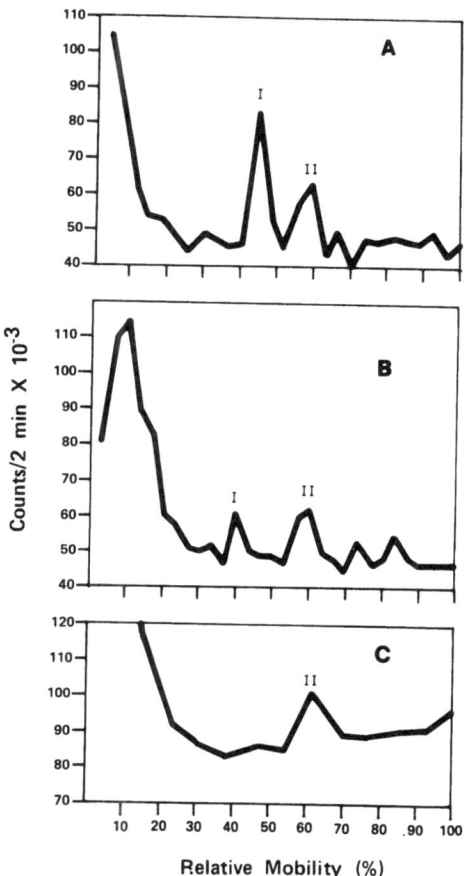

Figure 5. The effect of unlabeled dihydrotestosterone on the binding of ³H-dihydrotestosterone to androgen binding protein (I) and
albumin (II). Both incubation media and polyacrylamide gels contained 45 nM ³H-dihydrotestosterone and in addition 0 (A), 14 (B)
or 1400 (C) nM unlabeled dihydrotestosterone.

Legend to Table III.

a   DHT = Dihydrotestosterone, T = testosterone, SGE = Sephadex
    gel equilibration, PAGE = polyacrylamide gel electrophoresis,
    C/D = dextran-coated charcoal, UC = ultracentrifugation.

b   Five aged cytosols; K_a , n significantly different at $p < 0.05$.

c   Performed on same cytosol.

d   Analyzed by Scatchard plot analysis using increasing concen-
    trations of ³H-T in both incubation medium and gel.

Least squares analysis of a Scatchard plot of binding data obtained by polyacrylamide gel electrophoresis using increasing amounts of testosterone showed about the same number of binding sites as the dextran-coated charcoal method (Table III). The points were greatly scattered at low concentrations of bound hormone, however, and this may explain the differences in K_a .

The binding parameters obtained by the dextran-charcoal technique are reproducible using multiple cytosols and are quite similar to those reported by others using the same and other methods (Table III). For example, affinity constants for dihydrotestosterone in testis and epididymal cytosols have been reported by Ritzen et al. (9,18), French and Ritzen (10), and Hansson (28) to be 0.11 $- 0.4 \times 10^9$ M^{-1} as measured by Sephadex gel equilibration and dialysis, while we report values of 0.20×10^9 M^{-1} and 0.15×10^9 M^{-1} in epididymal and testicular cytosols, respectively. An apparent exception to these data is the affinity constant of 1.25×10^9 M^{-1} reported for dihydrotestosterone as measured by Sephadex gel equilibration duct fluid by French and Ritzen (11), a value which is ten fold higher than the affinity constants obtained by these authors in testis and epididymal cytosols using the same technique (9,18). As shown in Table III, the testosterone affinity constant in efferent duct fluid reported by French and Ritzen is 0.5×10^9 M^{-1} (11), a value which is comparable to what we obtained in testicular cytosol.

The testicular concentration of androgen binding sites in adult rats as measured by the charcoal technique and expressed per mg protein (0.54 + 0.08 pmoles for dihydrotestosterone) compares favorably with that reported by Hansson et al. in 2-36 week old rats as measured by polyacrylamide gel electrophoresis, 0.5 pmoles/mg protein (12). The levels in epididymis, 3.3 pmoles/mg protein or 10 pmoles/100 mg wet weight, compare well with the value of 2-3 pmoles/mg protein measured by Hansson et al. (12) and 7.6 pmole/100 mg wet weight reported by Ritzen et al. (18). The testicular content of binding protein expressed on a per testis basis as measured by Sephadex gel equilibration (10) is higher than we have reported (~50-60 pmoles/testis for dihydrotestosterone). We have found the Sephadex technique extremely difficult to employ with testis cytosol, especially in view of the fact that substantial nonspecific binding occurs. Our estimates of testicular androgen binding protein

TABLE IV. The Effect of Hypophysectomy and FSH Administration on the Levels of Androgen Binding Protein in Testis and Epididymis

Experimental conditions are described in the legend to Figure 6. The number of animals in the cytosol pools appear in parentheses. Control testicular content ranged from 13-18 pmoles/testis; K_a in all groups was within the range 2.7 - 9.0 x 10^8 M^{-1}. PAGE[a] = electrophoresis, ND = not determinable; †, based on control value at 0 d.

Treatment Group	Days of FSH Treatment	Relative Amount Per Organ		
		Testis (Scatchard)	Testis (PAGE)	Epididymis
Maintenance:	FSH treatment initiated 1 d after surgery			
Control (5)	1	1.00	1.00	1.00
Hypox (5)		0.89	0.39	1.20
Control (5)	10	1.00	1.00	1.00
Hypox (5)		0.59	0.24	0.33
FSH (5)		0.63	0.41	0.14
Control (5)	29	1.00	1.00	1.00
Hypox (6)		ND	ND	ND
FSH (5)		0.33	0.32	0.38
Control (5)	54	1.00	1.00	1.00
Hypox (7)		ND	ND	ND
FSH (7)		0.12	ND	0.03
Restoration:	FSH treatment initiated 30 d after surgery			
Control (5)	0	1.00	1.00	1.00
Hypox (6)		ND	ND	ND
Hypox (7)	11	0.06	ND	0.01†
FSH (7)		0.27	ND	0.03†
Control (5)	25	1.00	1.00	1.00
Hypox (7)		ND	ND	ND
FSH (6)		0.22	ND	0.15
Control (7)	53	1.00	1.00	1.00
Hypox (7)		0.02	ND	ND
FSH (6)		0.04	ND	ND

content are roughly equivalent using the charcoal, polyacrylamide (saturating and non-saturating hormone levels), and Sephadex gel equilibration methods.

Despite the differences detailed above, the properties (K_a for testosterone of 5×10^8 M^{-1} ; Rf 0.54, sedimentation coefficient 4S) for both the testicular and epididymal androgen binding activities are simiar enough to the numbers reported by others (8,9,18, 19,20), to make it highly probable that the same protein is being studied.

The Effect of Changes in the Hormonal Milieu on the Testicular and Epididymal Levels of Androgen Binding Protein

The control of testicular function has been shown to be exceedingly complex. The biochemical state of the tissue and the hormonal factors required for initiation, maintenance, and restoration of spermatogenesis may not be identical (1). Thus, one might anticipate that the hormonal control of biological parameters would be complex. The present study has borne this out.

Effect of Hypophysectomy

The level of high affinity androgen binding protein in the testis gradually declined following hypophysectomy. This decline was clearly visible when expressed per mg protein (Figure 6A) or per testis (Table IV), reaching undetectable levels (< 0.08 pmoles/mg protein) by 30 days. The low affinity component ($K_a \sim 10^7$ M^{-1}) declined more slowly and was essentially the only component left at 30 days. Testicular morphology, accessory organ weights, and plasma FSH levels showed changes consistent with hypophysectomy (17).

Ability of FSH Treatment to Maintain Binding Activity Following Hypophysectomy

FSH injected twice daily was able to prevent the gradual decline in high affinity androgen binding which followed hypophysectomy. However, it was not able to maintain the binding protein at the level in the testis of the intact rat, expressed either on a per testis (Table IV) or a per mg protein (Figure 6) basis. Prostate and seminal vesicle weights in this group were no different from untreated hypophysectomized controls.

The loss of testicular androgen binding protein (Rf 0.54) and its maintenance with FSH treatment was also observable by polyacrylamide gel electrophoresis in both the testis and epididymis

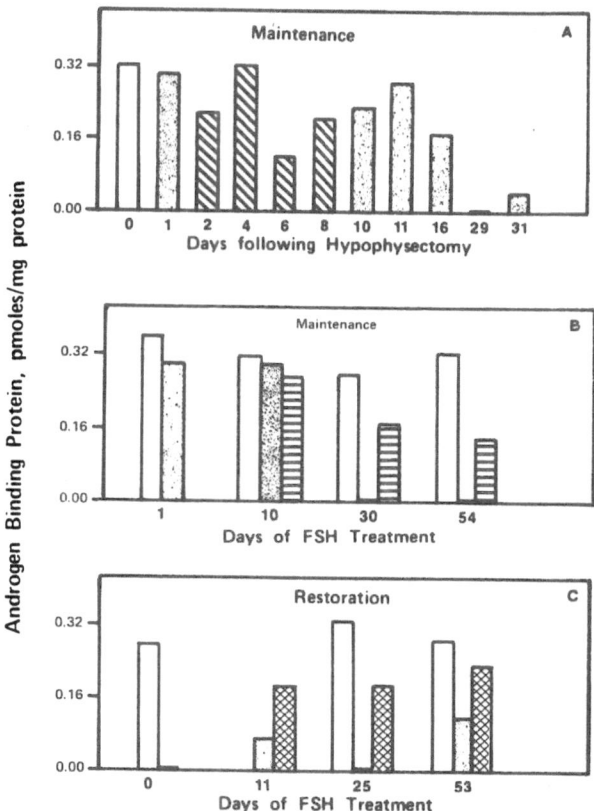

Figure 6. The effect of hypophysectomy and FSH treatment on the testicular concentration of high affinity androgen binding protein. Sprague-Dawley male rats (100 days old) were hypophysectomized (Hormone Assay Laboratories, Chicago) and injected twice daily with NIH-FSH-P1 (75 µg/rat, s.c. in 0.85% saline) beginning one day (maintenance) or thirty days (restoration) following hypophysectomy. (A) The binding protein concentration in the testis of rats 60 d ([symbol], unextracted cytosols) and 100 d ([symbol], extracted cytosols) at the time of surgery. (B) The level of binding protein in extracted cytosols from the testes of intact controls ([symbol]), untreated hypophysectomized rats ([symbol]), and rats given FSH daily from the day following hypophysectomy, ([symbol]). All rats were 100 d of age on the day of surgery. (C) The level of binding protein in testicular cytosols as in B except that FSH treatment ([symbol]) was started 30 d after hypophysectomy.

(Figure 7). Qualitative trends in the effect of hypophysectomy and FSH treatment, noted in testis using Scatchard plots or electrophoresis (Table IV).

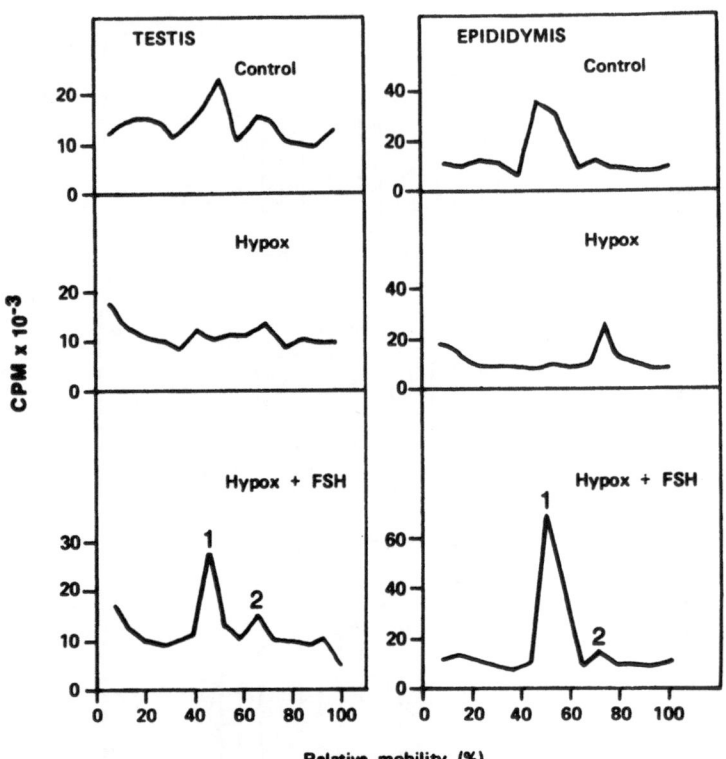

Figure 7. The effect of hypophysectomy and daily FSH treatment from day 1 on androgen binding activity in the testis and epididymides of rats 29 d after surgery as visualized by polyacrylamide gel electrophoresis. Testicular cytosols (0.25 ml) were incubated with 26.1 nM ^{3}H-dihydrotestosterone (12 hr, 4° C) and separated on polyacrylamide gels, prelabeled with ^{3}H-dihydrotesterone (3.9 nM). Peak 1 has been shown to be androgen-specific and saturable; Peak 1 migrates with albumin.

Ability of FSH Treatment to Restore Binding Activity After Post-Hypophysectomy Degeneration of the Germinal Epithelium

Thirty days after hypophysectomy, the germinal epithelium had regressed to such an extent that there were virtually no spermatids and few maturing spermatocytes. Under these conditions, the administration of FSH for 10 days resulted in an increase in high affinity binding protein (Fig. 6C, Table IV). On a per mg protein basis, the level reached almost half that in control testes, but on a per testis basis the levels were not restored.

Continuation of treatment did not further increase the binding protein content by either criterion. Qualitatively similar results were seen in the epididymis. The accessory organ weights throughout the time course of FSH treatment were close to those of untreated hypophysectomized animals indicating minimal testosterone production.

The fact that the concentration of binding protein per mg soluble protein never reached control level is unexplained but may be a reflection of a new "steady-state", the balance of synthesis and turnover, in the absence of testosterone. Preliminary results show that testosterone administration is also effective in both maintaining and restoring binding protein levels, expressed per mg protein or per testis.

Summary and Comments

In summary, the rat testicular androgen binding protein described here has properties (K_a = 5 x 10^8 M^{-1}, Rf 0.54, 4S) similar to those described by others for a protein formed in the testis and transported in tubular fluid into the epididymis (8-12, 18-20). The protein is highly specific; of the many steroids studied, only dihydrotestosterone and testosterone compete in the nM range for labeled testosterone.

An assay method has been developed for the measurement of this rapidly dissociating complex which allows measurement of the total number of binding sites in the presence of nM concentrations of endogenous testosterone. Polyacrylamide gel electrophoresis on prelabeled gels can be used as a quantitative as well as a qualitative tool, but it is a less sensitive technique under saturating conditions.

The influences of hormonal state on the testicular concentration of androgen binding protein have been shown to be quite complex. Hypophysectomy results in the gradual loss of high affinity binding material. FSH administration results in both maintenance and induction of this protein on a per mg protein basis relative to its concentration in the testes of hypophysectomized animals even though the advanced elements of the germinal epithelium are degenerating.

The function of the testicular androgen binding protein in testis and epididymis is as yet unclear. This protein differs from the more classical steroid "receptor" proteins in that, although of high affinity, it has a very rapid dissociation rate constant and is relatively stable to heat. This of course does not rule out the possibility that this protein, or at least some component of the androgen binding activity, has a testicular role. The use of carbon extraction to lower endogenous testosterone level gives reproducible results, but it may preclude study of any binding protein adsorbed or denatured by this procedure (19). The facts that testicular cytosol from 6-10 d hypophpysectomized animals show apparently no other high affinity components by Scatchard plot or electrophoresis and that the number of binding sites is essentially unchanged by carbon extraction (21) argue against this possibility, but a small proportion of such a component could be overlooked. The amount of slow dissociating androgen binding activity is exceedingly small and or equal or lower binding affinity.

Finally, the cell or cells or origin of this androgen binding protein is as yet unknown. We have found that 20 days cryptorchidism results in a doubling in the specific activity of high affinity binding activity per mg protein compared to normal testis. This finding has also been reported by others (22). We have presented evidence here that the testis is capable of producing androgen binding protein even after regression of the post meiotic elements of the germinal epithelium. These findings, together with evidence that this protein is found early in testicular development (12), support the contention that Sertoli cells may be the source.

Acknowledgments

This work was supported in part by Contract NO1-HD-3-2782, NICHD and a grant from the Ford Foundation to Emil Steinberger, M.D. The authors wish to thank NIAMD, Pituitary Hormone Distribution Program, for the NIH-FSH-P1, and acknowledge the excellent technical assistance of Ms. Hsu Kuo.

References

1. Steinberger, E., Physiol. Rev. 51, 1, 1971.

2. Greep, R. O., and Fevold, H. L., Endocrinology 21, 611, 1937.

3. Dufau, M. L., Catt, K. J., and Tsuruhara, T., Biochim. Biophys. Acta 252, 574, 1971.

4. Rommerts, F.F.G., Cooke, B. A., van der Kemp, J.W.C.M., and van der Molen, H. J., FEBS Letters 33, 114, 1973.

5. Means, A. R., and Vaitukaitis, J., Endocrinology 90, 39, 1972.

6. Mainwaring, W.I.P,., Mangan, F. R., Wilce, P. A., and Milroy, E.G.P., In O'Malley, B. W., and Means, A. R. (eds.), Receptors for Reproductive Hormones, Plenum Press, New York, 1973, pp. 197-231.

7. Williams-Ashman, H. G., and Reddi, A. H., Ann. Rev. Physiol. Rev. 33, 31, 1971.

8. Hansson, V., Djoseland, O., Reusch, E., Attramadal, A., and Torgersen, O., Steroids 21, 457, 1973.

9. Ritzen, E. M., Dobbins, M. C., Tindall, D. J., French, F. S., and Nayfeh, S. N., Steroids 21, 593, 1973.

10. French, F. S., and Ritzen, E. M., Endocrinology 93, 88, 1973.

11. French, F. S., and Ritzen, E. M., J. Reprod. Fert. 32, 479, 1973.

12. Hansson, V., Reusch, E., Trygstd, O., Torgersen, O., Ritzen, E. M., and French, F. S., Nature New Biol. 246, 56, 1973.

13. Layne, E., Methods. Enzymol. 111, 448, 1957.

14. Scatchard, G., Ann. N. Y. Acad. Sci. USA 51, 660, 1949.

15. Tanford, C., Physical Chemistry of Macromolecules, J. Wiley & Sons, Inc., New York, 1961, pp. 573-574.

16. Milgrom, E., Perrot, M., Atger, M., and Baulieu, E.E., Endocrinology 90, 1064, 1972.

17. Sanborn, B. M., Elkington, J.S.H., Tcholakian, R. K., Chowdhury, M., and Steinberger, E., unpublished, 1974.

18. Ritzen, E. M, Nayfeh, S. N., French, F. S., and Dobbins, M. C., Endocrinology 89, 143, 1971.

19. Hansson, V., Djoseland, O., Reusch, E., Attramadal, A., and Torgersen, O., Steroids 22, 19, 1973.

20. Danzo, B. J., Orgebin-Crist, M. -C., and Toft, D. O., Endocrinology 92, 310, 1973.

21. Sanborn, B. M., Elkington, J.S.H., and Steinberger, E. M., unpublished, 1973.

22. Vernon, R. G., Kopec, B., and Fritz, I. B., J. Endocr. 57, ii, 1973.

23. Frost, A. A., and Pearson, R. G., Kinetics and Mechanism, J. Wiley & Sons, New York, 1961, p. 162.

24. Davis, B. J., Ann. N. Y. Acad. Sci. USA 121, 404, 1964.

25. Korenman, S. G., Endocrinology 87, 1119, 1970.

26. Vernon, R. G., Dorrington, J. H., and Fritz, I. B., IV Int. Cong. Endocrinol. Abstr. 200, Washington, D. C., June 1972.

27. Hansson, V., Ritzen, E. M., French, F. S., Weddington, S. C., Nayfeh, S. N., Reusch, E., and Attramadal, A., Steroids 22, 185, 1973.

28. Hansson, V., Steroids 20, 575, 1972.

Effects of FSH on Levels of Androgen

Binding Protein in the Testis

Irving B. Fritz, Bozena Kopec, Kam Lam and Richard G. Vernon

Banting and Best Department of Medical Research
University of Toronto
Toronto, Canada M5G 1L6

Introduction

Preliminary observations reported at meetings held in 1972 (1, 2) indicated the existence of at least two classes of androgen binding proteins (ABP) in seminiferous tubules and in extracts from tubules isolated from testes of recently hypophysectomized rats. We observed that most of the androgen binding protein activity in testis was associated with the extracellular fractions, presumably in tubular fluid (2). We were somewhat disconcerted by the low values in germinal cells, since our initial motivation for performing these experiments was based upon hopes that we might identify those germinal cells which were potentially responsive to androgens by determining which cells contained the high affinity ABP.

Our interest was reawakened, however, when we discovered that the high affinity ABP activity was greatly diminished in testes from completely regressed hypophysectomized rats, and that treatment of these animals with FSH largely restored the ABP capacity in testis extracts (2). A detailed report of these observations is now in press (3). In the present communication, we wish to summarize the salient findings, and we shall be primarily concerned with interpretations of the basis for the decrease in the high affinity ABP (hereafter called ABP-I) in extracts of testes obtained from regressed hypophysectomized rats. The restoration by FSH treatment will be related to evidence indicating that Sertoli cells are probably the source of ABP-I. Finally, preliminary results will be presented which demonstrate a direct action of FSH in stimulating ABP-I formation by preparations of Sertoli cells maintained in culture.

II.   Summary of the Properties of ABP in Testis

A.   ABP in Seminiferous Tubules and Extracts from Seminiferous Tubules

Using methods described in detail elsewhere (3), we observed that the uptake of ^{3}H-testosterone by isolated seminiferous tubules obtained from testes of rats hypophysectomized 7-10 days previously (recently hypophysectomized rats) was proportional to testosterone concentrations ranging from 8×10^{-10}M to 4×10^{-8}M. Uptake was rapid, with maximum uptake occurring by 20 minutes, and this rate was essentially the same when tubules were incubated at either 4° or at 32° (3). Scatchard plots of the data obtained in experiments on the uptake of ^{3}H-testosterone by tubules from recently hypophysectomized rats and from totally regressed hypophysectomized rats are shown in Fig. 1. Component I (ABP-I), having a dissociation constant of 4.1×10^{-9}M, was present in tubule extracts from recently regressed rats but was

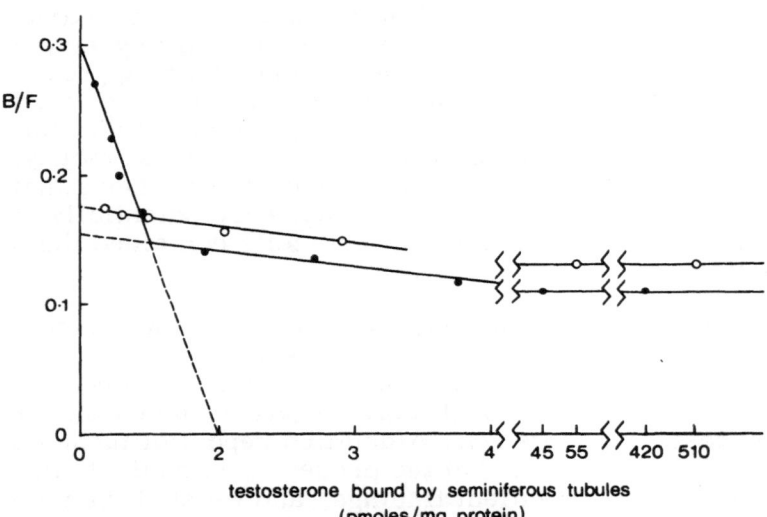

Figure 1.   Scatchard plot of ^{3}H-testosterone uptake by isolated seminiferous tubules from rats hypophysectomized either 8 days (●) or 36 days (o) before killing. Tubules were incubated for 20 minutes at 32°. The ordinate (B/F) is expressed as the ratio of pmoles bound per mg seminiferous tubule protein to pmoles testosterone per ml medium, while the abscissa is expressed as pmoles bound per mg tubule protein. For further details, see the original publication (3).

absent in tubule extracts from totally regressed animals. ABP-II, which had a lower affinity for androgen binding (K_d of 8.8 x 10^{-8}M), was present in tubules from both sets of animals.

Binding studies were also performed using 105,000 g supernatant fractions from extracts of isolated seminiferous tubules, and comparable results were obtained. A Scatchard plot of data obtained in an experiment on extracts from the tubules of rats killed 8 days after hypophysectomy is shown in Fig. 2.

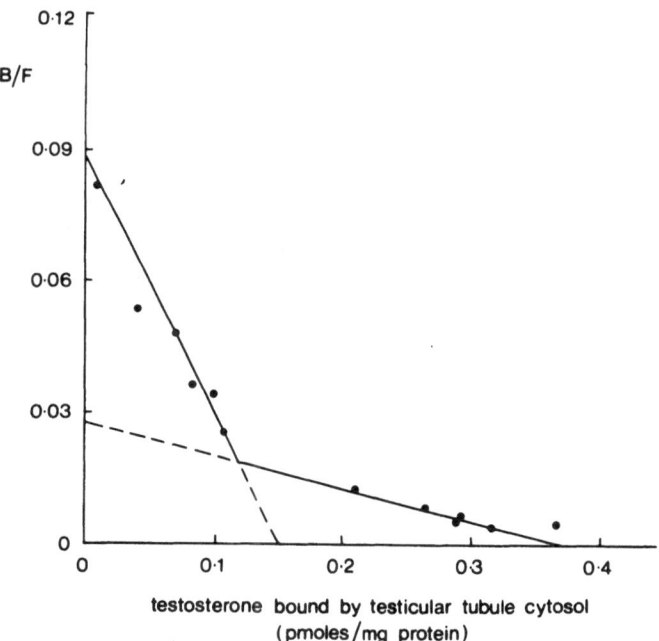

testosterone bound by testicular tubule cytosol
(pmoles/mg protein)

Figure 2. Scatchard plot of ^{3}H-testosterone uptake by 105,000 x g supernatant fractions from seminiferous tubules obtained from testes of rats hypophysectomized 8 days previously. The ordinate (B/F) is expressed as in Fig. 1.

Studies on the steroid specificity of ABP-I present in extracts from tubules isolated from testes of recently hypophysectomized rats indicated that testosterone and dihydrotestosterone were bound with equal avidity, and other steroids tested competed weakly for the androgen binding sites (column 1 of Table 1). In contrast, the binding of steroids by ABP-II present in extracts from tubules of totally regressed hypophysectomized rats was less specific. Labeled testosterone bound to ABP-II was readily

Table 1

Steroid Specificity of Androgen Binding Proteins in Extracts
from Isolated Seminiferous Tubules Prepared from Hypophysectomized Rats

Unlabeled Steroid Added	Relative Affinity of Steroid*	
	High Affinity ABP-I (10^{-9} M ^{3}H-Testosterone)	Low Affinity ABP-II (6×10^{-9} M ^{3}H-Testosterone)
Testosterone	100	100
Dihydrotestosterone	99 ± 7 (6)	109 ± 6 (5)
17β-Estradiol	37 ± 5 (6)	118 ± 10 (4)
5α-Androstane-3α,17β-diol	34 ± 6 (6)	86 ± 11 (6)
Pregnenolone	30 ± 7 (9)	57 ± 15 (8)
Estrone	28 ± 5 (9)	77 ± 10 (4)
Progesterone	20 ± 5 (9)	81 ± 10 (7)
17α-Hydroxyprogesterone	19 ± 3 (6)	36 ± 9 (8)
20α-Hydroxyprogesterone	15 ± 6 (6)	34 ± 10 (8)
Androsterone	15 ± 6 (6)	15 ± 7 (5)
Androstenedione	10 ± 7 (6)	24 ± 11 (8)

Table 1. Extracts from testes of rats hypophysectomized 7-10 days previously (ABP-I experiments), or from rats hypophysec-tomized 34-38 days previously (ABP-II experiments), were spun at 100,000 x g for 1 hr. Aliquots were incubated for 60 min at 4° C with 1 x 10^{-9}M ^{3}H-testosterone (ABP-I experiments), or with 6 x 10^{-9}M ^{3}H-testosterone (ABP-II experiments). Unlabeled steroids indicated were added (5 x 10^{-9}M for ABP-I experiments and 1 x 10^{-7} M for ABP-II experiments), and the solutions were allowed to equilibrate for an additional 60 min at 4°. The amounts of labeled steroid remaining bound to proteins were determined by the dextran charcoal adsorption technique (3). Values are ex-pressed as the mean + S.E.M., and the numbers within paren-theses denote the numbers of separate experiments performed with each steroid. In ABP-I experiments, 5 x 10^{-9} M cold testos-terone displaced 42% of 1 x 10^{-9} M ^{3}H-testosterone (designated as 100 for the relative affinity in this series of experiments). In ABP-II experiments, 1 x 10^{-7} M unlabeled testosterone reduced the amount of 6 x 10^{-9}M ^{3}H-testosterone bound by 45% (desig-nated as 100 in this series). Displacement of labeled testoster-one by other steroids listed is expressed as a percentage of these values in each series of experiments. It is assumed that pri-marily ABP-I is being examined in the ABP-I series of experi-ments because binding of 1 x 10^{-9} M ^{3}H-testosterone by ABP-II would be negligible. It is assumed that primarily ABP-II is being examined in the ABP-II series of experiments because ABP-I binding capacity diminishes greatly during regression after hypo-physectomy (Table 2).

---

displaced by 17ß-estradiol, 3α-androstanediol, estrone or by pro-gesterone (column 2 of Table 1). Adrenal cortical steroids did not compete with androgens for binding sites on either ABP-I or ABP-II.

B. ABP in Supernatant Fractions from Extracts of Whole Testes

Binding constants calculated from Scatchard plots of experi-ments on ^{3}H-testosterone uptake by 105,000 g supernatant frac-tions from extracts of total testis are summarized in Table 2. The ABP-I (K_d of approximately 10^{-9}M) binding capacity of 0.53 pmoles per mg protein in testis extracts from normal rats dimin-ished following hypophysectomy, reaching lowest values in totally regressed animals. The binding capacity per testis decreased even more pronouncedly because the testis weight was simultane-ously decreasing (Table 2).

Other studies on the general properties of ABP-I present in

Table 2

Testosterone Binding Protein Activity in Supernatant Fractions
Prepared from Whole Testes of Normal and Hypophysectomized Rats

Type of Rat	Testis wt (g/rat)	Binding Capacity		K_d (nM)	Number of Separate Experiments
		(pmoles/mg protein)	(pmoles/testis)		
Normal Adults	3.56 ± 0.14	0.53 ± 0.10	41.6 ± 1.8	1.26 ± 0.9	8
Hypophysectomized 7-10 days previously.	2.40 ± 0.16	0.31 ± 0.04	14.1 ± 2.5	1.50 ± 0.3	4
Hypophysectomized 34-38 days previously.	0.52 ± 0.02	0.08 ± 0.03	1.1 ± 0.5	.1.2 ± 0.5	8

Binding constants (K_d and binding capacity values) were calculated from Scatchard plots of the ratios of bound to free testosterone against the amounts of bound testosterone at various levels of 3H-testosterone in the media, ranging from 5 x 10-10 M to 1 x 10-7 M. Protein concentrations in the supernatant fractions were approximately 1 to 3 mg/ml. Full details are described elsewhere (3).

testis extracts indicated that binding activity was destroyed by preincubation with proteases but not with RNAase, DNAase, or phospholipase. It was partially inactivated (40%) during incubation at 32° for an hour, and almost totally inactivated (90%) by exposure to 80° for 15 minutes. In contrast, ABP-II binding activity was not impaired during incubation at 32° for an hour, and 67% activity remained after exposure to 80° for 15 minutes. ABP-I, frozen at -20° C, was stable for at least two weeks under conditions employed (3). As indicated above, preincubation of the testis extracts from hypophysectomized rats with dextran-coated charcoal did not alter the ABP activities.

III. Possible Sources of ABP-I in Testicular Extracts

In the course of our investigations on ABP-I in testis extracts, we observed that only a small fraction (about 10 to 20%) of the total binding capacity could be accounted for by that present in cells isolated from the tubules. The rest appeared to be present in the extracellular space, most probably in tubular fluid (3). Recent reports by others (4, 5) indicate that ABP in the testis appears in the rete testis fluid and can be transported to the epididymis. Since ABP-I levels decrease after hypophysectomy (Fig. 1 and Table 2), we considered the possibility that advanced germinal cells are required for the elaboration of ABP. However, this possibility has been ruled out. In cryptorchid regressed rats, spermatozoa and spermatids are absent, and the number of spermatocytes is diminished (6, 7). Yet, the binding capacity of ABP-I in extracts from cryptorchid testis is within normal levels, when expressed as pmoles per mg protein (Table 3). The amount per testis is reduced, in association with the decrease in testis weight.

Other data supporting the conclusion that germinal cells are not required to elaborate ABP in testis extracts have been obtained from analyses of extracts of testes from mice bearing the SXR or sex reversal translocation (8). In this mutant, the seminiferous tubules in the testis of the adult genotypic female animal contain Sertoli cells but no germinal cells (8). As shown in Table 3, the binding capacity for ^{3}H-testosterone per mg protein is as high in extracts from testes of SXR mice as in extracts from testes of normal mice. Again, the total amounts per testis are reduced, in association with a diminished testicular size.

IV. Effects of Hormonal Treatments to Regressed Hypophysectomized Rats on Testicular ABP-I Activity

The effects of administration of FSH and LH to regressed hypophysectomized rats on the binding activity of ABP-I in

Table 3

Testosterone Binding Protein Activity in 100,000 x g Supernatant
Fractions Prepared from Testes of Cryptorchid Rats and SXR Mice

Type of Animal	Testis Weight (g/animal)	Binding Capacity (pmoles/mg protein)	Binding Capacity (pmoles/testis)	K_d (nM)	Number of Separate Experiments
Normal Adult Rats	3.56 ± 0.14	0.53 ± 0.10	41.6 ± 1.8	1.26 ± 0.9	8
Cryptorchid Rats, 14 days Regressed	1.29 ± 0.02	0.67 ± 0.04	16.7 ± 1.2	1.0 ± 0.1	12
Normal Male Adult Mice*	0.14 ± 0.015	0.35 and 0.55	2.4 and 3.2	1.8 and 2.7	2
SXR Adult Mice**	0.026 ± 0.003	0.54 and 0.55	0.52 and 0.67	0.6 and 0.9	2

Data were obtained by the methods described in Table 2.

* In each of two experiments, testes from five mice were pooled. The teased preparations were washed twice, and homogenized in 4 volumes of buffer (3). The second wash was shown to be free of ABP activity. Testes from normal adult mice were from the Jackson Lab C3H-101-HeG strain rather than the more customary CBA strain because the former is more closely associated with the strain of animals from which the SXR translocation was derived.

** SXR mice were kindly provided by Drs. B. M. Cattanach and M. F. Lyon, of the MRC Radiobiology Unit. We have confirmed the observations of Cattanach (8) that the tubules from testes of adult SXR mice contained only Sertoli cells, but no germinal cells.

testis extracts are shown in Table 4 and Fig. 3. Treatment of
regressed hypophysectomized rats for three days with ovine FSH-
NIH-S-8 (100/μg/day) increased the binding capacity of ABP-I in
testis extracts from 0.08 to 0.59 pmoles per mg protein. Comparable in vivo administration of ovine luteinizing hormone (LH-
NIH-S-16) for a similar time period also increased ABP-I binding
capacity for testosterone, but to a lesser extent (Table 4). Treatment for longer periods with either FSH or LH increased ABP-I
levels to a nearly comparable extent (Fig. 3).

     In testis extracts prepared from hypophysectomized regressed
rats treated with 50 μg FSH for only 24 hours, the ABP-I binding
capacity was increased nearly three-fold. In contrast, LH treatment for 24 hours increased the binding capacity only slightly in
these regressed animals (Fig. 3). Administration at shorter
intervals over a 24 hour period of lesser amounts of a partially

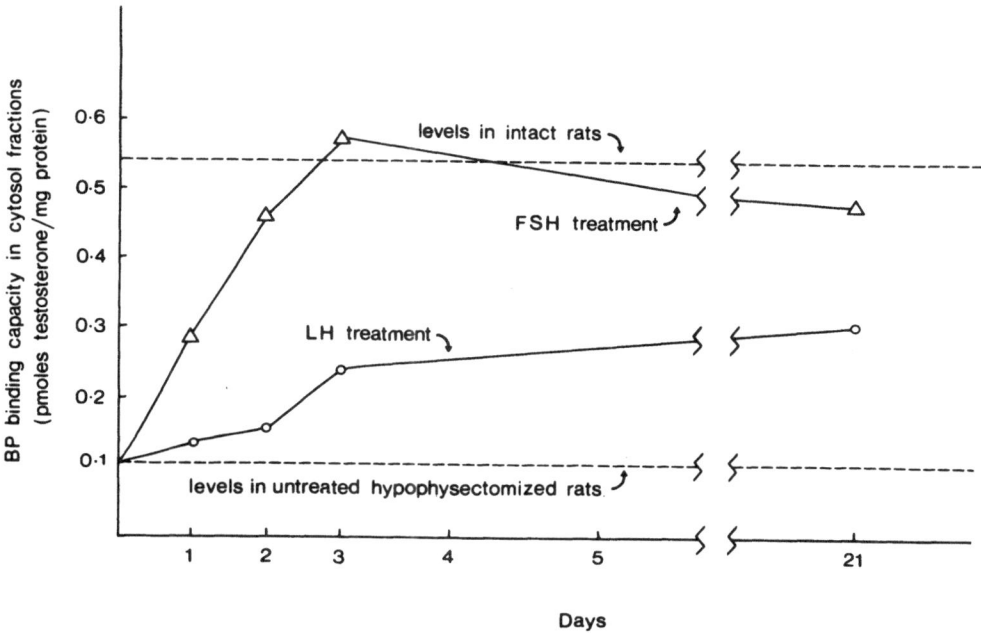

Figure 3. Effects of administration of ovine NIH-FSH and LH
to fully regressed hypophysectomized rats on ABP binding
capacity in supernatant fractions of rat testis. Hormones
50 μg/day) were injected subcutaneously for periods of time
indicated. Rats (8 per group) were killed 24 hours after the
last injection, and 105,000 x g supernatant fractions of whole
testis were prepared and assayed for ABP binding capacity
of ^{3}H-testosterone by methods described elsewhere (3).

Table 4

Effects of Administration of Gonadotropic Hormones for Three Days to Regressed
Hypophysectomized Rats on Testosterone Binding Protein
Activity in Supernatant Extracts from Testes

Treatments to 30 Day Regressed Hypophysectomized Rats.	Testis wt (g/rat)	Binding Capacity*		K_d (nM)	Number of Separate Experiments
		(pmoles/mg protein)	(pmoles/testis)		
None	0.52 ± 0.02	0.08 ± 0.03	1.1 ± 0.5	1.2 ± 0.5	8
FSH**	0.82 ± 0.20	0.59 ± 0.04	5.2 ± 1.1	1.49 ± 0.6	6
LH**	0.67 ± 0.07	0.23 ± 0.08	2.5 ± 2.2	1.68 ± 0.3	6

* For details see the legend to Table 2 and our previous publication (3).

** Ovine FSH and LH (100 µg/day for 3 days, administered subcutaneously) were obtained from
NIH (NIH FSH-S 8 and LH-S 16), courtesy of Dr. R. W. Bates.

purified ovine FSH preparation (LER-886-3, having an activity 26 times that of NIH FSH S-1) gave results similar to those obtained with the less purified NIH FSH-S-8 (Table 5). The effects obtained at these intervals demonstrate an influence of FSH on existing cell populations, and it is unlikely that the formation of new populations of germinal cells is involved. Treatment with low doses of LH during the shorter time period had no discernible effects on ABP-I binding capacity. The effects of high doses of LH at longer time intervals have not been explored further. In all cases, the K_d for testosterone and ABP-I remained unchanged at $1-2 \times 10^{-9}$ M.

Hansson et al. (13) have recently reported that administration of a highly purified FSH preparation for 10 days to rats hypophysectomized at 5 weeks of age increased concentrations of ABP in testicular and epididymal extracts. These findings confirm and extend our previously reported observations that FSH treatment to regressed hypophysectomized adult rats results in increased ABP capacity in testis extracts (2). From results just summarized in the presentation by French (14) and Sanborn (15), general agreement is evident that FSH treatment does increase ABP-I activity in extracts of testes from hypophysectomized rats, as shown above (Fig. 3, Tables 4 and 5). Apparent differences do exist with respect to the time after hypophysectomy required for disappearance of testicular ABP-I reported by French (14), but it should be noted that these workers employed 5 week old rats while we used adult hypophysectomized animals.

V. Evidence that Sertoli Cells are Involved in ABP-I Formation

ABP-I levels in extracts from cryptorchid testes and from testes of SXR mice were as high as those in extracts from normal testes, when expressed as binding capacity per mg protein (Table 3). Imai (16) also reported the presence of a high affinity ABP which remains in extracts from cryptorchid testes. Since testes from SXR adult mice do not contain germinal cells (8), it may be concluded from the high ABP-I levels observed in testes from these animals, that the source of ABP-I must be derived from testicular cells other than germinal cells.

Interstitial cells appear to be an unlikely source of testicular ABP-I. We were unable to detect evidence for ABP-I in extracts from interstitial cell preparations (3). Extracts of interstitial cells are reported to bind 17ß-estradiol (17), and the estradiol receptor has a very low affinity for androgens (18,19).

Normal ABP-I levels in testes from SXR and cryptorchid animals, the low levels in regressed hypophysectomized rats and the increase in ABP-I capacity after treatment with FSH

Table 5

Effects of Administration of Partially Purified FSH on Testosterone Binding Protein Activity in Supernatant Extracts from Testes of Regressed Hypophysectomized Rats

Treatments to Regressed Hypophysectomized Rats.	Binding Capacity*		K_d	Number of Separate Experiments
	(pmoles/mg protein)	(pmoles/testis)	(nM)	
Saline	0.081 + 0.02	1.05 + 0.5	1.08 + 0.08	8
FSH**	0.31 + 0.03	3.25 + 0.80	1.75 + 0.11	8

* For details, see the legend to Table 2 and our previous publication (3).

** Ovine FSH (1 µg of ovine LER-886-3, courtesy of Dr. L. Reichert, having an activity 26 times that of NIH FSH-SI) was injected subcutaneously four times in 100 µl of 0.9% NaCl solution, or the NaCl solution was injected alone, in approximately 8 hour intervals over a 24 hour period, and rats were killed 4 hours after the last injection.

combine to suggest that Sertoli cells are probably involved in ABP formation. The finding that approximately 80% of the total testicular ABP capacity is in extracellular compartments, presumably in tubular fluid, suggests the possibility that Sertoli cells are also implicated in ABP secretion.

It is generally accepted that Sertoli cells play a major role in forming the blood-testis barrier (20), and in generating tubular fluid (21,22). It now also appears increasingly probable that Sertoli cells are directly responsive to FSH. In vitro addition of FSH increases adenylate cyclase activity in isolated seminiferous tubule preparations obtained from regressed hypophysectomized or cryptorchid rats (7,10). In contrast, FSH addition to isolated germinal cell or interstitial cell preparations does not influence cyclic AMP production (10,23) whereas treatment of isolated Sertoli cell preparations with FSH does increase adenylate cylcase activity (24). From combined observations, the conclusion has emerged that the most FSH-responsive cells in the testis, with respect to increased adenylate cyclase activity, are the Sertoli cells.

Using the cultured Sertoli cell preparation described at these meetings by Dorrington et al. (24), we have recently investigated the possible effects of FSH on ABP-I formation. During incubation periods of 24-48 hours, FSH addition increased the appearance of ABP-I in the medium (Table 6). These data demonstrate that FSH acts directly on Sertoli cells to increase the production and secretion of ABP-I. The production of ABP-I by Sertoli cells thereby provides a specific response of potential physiological significance with which to follow FSH actions on the Sertoli cell.

What are the relations, if any, of this phenomenon to the increased cAMP production by Sertoli cells in response to FSH stimulation? Is either of these phenomena related to the effects of FSH administration in vivo on the enhancement of protein synthesis by testicular preparations (25)? Most importantly, does any of these findings give promise to providing insight into the requirement for FSH for efficient spermatogenesis to proceed (26)?

At other levels of inquiry, which germinal cells of the tubule contain intracellular androgen receptors which may be required for mediating direct androgen actions on the germinal cells? It is unlikely that ABP-I has the properties required for such receptors. Yet if ABP-I can be extracted from certain germinal cells, it remains possible that ABP-I may be indirectly involved in mediating androgen effects on these cells. Data on ABP-I levels in extracts from isolated preparations of spermatozoa, spermatids and spermatocytes are presented in Table 7. While extracts of spermatozoa and spermatids are apparently deficient

Table 6

Effects of FSH on ABP-I Activity
in Cultured Sertoli Cell Preparations

Hours Incubation at 32°	Activity of ABP-I (Percentage DHT* Bound per 200 µl)	
	Control	FSH
0 - 24	7.8%	13.0%
0 - 24	8.1%	14.8%
0 - 48	27.6%	43.4%
0 - 48	24.2%	47.8%
48 - 96	15.1%	37.2%
48 - 96	14.4%	48.8%

Sertoli cells were prepared from testes obtained from 20 or 21 day old rats by the procedures described by Dorrington et al. (24). Ovine FSH (NIH S-8) was added to the protein-free culture medium at concentrations of 10 µg/ml each day. Each flask contained Sertoli cells equivalent to approximately 2.0 mg protein in 5.0 ml of medium. The protein concentration at the end of incubation of the supernatant cell-free medium was less than 0.01 mg/ml by the Lowry procedure. Results shown represented binding at 0° of ^{3}H-dihydrotestosterone (2 to 4 x 10^{-9}M) by 200 µl aliquots, measured by the dextran coated-charcoal procedure (3). The K_d was 2·x 10^{-9}M, and the binding capacities were respectively 1.5 pmoles/ml control medium and 2.6 pmoles/ml medium from FSH-treated cells, as calculated from Scatchard plots of the data. Binding activity in the medium was destroyed by heating. The ABP-I showed the same steroid specificity as that described in Table 1. The pmoles DHT bound per unit volume at a fixed DHT concentration were equivalent when 100, 200 and 400 µl aliquots were assayed. Each figure shown is the average of duplicate determinations on media from a single flask in which cells had been incubated for either 24 or 48 hours, as indicated.

in ABP-I, the spermatocyte preparations contain measurable amounts. Among populations of germinal cells thus far examined, spermatocytes have also proved to be richest in the ability to convert testosterone to dihydrotestosterone (28). By these two criteria, spermatocytes would appear to be likely candidates as targets for androgen action.

Table 7

Dihydrotestosterone Binding by ABP-I in Cytosol Fractions
From Rat Testis Germinal Cell Preparations

Cell Type*	K_d (nM)	Binding Capacity (pmoles per mg protein)
Spermatozoa	-	Not detectable **
Spermatids	-	Not detectable **
Spermatocytes	0.49 and 0.84	0.39 and 0.44

* Spermatozoa were obtained from the cauda epididymides of normal adult rats. Spermatids were obtained from the caput epididymides of rats injected 48 hrs previously with 100 mg/kg U-20, 409 by the procedure of Ericsson (27). Spermatocytes were obtained from the pooled testes of 10 to 12 24-25 day old rats by procedures described by Dorrington and Fritz (28). Data are shown as averages obtained from separate experiments.

** No binding was observed at dihydrotestosterone levels of 1 to 3 x 10^{-9} M.

Acknowledgement

Research reported was supported by grants from the Canadian Medical Research Council and the Banting Foundation.

References

1. Vernon, R. G., Dorrington, J. H., and Fritz, I. B., IV International Congress of Endocrinology, Washington, D. C., Abstract 200, 1972.

2. Vernon, R. G., Kopec, B. and Fritz, I. B., J. Endocrinol. 57:IIp, 1973. (Proceedings of the Society for Endocrinol., D. Hull, 4-7 Sept. 1972.)

3. Vernon, R. G., Kopec, B., and Fritz, I. B., Molec. and Cellular Endocrinol., in press, 1974.

4. French, F. S. and Ritzen, E. M., Endocrinol., 93:88, 1973.

5. French, F. S., and Ritzen, E. M., J. Reprod. Fertil 32: 479, 1973.

6. Van Demark, N. L. and Free, M. J. In: The Testis, Johnson, A. D., Gomes, W. R. and Van Demark, N. L. (eds) Vol. III, Academic Press, New York, 1971, p. 233.

7. Dorrington, J. H., and Fritz, I. B., Endocrinol. 94: 395, 1974.

8. Cattanach, B. M., Pollard, C. E., and Hawkes, S. G., Cytogenetics 10: 318, 1971.

9. Murphy, H. D., Proc. Soc. Exptl. Biol. Med. 118: 1202, 1965.

10. Dorrington, J. H., Vernon, R. G. and Fritz, I. B., Biochem. Biophys. Res. Commun. 46: 1523, 1972.

11. Castro, A. E., Seiguer, A. C., and Mancini, R. E., Proc. Soc. Exptl. Biol. Med. 133: 582, 1972.

12. Castro, A. E., Alonso, A., and Mancini, R. E., J. Endocrinol. 52:129, 1972.

13. Hansson, V., Reusch, E., Trygstad, O., Torgerson, O., Ritzen, E. M., and French, F. S., Nature New Biology 246: 56, 1973.

14. French, F. S., This volume, p. 258.

15. Sanborn, B. M., This volume, p. 283.

16. Imai, K., Gunma Symposium Endocrinol. 7: 169, 1970.

17. Brinkman, A. O., Mulder, E., Lamers-Stahlhofen, G.J.M., Mechielsen, M. J., and van der Molen, H. J., FEBS Letters 26: 301, 1972.

18. van Buerden-Lamers, W.M.O., Brinkmann, A. O., Mulder, E., and van der Molen, H. J., Biochem. J., in press.

19. van der Molen, H. J., This volume, p. 333.

20. Dym, M. and Fawcett, D. W., Biol. Reprod. 3: 308, 1970.

21.   Setchell, B. P. In: The Testis. Edited by Johnson, A. D., Gomes, W. R. and Van Demark, N. L., Vol. I, Academic Press, New York, N. Y., 1970, p. 101.

22.   Setchell, B. P., and Waites, G. M. H., J. Reprod. Fertil. Suppl. 13:15, 1971.

23.   Dorrington, J. H., and Fritz, I. B. In: Chemistry, Biology and Immunology of Gonadotropins. Edited by Moudgal, N. R., Academic Press, New York, N. Y., in press.

24.   Dorrington, J. H., Roller, N., and Fritz, I. B., This volume, p. 231.

25.   Means, A. R., and Hall, P. F., Biochemistry 8: 4293, 1969.

26.   Steinberger, E., Physiol. Revs. 51: 1, 1971.

27.   Ericsson, R. J., Exper. Biol. Med. 137: 532, 1971.

28.   Dorrington, J. H., and Fritz, I. B., Biochem. Biophys. Res. Commun. 54: 1425, 1973.

STUDIES ON THE CORRELATION BETWEEN ANDROGEN BINDING AND ACTIVATION OF RAT EPIDIDYMAL TUBULES IN CULTURE

Jorge A. Blaquier, Monica S. Cameo and Ricardo Calandra

The Population Council, The Rockefeller University, New York

and

Laboratorio de Esteroides
Instituto de Biologia y Medicina Experimental
Buenos Aires, Argentina

Introduction

We have recently reported that rat epididymal tissues maintained in organ culture responded to androgens added to the culture media by stimulating the incorporation of radioactive amino acids into protein (1). Similarly, the incorporation of radioactive uridine into RNA was also increased. However, in contrast to the rapid effects induced by androgens when injected into animals, the response of cultured tissues to added hormone occurred after a rather prolonged time lag.

This finding prompted us to undertake the present study in which we have attempted to correlate the time course of binding of androgen to intracellular receptors with the activation of the system.

Materials and Methods

Adult Holtzman rats were used throughout. The efferent ducts on the right side were ligated and the animals caged with normal females for 2 to 3 weeks. When indicated, castration was performed by the scrotal route 24 hours prior to sacrifice.

The animals were anesthesized with ether and the right epididymides, empty of spermatozoa, were removed under sterile conditions and cultured as previously described (1) in Eagle's minimum
essential medium supplemented with 10% fetal calf serum.

Protein and RNA synthesis were followed by measuring the
amounts of incorporation of radioactive precursor, [^{14}C] amino
acid mixture and [^{14}C] uridine (New England Nuclear Corp.)
respectively, over a 2-hour incubation of the minced tissue in Earle's
balanced salt solution, supplemented with 0.1 mM methionine, at
31° C in an atmosphere of 95% air, 5% CO_2 .

The tissues were homogenized, aliquots withdrawn for protein
determination, and precipitated with trichloroacetic acid. The precipitates were collected over glass fiber filters, extensively washed
with TCA and ethanol, dried with ether and counted. Results are
expressed as cts/min incorporated into acid insoluble material/mg
of protein. The binding of testosterone to fetal calf serum was determined by equilibrium dialysis for 24 hours at 31° C, as previously
described (2).

In the receptor studies, tissues of rats castrated 24 hours before
sacrifice were cultured for 3 days. At the end of this period, 0.5 μ
Ci of [1-2-6-7 ^{3}H] testosterone (S.A.: 91 Ci/mmole, New England
Nuclear) were added to the culture medium at a final concentration
of 5 x 10^{-9} M. Labelling was allowed to take place for various
periods of time from 30' to 24 hours. At the completion of the labelling period, the tissues were transferred to beakers containing chilled MEM made 10^{-7} with respect to non-radioactive testosterone.
After washing, the tissues were blotted, weighed and homogenized
in 0.32 M sucrose prepared in Earle's balanced salt solution containing 10% glycerol and buffered with 50 mM TES, pH 7.35 at 4° C.
Cytosol fraction and purified nuclei were prepared as described in
a previous report (3,4). The binding to cytoplasmic receptors was
investigated using acrylamide gel electrophoresis (3.5% acrylamide,
0.5% agarose) as described by Tindall et al. (5). Nuclear receptors
were studied by sucrose gradient ultracentrifugation (4).

Results

I. Protein Synthesis

The rate and total amount of radioactive amino acids incorporated into acid insoluble material are higher in rat epididymal tubules
cultured in media containing androgen than in the respective control
tissue. This increase is statistically significant in tissues cultured
for 24 hours in the presence of androgen and is substantially enhanced

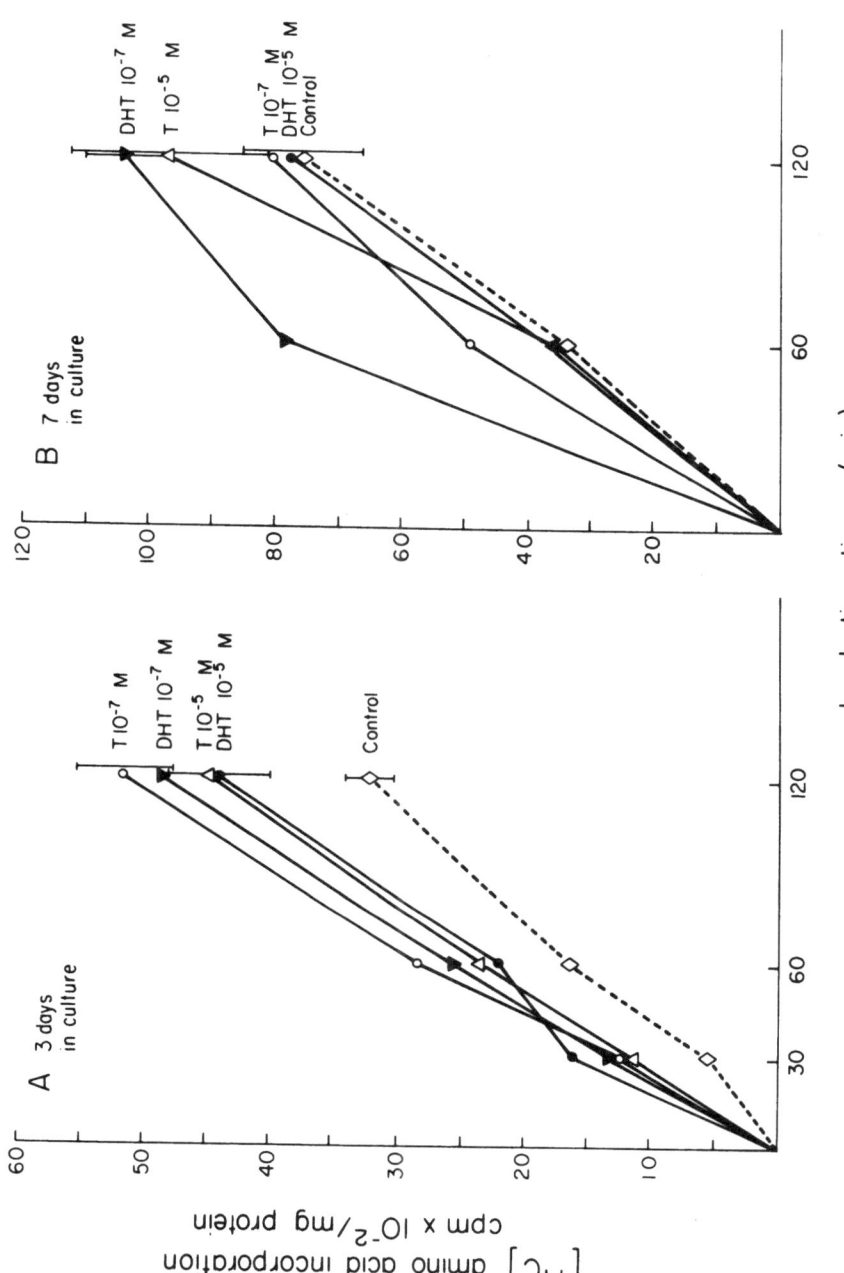

Figure 1. The effect of androgens added to the culture media at concentrations of 1 x 10-5 M or 1 x 10-7 M on [14C] amino acid incorporation into acid insoluble material by epididymal

tubules maintained in organ culture. At the end of the culture period the tissues were minced and incubated with $0.01 \, \mu Ci$ $[^{14}C]$ amino acid mixture for 0, 30, 60 and 120 min in 1.0 ml of Earle's balanced salt solution containing 0.1 mM methionine, at 31° C under an atmosphere of 95% air, 5% CO . Panel A = epididymal tubules cultured for 3 days in the presence or absence of different androgens. Panel B = epididymal tubules cultured for 7 days in the presence or absence of different androgens. T = testosterone; DHT = dihydrotestosterone.

after 3 or 7 days in culture (Figure 1). Testosterone and dihydrotestosterone at concentrations of 1×10^{-5} M and 1×10^{-7} M were used in these experiments. Subsequent evidence indicated that these steroids were also active when the concentration was reduced to 1×10^{-8} M. Under similar conditions, dihydrotestosterone-3-hemisuccinate linked to bovine serum albumin (Steraloids, 20 moles of steroid per mole of albumin) was inactive.

The time course of the early response was followed after the addition of DHT at a final concentration of 1×10^{-5} M to the medium in which tubules were previously cultured for 3 days. As depicted in Figure 2, the initial response was a marked inhibition of the incorporation of amino acids. A 30% decrease in the incorporation with respect to the controls was observed 2 hours after the addition of the androgen. The inhibitory effect gradually diminished, such that after 16 hours of exposure to the hormone, the incorporation was identical to the control value. Subsequently, a stimulation of the incorporation occurred and the value obtained at 24 hours (19%, $P < 0.05$) was statistically significant.

II. RNA Synthesis

The results of the experiments on protein synthesis directed us to study RNA synthesis in tissues cultured for 3-4 days. Androgen in the media for the duration of the culture increased markedly the rate and overall amount of radioactive uridine incorporated into acid insoluble material (Figure 3). The difference between control and DHT-treated tissue was highly significant ($P < 0.005$ for DHT 10^{-7} M and $P < 0.001$ for DHT 10^{-5} M). Stimulation of RNA synthesis appeared to be a more sensitive measurement of response to androgen than the incorporation of amino acids into protein. This conclusion is supported by the finding that a stimulation of the incorporation of uridine, adding 5×10^{-9} M dihydrotestosterone to the media of tissues cultured for 3 days, was consistently observed. Testosterone and 5α-androstane-3α, 17-ß diol at the same

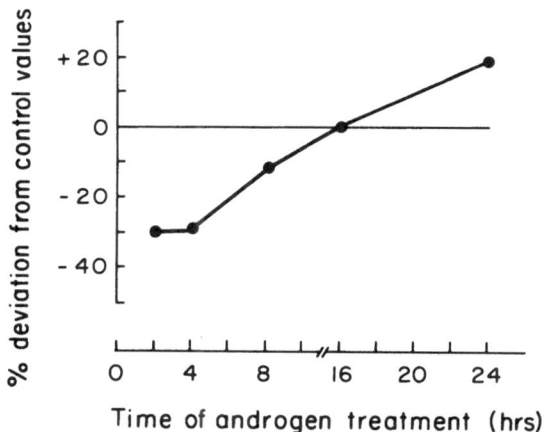

Figure 2. Time course of the androgen effect on amino acid incorporation into acid insoluble material by epididymal tubules in organ culture. Tissues were cultured for 3 days. At the end of this period dihydrotestosterone was added to the culture media at a concentration of 1 x 10^{-5} M. Androgen treated and control tissues were withdrawn from culture at different times after the addition of the hormone and tested for their capacity to incorporate [^{14}C] amino acid. Incubation conditions as described in Figure 1, except that incubations were carried out for 0 and 120 only. Results are expressed as the percentage of deviation from the corresponding control value.

concentrations produced the same stimulatory effect.

The time course of RNA synthesis in response to androgen was similar to that described for protein synthesis. Figure 4 shows that in this case, the initial effect was also inhibitory, reaching a maximal block at 4 hours after androgen (41%) followed by a return to control values at a rate such that the values exceeded the control at 8 hours and rose to a significant level 16 hours after addition of the hormone (P < 0.01).

III. Androgen Binding by Serum Proteins

The necessity of using androgen concentrations of the order of 10^{-5} M and 10^{-7} M in the culture media in order to elicit rapid responses of the tissues led us to investigate the possibility that the steroids might be bound to the proteins of the fetal calf serum and, therefore, not readily available to the cultured tissues. The

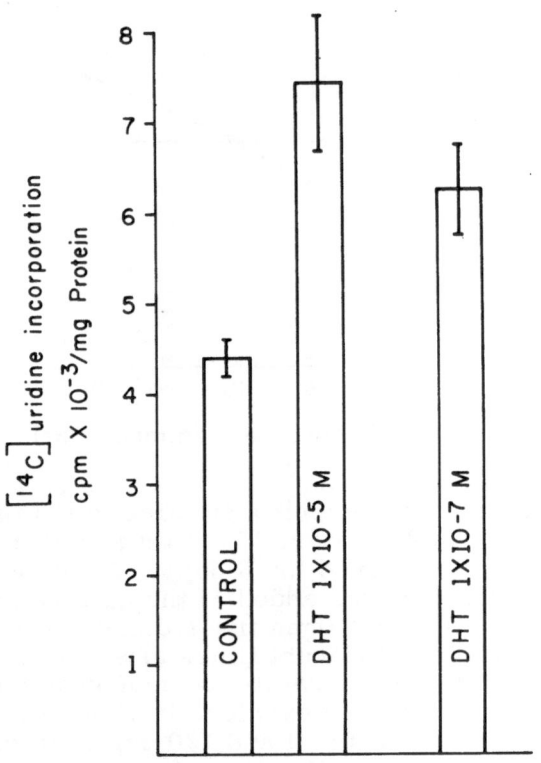

Figure 3. The effect of dihydrotestosterone added to the culture media at concentrations of 1 x 10^{-5} M and 1 x 10^{-7} M upon the incorporation of [^{14}C] uridine into acid insoluble material. Tissues cultured in the presence or absence of androgen for 4 days. Incubation conditions as in Figure 1, except that 0.1 μCi of[^{14}C] uridine replaced the radioactive amino acids.

technique of equilibrium dialysis was employed to determine the binding of testosterone at different concentrations by fetal calf serum at several dilutions. The results are summarized in Figure 5 which shows that with 10% serum, 57% of the steroid present at 1 x 10^{-5} M and 61% at 1 x 10^{-7} M were bound. To detect the presence of receptors in serum with high affinity for

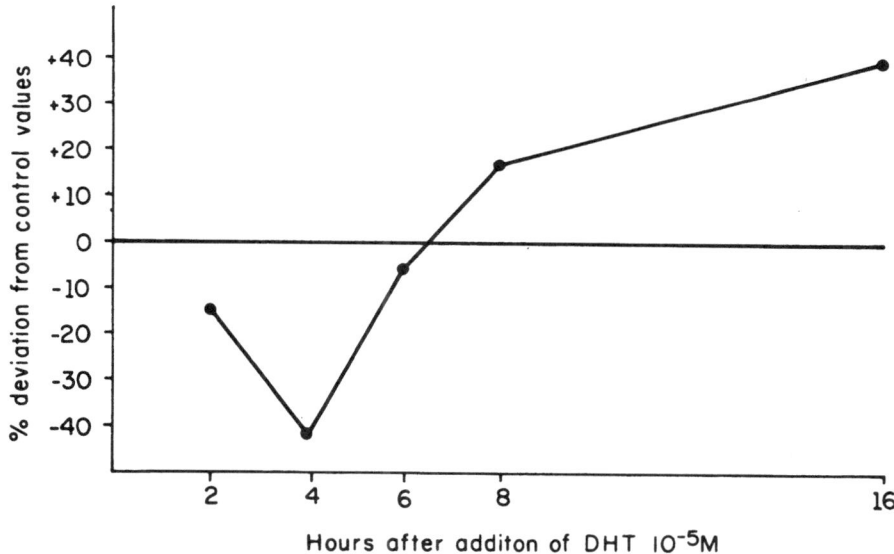

Figure 4. The time course of androgen effect on uridine incorporation into acid insoluble material by rat epididymal tubules in organ culture. Tissues were cultured for 3 days and at the end of this period 1 x 10^{-5} M DHT was added to the media. Control and androgen treated tissues were withdrawn from culture at different times after the addition of the hormone and tested for their capacity to incorporate [14C] uridine on a 2 h incubation, as described in Figure 3. Results are expressed as the percentage of deviation from the corresponding control value.

testosterone, dialysis was performed adding to the external solution enough bovine serum albumin to equal the protein concentration of the 10% serum placed inside the dialysis bag. Under this condition, 10% fetal calf serum bound 57% of the testosterone present at a concentration of 1 x 10^{-9} M as compared to 75% of the steroid bound on standard dialysis at this steroid concentration (Figure 5). A Scatchard plot was drawn with the data obtained from these experiments, showing the presence of at least two different binding components in the fetal calf serum (Figure 6).

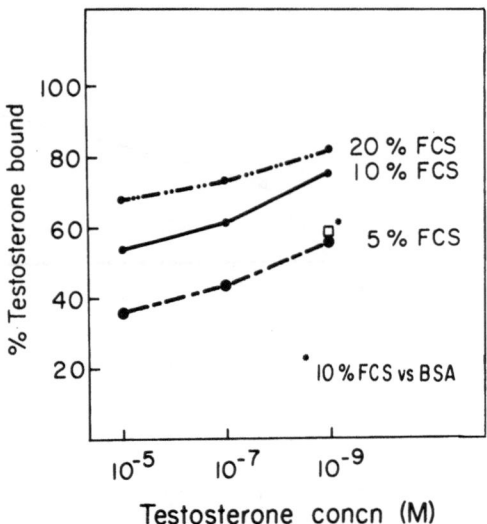

Figure 5. Binding of testosterone to fetal calf serum components:
The percentage binding of [^{3}H] testosterone at 10^{-5}, 10^{-7} and 10^{-9} M
by different dilutions of fetal calf serum (FCS) was determined by
equilibrium dialysis. One ml of the desired dilution of FCS was
dialyzed against 50 ml of Earle's balanced salt solution containing
1 μCi of [1-2-6-7 ^{3}H] testosterone and sufficient amounts of non-
radioactive testosterone to yield the desired molar concentrations.
   10% FCS was dialyzed as described except that enough bovine
serum albumin (BSA) was added to the dialyzing solution to equal
the protein concentration of the diluted serum.

IV. Binding of Androgen to Cellular Receptors

   Tritiated testosterone was added to the media of epididymal
tubules which had been maintained in culture for 3 days, and the
binding of the androgen to intracellular receptors was followed
at different intervals, ranging from 30 min to 24 hours. Figure
7 illustrates the results obtained with the cytoplasmic receptor.
After 24 hours of exposure of the tissue to radioactive testosterone,
a well-defined peak of radioactivity which moved with an approximate
Rf of 0.4 with respect to the tracking dye, bromophenol blue, was
detected. The amount of radioactivity bound to this peak decreased
with shorter times of exposure. Integratig the area under the peak,
we found that after 12 hours of androgen treatment, the zone contained only 1/3 of the radioactivity found at 24 hours, while the amount
accumulated after 6 hours was barely detectable. No radioactivity
was found associated with this region of the gel at shorter periods.
Under these conditions we were unable to locate any significant

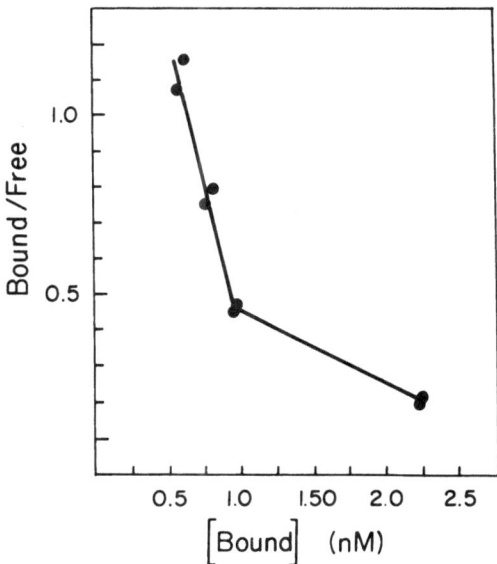

Figure 6. The presence of two testosterone binding components in fetal calf serum: Scatchard plot of the data for testosterone binding by 10% fetal calf serum.

radioactivity in the zone where the intraluminar ABP should flow to (RF = 0.65-0.7) (5). Only in tissues after 24 hours of labelling was a discrete peak of radioactivity associated with the intermediate 5S receptor observed. It should be emphasized that the present experiments were performed with small amounts of tissue approximately 100 mg per sample (4 to 5 culture plates). The limiting factor accounting for the small size of the samples is the time required to prepare the cultures.

Discussion

It is our current hypothesis that androgens exert their action on target tissues by a mechanism involving the stimulation of the transcription of genetic material (6). This process seems to be mediated by specific intracellular receptors which convey the steroid from the cytoplasm into the acceptor sites in the nuclear chromatin. Therefore, it appears reasonable to postulate that a given androgen-dependent system will not be activated until binding of the hormone to the receptors has occurred.

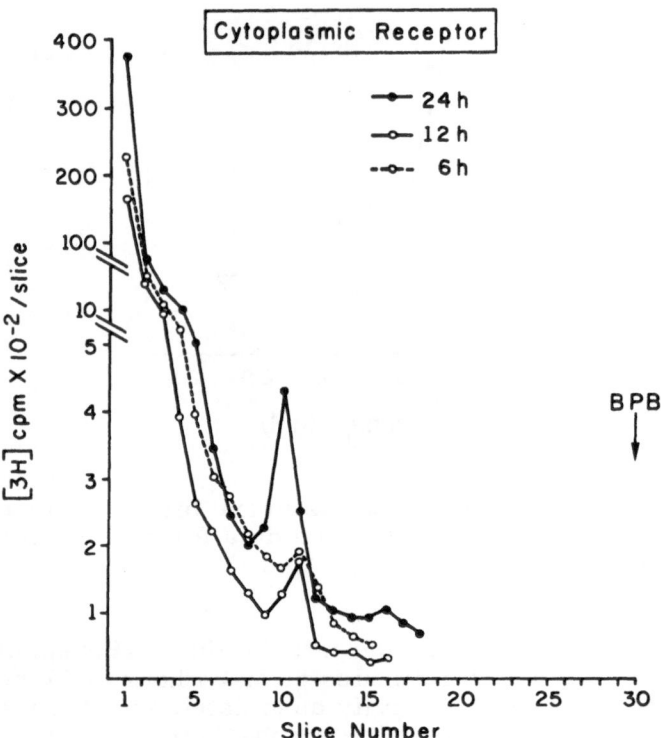

Figure 7. The binding of ^{3}H testosterone to cytoplasmic receptor
from rat epididymal tubules maintained in organ culture. Epididy-
m/l tubules, free of spermatozoa by efferent duct ligation, were
obtained from rats castrated 24 hr prior to the experiments. The
tissues were cultured for 3 days and at the end of this period 0.5
μCi of [1-2-6-7^{3}H] testosterone were added to each culture dish.
The tissues were removed from culture at 6, 12 and 24 hr after
the addition of the hormone, washed in media containing 1 x 10^{-7} M
non-radioactive testosterone, homogenized and centrifuged at
105,000 g x 1 hr. Aliquots of the cytosol containing equal amounts
of protein were run on 3.5% acrylamide gels prepared in 0.5%
agarose, as described by Tindall et al. (5). Radioactivity was
counted after allowing the gel slices (2 mm) to stand over night
at room temperature in toluene based scintillation fluid.

The delayed response of rat epididymal tubules maintained in organ culture to added androgen presented a suitable preparation to test this hypothesis. The correlation in time between the stimulation of RNA synthesis (16 hours) and protein synthesis (24 hours) with detectable levels of binding of tritiated testosterone to the cytoplasmic receptor supports this notion. Nevertheless, the early inhibitory effect which is clearly attributable to the hormone is real, since the control samples contained identical amounts of alcohol and were manipulated in a similar fashion. It is possible that the detection techniques available to us at present lack the necessary sensitivity and resolution to detect minute amounts of receptor-bound steroid, especially when the starting material is complete cytosol which contained a large amount of different proteins and free steroid. The early inhibitory effect might be due to the mobilization, under the influence of the hormones, of amino acids or bases from a pool which was not readily accessible to the added radioactive precursors. The finding that the kinetics of amino acid incorporation into cell proteins deviate from predicted values based on the assumption that the total intracellular amino acid pool was an obligatory intermediate in protein synthesis, thereby indicating a functional compartmentalization (7-8), supports this contention. Our results are analogous to those reported by Means and Hamilton (9). After the injection of estradiol-17ß into the female rat, these authors found a significant decrease in the amino acid incorporation into nuclear protein 30 min after administration of the hormone, subsequently followed by a stimulation. They hypothesized that this initial inhibition might be due to the preferential utilization of ATP for RNA synthesis during the early stage of hormone action.

Upon further inquiry into this problem, carried out presently at our laboratories, it appears that androgen modulates the synthesis of some specific proteins present in the epididymal cytosol of the rat (10). Some protein bands, easily detected by absorption at 280 nm or staining on disc electrophoresis, present in the cytosol of the intact rat, gradually decrease after castration, reaching undetectable levels 10-12 days after castration (in gels containing equal amounts of total protein) and are re-induced by short treatment with testosterone propionate (0.5 mg/day/4 days).

This evidence supports our preliminary findings obtained with cultured epididymal tubules. Labeled proteins synthesized under control conditions or in the presence of 10^{-6} M DHT using ^{14}C or ^{3}H aminoacids respectively were analyzed by disc electrophoresis. The ratio of the isotopes in different parts of the gel shows deviations, favoring the isotope present in the androgen-treated tissue. After relatively short periods of androgen action, between 1 and 6 hours, the deviation in the ratios was found to be confined to a zone with a relative mobility of about 0.85 with respect to the tracking dye, while after longer exposure to the hormones, several

regions of the gel showed evidence of induced proteins. These
results, although preliminary, raise the possibility that the early
effect of androgens may be the induction of a few proteins, apparently of low molecular weight, which may play a role in
the amplification of the response. It is possible that the early response is too minute to be detected by our conventional incorporation
techniques but could be responsible for the preferential utilization of
the cellular resources for the production of that substance, resulting
in the overall inhibitory effect that we had observed.

Some of our most recent experiments indicate that the binding
of androgens to the epididymal cytoplasmic receptor was demonstrated in the 20-day old rat, which corresponded roughly with the
finding of detectable tissue levels of DHT in that organ, and also
with the first meiotic division of the spermatogenic process. We
hope that this system will prove useful in our quest to trace the
initial events of the androgen activation of the epididymis.

The effect of androgen on amino acid and uridine incorporation
appears to be specific for these hormones since it is not elicited by
estradiol 17ß, corticosterone or progesterone and, furthermore, it
is blocked by the simultaneous presence of cyproterone acetate
(1). The addition of actinomycin D to the culture media suppressed
the effect of added androgens, suggesting that the hormones exert
their action through the synthesis of RNA (1). Finally, we presume
that binding of androgens to the proteins of fetal calf serum, perhaps to the same androgen binding globulin present in adult bovine
plasma, may explain the requirement of having concentrations of
steroid of the order of 1×10^{-5} M in the media in order to elicit rapid
responses.

Summary

Rat epididymal tubules maintained in organ culture for 3 or 7
days in media containing androgen showed a marked increase in
the incorporation of radioactive amino acids and uridine into acid
insoluble material. When the tubules were exposed to these
hormones for brief periods, the incorporation of precursors was
inhibited initially. In studying the time course of binding of ^{3}H
testosterone to the cytoplasmic receptor, a significant amount of
radioactivity bound to the receptor was detected only after 12 hr of
exposure to the hormone which increased three-fold after 24 hr.
The time lag in the binding corresponded closely to the shortest
times of observed hormone action wherein a significant increase
in the incorporation of uridine (16 hr) and amino acids (24 hr) was
produced. Evidence is presented demonstrating that testosterone
is bound with high affinity by components of the fetal calf serum
present in the culture medium.

Acknowledgements

The excellent technical assistance of Mrs. Debora Breger and Miss Elsa Millar is gratefully acknowledged.

References

1. Blaquier, J.A., Biochem. Biophys. Res. Commun. 52, 1177, 1973.

2. Blaquier, J.A.: J. Steroid Biochem. 1, 319, 1970.

3. Blaquier, J. A.: Biochem. Biophys. Res. Commun. 45, 1076, 1971.

4. Blaquier, J. A. and Calandra, R. S., Endocrinology 93, 51, 1973.

5. Tindall, D. J., Hansson, V., McLean, W. S., Nayfeh, S. N., and French, F. S., J. Biol. Chem. (in press).

6. Williams-Ashman, H. G., and Reddy, A. H., in Litwack, G. (ed.), "Biochemical Actions of Hormones", Vol. II, Academic Press, New York, pp. 257-294.

7. Kipnis, D., Reiss, E., and Helmreich, E., Biochim. Biophys. Acta 51, 519, 1961.

8. Rosenberg, L. E., Berman, M., and Segal, S., Biochim. Biophys. Acta 71, 664, 1963.

9. Means, A. R., and Hamilton, t. H., Proc. Natl. Acad. Sci. USA 56, 686, 1966.

TESTICULAR ESTRADIOL RECEPTORS IN THE RAT

E. Mulder, W. M. O. van Beurden-Lamers, W. De Boer,
A. O. Brinkman and H. J. van der Molen

Department of Biochemistry (Division of Chemical Endocrinology)
Medical Faculty, Erasmus University Rotterdam
Rotterdam, The Netherlands

Introduction

Investigations concerning a biochemical explanation for the mechanism of action of steroids have revealed the presence of specific receptors for steroids in target tissues. Specific steroid binding receptors in testicular tissue have only recently been studied, although in 1969 Stumpf (1) presented autoradiographic evidence for a nuclear localization of radioactivity in interstitial cells of the immature rat testis after administration of radioactive oestradiol. In the course of a study on steroid receptors in the testis we observed specific binding of oestradiol by the cytoplasm of the rat testis tissue (2, 3). It appeared of interest to investigate if the binding for this steroid fulfills the criteria for a true steroid receptor, i.e. high affinity binding of steroid, saturability, steroid specificity and tissue specificity. Data will be given on the specific localization of this receptor in interstitial tissue obtained after wet dissection of mature rat testis and on the characterics of oestradiol binding by the cytoplasmic macromolecule. In addition, it will be reported that after in vivo or in vitro administration of oestradiol, this steroid can be bound by nuclear fractions isolated from rat testis interstitial cells (4). The distribution of high affinity oestradiol binding components in the different tissues of the male rat was also studied. The highest amount of specific oestradiol binding macromolecules per cell were found in testis interstitial cells and in the pituitary, smaller amounts were present in epididymis, prostate, adrenal and liver. Finally, results will be presented on agar gel electrophoresis of the oestradiol receptor, a specific androgen receptor and androgen binding protein from rat testis.

High Affinity Binding of Oestradiol by Testicular Interstitial
Tissue

Testis tissue of mature rats was separated in interstitial
tissue and in seminiferous tubules by wet dissection at 4°. The
tissues were homogenized in 10 mM Tris buffer, pH 7.4, and
centrifuged at 105,000 x g. For in vitro labelling 105,000 x g
supernatant was incubated for 2 hours at 0° C with ^{3}H-oestradiol.
This supernatant was called the "cytosol" fraction and was subjected to density gradient analysis on linear 5-20% sucrose gradient. A sharp peak of radioactivity was observed in the 8S region
when the cytosol obtained from interstitial tissue was labelled

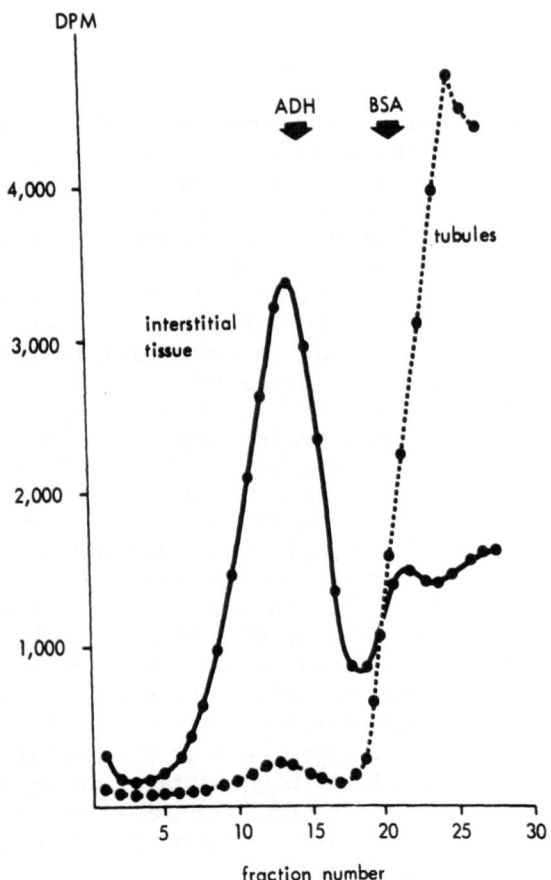

Figure 1. Sucrose gradient analysis of oestradiol binding by
cytosols of interstitial tissue (solid lines) and seminiferous
tubules (dashed lines). Cytosols were labelled by in vitro incubation with 0.7 x 10⁻¹⁰ M ^{3}H-oestradol.

either by in vitro incubation (Fig. 1) or during in situ perfusion
of the testis with ³H-oestradiol. The sedimentation profile of the
tubular cytosol preparation showed only a very small elevation in
the 8S region, possibly due to a contamination by interstital
tissue.

Quantitative analysis of the binding of oestradiol with the cytoplasmic receptor has been investigated using a Scatchard-type
plot as shown in Figure 2. The binding was studied by adsorption
of the free steroid on dextran coated charcoal at 4° C. Analysis
of these results gave an association constant in the order of 10^{10}
(M^{-1}). The concentration of binding sites in total testis cytosol
was calculated to be in the order of 2×10^{-14} mole/mg protein.

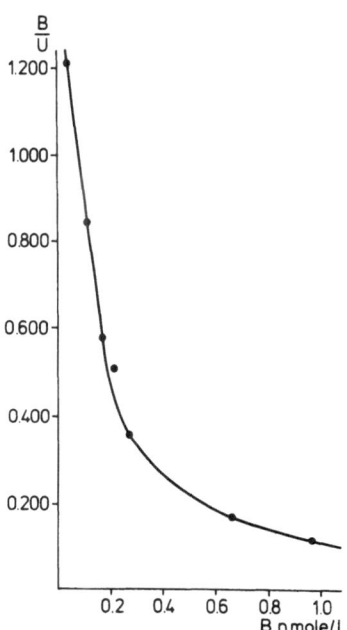

Figure 2. Scatchard plot of oestradiol binding in vitro by testis
cytosol from immature rats as determined by the dextran coated
charcoal adsorption method. B/U represents the amount of
bound (B) over unbound (U) steroid at equilibrium. Protein
concentration: 14.8 mg/ml.

The oestradiol binding macromolecule showed the characteristics
of a protein with respect to treatment with different enzymes and
temperature sensitivity (Table I).

Table I

Characteristics of Testicular Cytoplasmic Oestradiol Receptor

---

sedimentation coefficient $S_{20,w}$: 8S

association constant K_a : 10^{10} M^{-1}

concentration in total testis   : 2×10^{-14} moles/mg cytosol
                                     protein

localization   : interstitial tissue

heat treatment (30' at 37°)   : disappearance 8S macromolecules

pronase treatment   : disappearance 8S macromolecules

DNA-ase treatment   : no disappearance 8S macromolecules

RNA-ase treatment   : no disappearance 8S macromolecules

The presence of a specific 8S oestradiol receptor in testicular cytosol fractions could also be demonstrated in total testis tissue from mice and monkeys.

Specific Binding of Oestradiol by Different Tissues of the Male Rat

Cytosols of 13 different tissues of the male rat have been studied in order to investigate if the presence of an oestradiol receptor was restricted to testis interstitial tissue. Cytosols of all tissues were incubated with $4 \times 10^{-9}M$ labelled oestradiol and specific binding was determined using agar electrophoresis. The presence of an 8S binding protein was checked by sucrose gradient centrifugation of each cytosol. The uterus of the female rat was used as a control tissue. The results (Table II) show that a specific binding protein with a sedimentation coefficient of 8S could be demonstrated in testis interstitial tissue, prostate, epididymis, pituitary, adrenal and liver. Such a protein, however was absent in seminiferous tubules, seminal vesicle, hypothalamus, kidney, muscle and plasma. The amount of specific binding in the uterus was 240 fmole/mg protein. The highest amount of oestradiol binding macromolecules in male rats was found in the testis in interstitial tissue (140 fmole/mg protein) and in pituitary (75 fmole/mg protein).

Table II

Specific Binding of Oestradiol by Different Tissues of the Male Rat

Tissue	specific binding $(10^{-15}$ mole/mg protein)	8S-protein
Total testis tissue	9.8	+
Seminiferous tubules	0.1	-
Testis interstitial tissue	140	+
Epididymis	8.7	+
Prostate	11.4	+
Seminal vesicle	0.1	-
Pituitary	75.6	+
Hypothalamus	2.6	-
Adrenal	22.2	+
Liver	2.3	+
Kidney	1.4	-
Skeletal muscle	0	-
Plasma	0	-

Cytosols of different tissues and plasma of the male rat were incubated either with $4 \times 10^{-9}M$ labelled oestradiol or with $4 \times 10^{-9}M$ labelled plust $4 \times 10^{-7}M$ unlabelled oestradiol. Specific binding was determined using agar electrophoresis and is expressed as 10^{-15} mole oestradiol binding/mg protein of the cytosol. The presence (+) or absence (-) of a binding protein with a sedimentation value of 8S after sucrose gradient centrifugation is indicated in the last column.

Uptake of Oestradiol by Nuclei Obtained from Testis Interstitial Tissue

In most steroid target tissues the steroids can be bound by specific receptors in the cytosol and in the nuclear fraction. Therefore, we have considered the possibility that a comparable situation exists in testis interstitial tissue and whether in addition to cytoplasmic binding, oestradiol can also be bound by the nuclear fraction.

Testis was labelled either in vivo by subcutaneous injection of oestradiol, or by in vitro incubation of decapsulated testis tissue in a medium with labelled oestradiol. After the labelling procedure the tissue was dissected into tubules and interstitial tissue. The

interstitial tissue was homogenized and centrifuged at 700 g for
the preparation of a crude nuclear fraction. In some experiments
this nuclear fraction was further purified on a discontinuous
sucrose gradient with a bottom layer of 2.0 M sucrose. Through
this purification procedure the crude nuclear fraction was divided
in a precipitate of N_1 and a residue of N_2 on top of the 2.0 M sucrose (Fig. 3). After this purification the distribution of marker

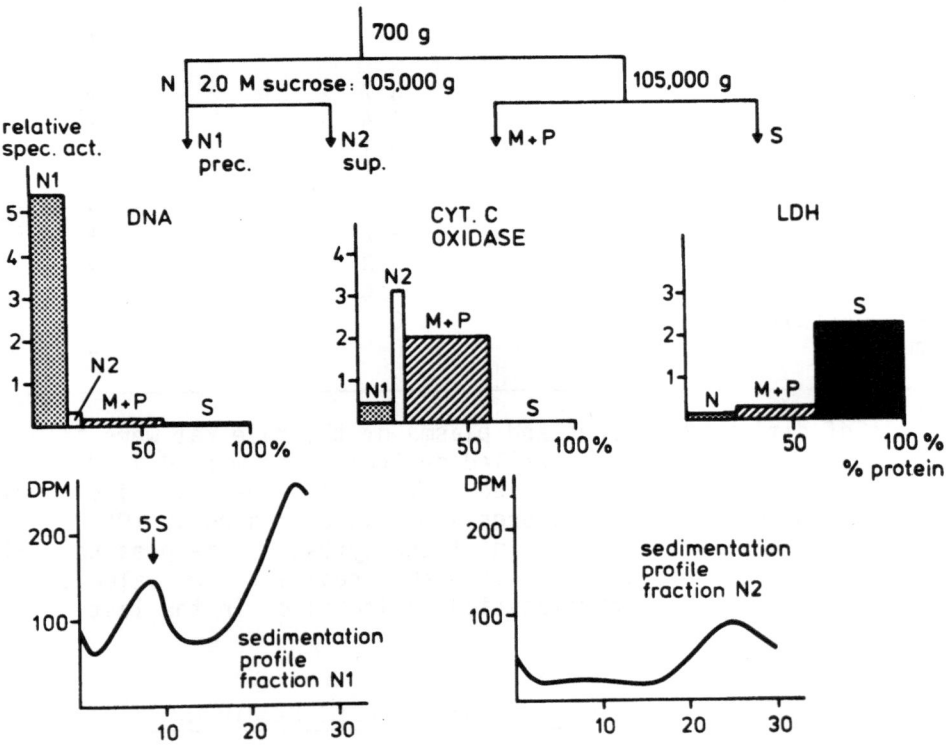

Figure 3. Marker enzymes and sedimentation profiles of [3]H-
oestradiol in subcellular fractions of isolated interstitial tissue.
Total testis tissue was incubated with 6 x 10^{-9}M ^{3}H-oestradiol for
30 min at 32° in Eagle's tissue culture medium before the dissection. The block diagrams show relative specific (enzyme) activities of marker molecules. DNA was used as a marker for nuclei,
cytochrome-C oxidase as a marker for mitochondria, lactate dehydrogenase (LDH) as a marker for cytoplasm, N_1 and N_2 : nuclear fractions; M + P: mitochondria and microsomes; S: cytosol.
The lower part of the figure shows sedimentation profiles of oestradiol after centrifugation of nuclear extracts in sucrose gradients after centrifugation of nuclear extracts in sucrose gradients
containing 0.4 M KCl.

molecules in the different fractions was also measured (middle part of Fig. 3). DNA was mainly present in the N_1 fraction. There was little contamination of this fraction with mitochondrial cytochrome-C oxidase and cytoplasmic lactate dehydrogenase. The sedimentation profile of ^3H-oestradiol in extracts from the N_1 nuclear fraction, obtained by treatment with a 0.4 M KCl solution, showed radioactivity in the 5S region. This 5S ^3H-oestradiol-macromolecule complex was not present in the extract from fraction N_2 (Fig. 3). Only in the nuclear fraction of interstitial tissue was oestradiol radioactivity observed in the 5S region after gradient centrifugation. Labelled oestradiol binding macromolecules could not be extracted from nuclear fractions of either seminiferous tubules or muscle (Fig. 4).

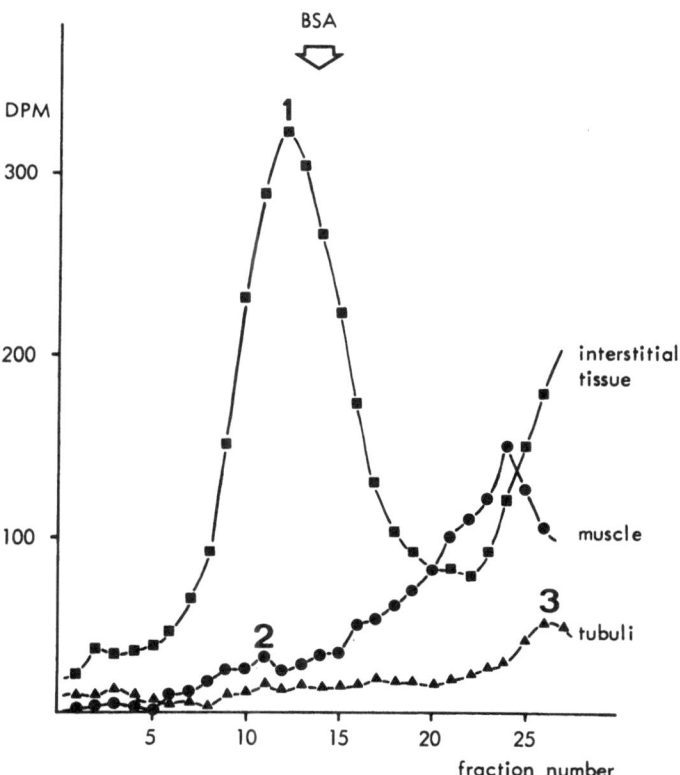

Figure 4. Sedimentation profile of oestradiol in the nuclear extract after in vivo labelling of testis interstitial tissue (curve 1), seminiferous tubules (curve 2) and muscle (curve 3) from a mature rat, injected with 6 pmole ^3H-oestradiol per g body weight 90 min before decapitation. The sucrose gradient contained 0.4 M KCl, and bovine serum albumin (BSA) was used as sedimentation marker.

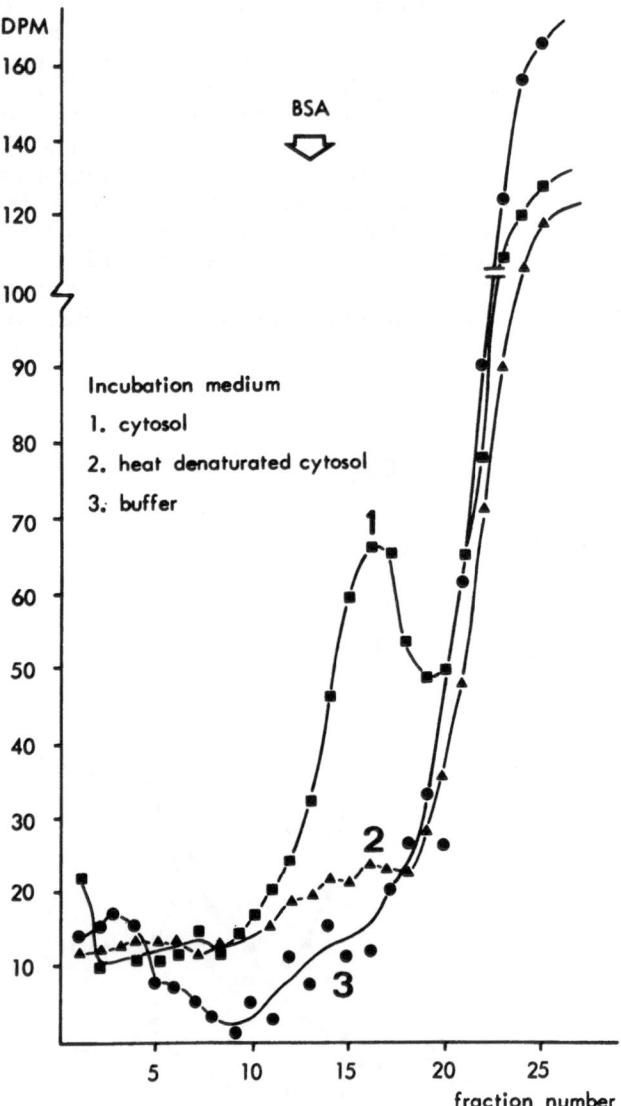

Figure 5. In vitro labelling of isolated nuclear fractions from testis interstitial tissue. Sedimentation profiles of oestradiol in nuclear extracts after incubation of isolated nuclear fractions in different media containing 0.06 μC ^{3}H-oestradiol/ml and either cytosol (curve 1), heat denatured cytosol (curve 2) or 10 mM Tris-EDTA buffer, pH 7.4 (curve 3). Before incubation with nuclear fractions the cytosol or heat denatured cytosol (20 min 60° C) was incubated with H-oestradiol for 90 min at 0° C. Subsequently nuclear fractions was mixed with the labelled cytosols or buffer and incubated for 45 min at 0° followed by 15 min at 25°. After incubation the nuclei were washed with 10 mM Tris buffer.

Incubation experiments with isolated subcellular fractions demonstrated that labelling of the nuclear fraction could be achieved only in the presence of the cytosol fraction (Fig. 5). This suggests that the steroid molecule after binding by cytoplasmic proteins is transferred to nuclear binding sites. In this respect the uptake of oestradiol by nuclei of testis interstitial tissue might require a similar mechanism as several other target tissues for steroid hormones. The sedimentation coefficients obtained for the oestradiol receptors in the nuclear extracts after labelling in vivo or in vitro of whole tissue (approximately 5S, Fig. 4) were different from those obtained for the receptors isolated from a reconstituted system containing cytosol and nuclei approximately 4S; Fig. 5). It is conceivable that during incubation of the isolated nuclear fraction the conversion of a cytoplasmic 4S receptor (in 0.4 M KCl) to a 5S complex might not have occurred.

Comparison of Receptors for Oestrogens and Androgens in Testis Tissue

Relative affinities of a number of steroids for the oestradiol receptor in the testis cytosol are presented in Figure 6. These experiments were carried out by incubation of 200 μl of cytosol

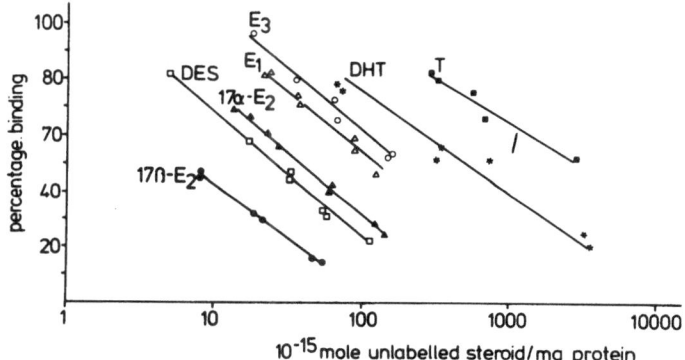

Figure 6. Binding affinity of various steroids for the testis cytosol oestradiol receptor (Percentage bound ^{3}H-oestradiol vs. nmole steroid). Testis cytosol was incubated with 0.7 x 10^{-10} M oestradiol and increasing amounts of unlabelled steroid. After 2 hr incubationa the percentage binding was estimated using the charcoal technique.

17ß-E : 17ß-oestradiol; DES: diethylstilboestrol;
17α-E : 17α-oestradiol; DHT: dihydrotestosterone;
E$_1$: oestrone; E$_3$: oestriol; T: testosterone.

with 3, 500 dpm (0.7 x 10^{-10}M) ^{3}H-oestradiol and increasing
amounts of the different unlabelled steroids. The percentage
binding was estimated using the dextran coated charcoal adsorption method. In the competition experiments with testosterone and
dihydrotestosterone it was necessary to hypophysectomize the
animals 8 days before the experiment in order to reduce the level
of endogenous androgens. The highest competition for the binding
sites was achieved with oestradiol-17ß, DES (diethylstilboestrol)
and oestradiol-17α. The decrease in percentage binding after
incubation with increasing amounts of unlabelled oestradiol was
the same for testis cytosols prepared from normal and hypophysectomized animals.

Specific binding of oestradiol by testis cytosol can also be demonstrated using agar gel electrophoresis as introduced by
Wagner (5) (Fig. 7). Free steroid moves to the cathode as a
result of the electro-endosmotic effect, while receptor-bound

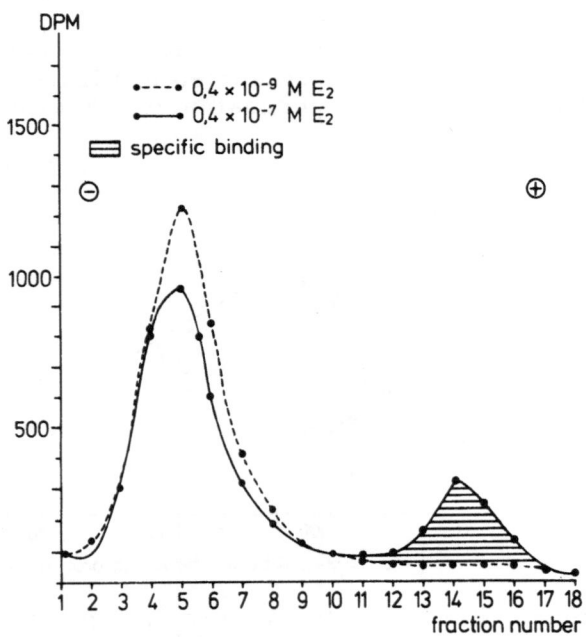

Figure 7. Agar gel electrophoresis of oestradiol binding proteins
of testis tissue. Testicular cytosol was incubated either with 0.4
x 10^{-9} M labelled oestradiol (curve 1) or with 0.4 x 10^{-9}M labelled
oestradiol plus 0.4 x 10^{-7} M unlabelled oestradiol (curve 2). The
sample was applied in the middle of the agar plate (fraction 10).
The peak at the left (cathodic) side represents unbound radioactive
steroid.

steroid at pH 8.5 moves to the anode. At this pH-value the
testicular androgen binding protein (ABP) found by Ritzen et al.
(6) and Hansson et al. (7) remains close to the application site on
the agar plate and can be clearly distinguished from the oestradiol
receptor (Fig. 8A). Preliminary experiments using agar electrophoresis indicate that in addition to ABP another binding protein
with a high affinity for androgenic steroids (testicular androgen
"receptor") is present in testis tissue extracts. This protein was
recovered from the 0.4 M KCl extract of nuclei obtained from total
testis tissue of 8 days hypophysectomized rats injected with testosterone (Fig. 8A, nuclear extract).

When a 100-fold excess of non-radioactive testosterone was
injected together with the labelled testosterone, hardly any radioactivity was present at the site of the androgen receptor after
agar electrophoresis of the nuclear extract. However, this receptor could be labelled when a 100 times higher amount of non-
radioactive oestradiol was injected together with the radioactive
testosterone (Fig. 8B).

Therefore it appears that androgens in the rat testis can be
bound by a specific androgen receptor different from the oestradiol receptor and ABP.

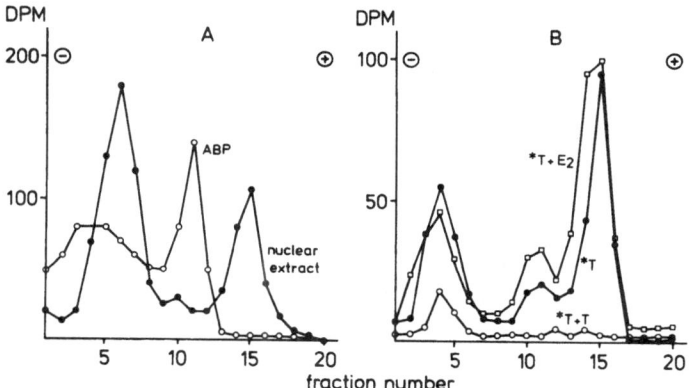

Figure 8. Agar electrophoresis of androgen binding proteins in
nuclear extracts of testis tissue. (A) Electrophoretic patterns of
the nuclear extract of testicular tissue of an 8 days hypophysectomized rat injected with labelled testosterone (nuclear extract) and
of purified dihydrotestosterone labelled androgen binding protein
(ABP) prepared according to Ritzen (6). (B) Electrophoretic
patterns of the nuclear extract of testicular tissue of 8 days hypophysectomized rats injected with either 100 μCi testosterone (*T),
100 μCi testosterone + 100 fold excess of unlabelled testosterone
(*T + T) or 100 μCi testosterone + 100 fold excess of unlabelled
oestradiol (*T + E$_2$).

Discussion

The physiolgoical meaning of the uptake of oestradiol by the testis interstitial cells is not yet clear. The presence of these receptors is not limited to rat testis tissue. In some preliminary results we also observed oestradiol receptors in mouse and monkey testis tissue. The concentration of oestradiol used for in vitro incubation of rat tissue in this study (6×10^{-9} M) was in the order of the concentration normally present in uterine tissue and rat testis interstitial tissue, but higher than that present in total testis (10^{-10} M) (8). Also, studies of de Jong (8, 9) have shown tht oestradiol concentrations in rat testis interstitial tissue ($0.5 - 1 \times 10^{-9}$ M) are higher than those in seminferous tubules. Actions of oestradiol in the testis on DNA, RNA and protein synthesis have been reported for Blab/c mice (10). Steinberger et al. (11) and Danutra et al. (12) have observed an effect of oestradiol on testosterone concentrations in the rat, without a concomitant change in LH level, which might imply a direct effect of oestradiol on steroidogenesis in testicular tissue. In other experiments carried out in our laboratory, a simultaneous fall in both testosterone and LH levels in the rat was observed after oestradiol benzoate injections (13). Further studies are clearly requird to find out whether oestradiol has a direct regulatory effect on testis steroidogenesis or spermatogenesis. It is of interest to investigate if the occurrence of oestradiol receptors in interstitial tissue are relevant in this respect. We have some results indicating that oestradiol injections into male rats do have an effect on the amount of the receptor for oestradiol itself.

Summary

Specific high affinity saturable binding proteins for oestradiol-17ß have been demonstrated in the cytoplasm of liver, adrenal, pituitary, prostate, epididymis and testis interstitial tissue of the rat. Specific testicular oestradiol receptors were present in cytoplasmic and nuclear fractions of interstitial tissue, but not in seminiferous tubules of rat testis.

After in vivo or in vitro administration of oestradiol the steroid was bound by the nuclear fraction of interstitial tissue only in the presence of the cytoplasmic receptor. Using agar gel electrophoresis the cytoplasmic oestradiol receptor from rat testis could be separated from the testicular androgen binding protein (ABP) and from a specific androgen receptor.

REFERENCES

1. Stumpf, W. E., Endocrinology 85:31, 1969.

2. Brinkmann, A. O., Mulder, E. and van der Molen, H. J., Compt. Rend. D 274:3106, 1972.

3. Brinkmann, A. O., Mulder, E., Lamers-Stahlhofen, G. J. M., Mechielsen, M. J., and van der Molen, H. J., FEBS Letters 26:301, 1972.

4. Mulder, E., Brinkmann, A. O., Lamers-Stahlhofen, G. J. M. and van der Molen, H. J., FEBS Letters 31:131, 1973.

5. Wagner, R. K., Hoppe-Seyler's Z. Physiol. Chem. 353:1235, 1972.

6. Ritzen, E. M., Dobbins, M. C. and Tindall, D. J., Steroids 21:593, 1973.

7. Hansson, V., Djøseland, O., Reusch, E., Attramdal, A. and Torgersen, O., Steroids 21:457, 1973.

8. de Jong, F. H., Hey, A. H. and van der Molen, H. J., Acta endocr. (Kbh) Suppl. 177:345, 1973.

9. de Jong, F. H., Hey, A. H. and van der Molen, H. J., J. Endocrinol, 1974, In Press.

10. Samuels, L. T., Uchikawa, T. and Huseby, R. A., Coll. Endocrinol. 16:211, 1967.

11. Steinberger, E., communicated at the 9th Acta Endocrinologica Congress, Oslo, 1973.

12. Danutra, V., Harper, M. E., Boyns, A. R., Cole, E. N., Brownsey, B. G. and Griffiths, K., J. Endocr. 57:207, 1973.

13. Verjans, H. L., de Jong, F. H., Cooke, B. A., van der Molen, H. J. and Eik-Nes, K. B., Acta endocr. (Kbh), 1974, submitted for publication.

CONFERENCE SUMMARY

William T. Schrader and Bert O'Malley

Department of Cell Biology
Baylor College of Medicine
Houston, Texas

This Symposium was held at the Department of Cell Biology at Baylor College of Medicine, Houston, Texas, on February 11-13, 1974. The conference was sponsored jointly by the National Institute of Child Health and Human Development (NICHD) and the Baylor Center for Population Research and Reproductive Biology. The Symposium was intended to focus on interactions of gonado-tropins and sex steroids with specific testicular receptor proteins and the subsequent events coupled to this process such as fluctuations in levels of cAMP or protein kinase.

This enlightening symposium gave evidence for the significant progress made recently in understanding the early events of hormone interactions in the testis. It is noteworthy that there was substantial agreement among the various laboratories on several key points, hotly debated only a year ago. Some novel approaches were outlined that provide enriched cell fractions and specific end-points for future studies. It was evident that there has been, and continues to be, close cooperation among research-ers at the molecular and morphological levels. The testis, which incontrovertibly displays the importance of cell-cell interactions, surely cannot be understood without this type of multidisciplinary approach.

A good case in point is the interaction of LH with the testis. Drs. Catt and Desjardins described their studies of LH and hCG binding to cell membrane receptors. The receptors show

specificity for homologous hormone preparations; binding of the
hormone from another species can occur, but frequently these
heterologous sources fail to compete effectively. The receptors
were shown to exist in the cell membranes of the Leydig cell -
enriched testis preparations used by Dr. Catt's laboratory. This
result was as predicted from the known stimulatory effects of LH
on testosterone secretion by these cells. Their findings were in
concert with the autoradiographic results of Dr. Desjardins. By
exposing consecutive tissue sections of testis to ^{125}I-hCG or
^{125}I-FSH, he could assign hCG binding to interstitial Leydig
cells, and FSH to Sertoli cells. There appeared to be little
overlap of the two classes of gonadotropin receptors on the same
cell types. Essentially all of the labeled hormones could be
competitively displaced by non-radioactive hormone in both
methods, thereby establishing the restriction of binding to receptors rather than nonspecific sites on the membranes.

A correlation of receptor occupancy with the biologic effect
of LH was reviewed by Dr. Catt. He showed by dose-response
relationships that secretion of testosterone and cyclic AMP were
maximum at doses of hCG far below those necessary to saturate
the receptors. There are thus many more receptor sites than
are necessary for these end-point events to occur.

Dr. Dufau described the characterization of solubilized hCG
receptors from testis homogenates, and showed that the kinetic
and specificity data were consistent with those values obtained
for the receptors in situ on membranes. The receptors were
solubilized with detergents, without which the isolated receptors
aggregated. Sedimentation and gel filtration data indicated
the asymmetrical protein nature of the receptors, and gave a
molecular weight of about 194,000 daltons for the nascent receptor
and 224,000 daltons for the complexes. These values are consistent with binding of a single ligand per receptor. Hormone
binding was destroyed by trypsin treatment and, significantly,
by phospholipase A. These findings may indicate important roles
for lipid and carbohydrate moieties in the receptor molecules,
an idea supported by Dr. Dufau's observation that the receptors
bind to concanavalin A-Sepharose columns. Initial attempts to
reconstitute binding of the phospholipase-treated receptors by
addition of phospholipids were unsuccessful.

Complementing these studies of the receptors were four
contributions on the chemistry of LH-like hormones. Receptor
binding was used frequently as an index of activity for deri-
vations and generally agreed with bioassay and radioimmunoassay determinations. Dr. Ward reported on the effects of
various chemical modifications on hormone activity. Nitration
of the exposed tyrosines of native LH decreased both biologic
potency and receptor binding of the hormone. All of the exposed

tyrosines were on the α-subunit, and were required for recombination with ß-subunits. However, reaction of both ß-subunit tyrosines did not destroy recombining activity. He also demonstrated the relative importance of the amino groups on both subunits. Carbamylation, which neutralizes an existing -NH +, reacts with both amino groups on the ß-subunit and with 9 of 10 amino groups on the α-subunit. Complete carbamylation of the subunits does not prevent their reassociation, and the complexes retain good biological activity. Maleation, on the other hand, reacts with charged amino groups to yield a negative group. These derivatives of the subunits or the native complex largely destroy the recombination capacity of the subunits and destroy the biologic activity of the native material. Through these measurements, he was able to distinguish surface reactive groups on the two subunits and to assess their importance to different aspects of the hormone's activity.

Dr. Puett described his conformational studies of gonadotropins and the assignment of various bands in the circular dichrosim spectra to specific structural features of native hormones and subunits of several LH's and hCG. A band at 208-210 nm was assigned to the glycopeptides of the molecules, thereby constituting a method for studying these functional groups in the hormones. Extensive studies have been done using hCG. Assessment of protein structure in the native hormone and subunits showed no evidence for α-helicity in keeping with their high proline content, but 15-30% ß-structure depending upon the subunit. The ß-structure diminished with dissociation of the subunits. He then turned his attention to longer wavelength CD spectra of growth hormone, showing how the technique could reveal important disulfide linkages and monitor the environment of aromatic residues. Again, the native hormone showed more ordered structure than either subunit. A disulfide bridge in the ß-subunit and at least one tyrosine were perturbed upon dissociation to subunits.

Dr. Puett's laboratory has also studied gonadotropin metabolism, and the role of carbohydrate moieties in the processes. Removal of terminal sialic acid residues caused human LH to be cleared rapidly, presumably by recognition of terminal galactose by liver cells. This explanation is not universal, however, since ovine LH, which contains no sialic acid, has a dual half-life. Although some of the protein is cleared with a half-life measured in minutes, some of the LH molecules have a half-life measured in hours. Thus the system for hCG clearance may be atypical of gonadotropins in general.

Dr. Bahl's laboratory has been involved in analysis of the carbohydrate residues of hCG. There are two carbohydrate moieties on the α-subunit, and 5 on the ß-subunit. He has

used extensive treatment with neuraminidase and specific glycosidases to remove as much carbohydrate as possible from the
hormones without prior hydrolysis to glycopeptides. Up to 100%
of the sialic acids, 60% of galactose and 20% of the mannose residues could be removed. Hormones treated in this fashion were
assayed in four separate ways for retention of activity. These
were radioimmunoassay and receptor-binding assays for conformational analysis, and the accumulation of cAMP and steroidogenesis assays for analysis of hormone biologic function. His
results in vitro clearly indicate that the carbohydrate residues
of the hormone play a more important role in its function than
mèrely to define its half-life in the circulation. Removal of
carbohydrate to different degrees yielded hormone preparations
which had varying degrees of similarity to the native gonadotropin
in the four assays. Radioimmunoassays showed only about a 50%
reduction in cross-reactivity of the highly-digested preparations
compared to native hCG, indicating that the carbohydrate removal
had little effect on conformation. Binding of the iodinated hormones to rat testis homogenates in a receptor-binding assay
showed that binding was reduced when mannose was removed, but
increased if only sialic acid was removed. This was an important result in a conceptual sense. Addition of free carbohydrate
to the binding reaction had no effect. Accumulation of cAMP and
induction of steroidogenesis showed significant decreases when
various carbohydrates were removed. However, even the most
highly reacted hormone preparation was active to some extent.
A preparation in which mannoses were removed bound poorly in
the receptor assay, but elevated cAMP levels to 20% that of native
hormone. Thus there appeared to be a potential for differential
response at the level of receptor-binding and biological activity,
similar to that observed through the dose-response curve comparisons described by Dr. Catt.

Dr. Papkoff described work on the structure of PMSG, a
hormone having both LH and FSH activities in a single protein.
The protein has a high proline content and no helical structure,
similar to ovine LH and FSH, but the tryptic peptide maps show
no obvious overlaps with either of these hormones. End-group
analysis revealed N-terminal heterogeneity. The PMSG subunits
are very tightly coupled, since the sedimentation coefficient of
the hormone does not change dramatically under extremes of
pH. Counter-current distribution methods can be used to separate two subunits with differing amino acid compositions. When
the subunits were recombined, the LH-like activity of the
recombinant was found to vary with the input ratio of α - and
ß-subunits. Recombinants also recovered FSH-like activity.

This protein, like LH and FSH, is also a glycoprotein. It
contains 45% carbohydrate by weight, and these residues affect
the clearance of the hormone from the circulation.

Studies concerning the molecular action of FSH have been hindered in the past by two key issues, lack of agreement on a specific testis target cell and lack of an end-point for quantitative work. By comparison, LH stimulation of steroidogenesis in Leydig cells had offered considerable advantages for study. Several laboratories have approached these two problems, and results of their work was presented.

Dr. A. Steinberger discussed the FSH receptors in low-speed pellets from rat testis homogenates. Specificity of binding of FSH was demonstrated by competition studies using hCG and LH. Binding activity per unit testis weight increased up to 15 days of postnatal life, in parallel to the increasing Sertoli cell titer in the tissue. Tissue levels of receptors varied with the serum levels of FSH, but the receptors persisted in the tissue of animals 37 days after hypophysectomy. Binding of FSH was shown to occur in a Sertoli-cell enriched fraction prepared by culturing testis tubules for up to 4 weeks, whereas a peri-tubular cell fraction devoid of Sertoli cells was shown not to contain these specific FSH-binding sites.

Dr. Rabin's laboratory has been studying FSH binding to testis homogenate receptor preparations. He described the effects of the degree of iodination of FSH by the chloramine-T method on the activity of ^{125}I-FSH. Iodination of FSH was followed by a size separation step on Sephadex columns which could distinguish aggregates from FSH monomers and subunits. As the degree of iodination increased, up to 20% of the hormone chromatographed as an aggregate excluded by G-100. Only at the lowest degree of isotopic labeling was the expected FSH monomer the labeled product. When the peaks were examined for FSH activity by radioimmunoassay and a specific receptor-binding assay, FSH aggregate fraction had the highest activity by both methods.

Dr. Bhalla reported the studies of the Emory group on FSH binding to testis receptors. A lightly iodinated preparation found to retain full biological activity in vivo was used to study binding of the hormone to a filtrat e of a testis homogenate. The 1000 x g particulate fraction contained receptors. The binding constant of 6 x 10^{-10} M (Kd) was consistent with other reported values, and with the expected biologic role in vivo. The receptors were unusually heat-stable, since 70° C treatment for 15 min only reduced binding by 50%. Microdissection of seminiferous tubules yielded a preparation which bound both FSH and LH, apparently at independent loci. The receptor binding to tubules was destroyed by treatment with 40% ethanol. Existence of an ethanol solubilized membrane factor was postulated from these experiments. The ethanol wash promoted elution of labeled FSH-receptor complexes from Sepharose columns.

Dr. Means reported on the experiments of his laboratory in studying FSH binding to receptors coupled to subsequent molecular events. The receptor for FSH was shown to be localized in tubular cells rather than interstitial cells, which bind FSH only nonspecifically. Tubule membrane preparations contained enhanced binding activity compared to the crude homogenate, suggesting receptor localization in this fraction. Adenyl cyclase activity was stimulated in vitro in those membranes by FSH, but not LH, 5 min after addition of the hormone. Tubular protein kinase activity was altered over the same time interval by the elevated levels of cAMP produced in response to the FSH. Preparation of tubules from immature animals with low endogenous cAMP levels showed the highest degree of FSH stimulation of active kinase; older animal preparations were less sensitive to FSH due to already elevated cAMP levels before hormone administration. Hypophysectomy caused protein kinase levels to decline by 35 days, which could be restored by FSH administration. In a manner similar to that for LH studies in the Leydig cells, the cAMP and kinase levels reached a maximum in vitro at doses of FSH far below those necessary to saturate all the receptors. This implied the existence of either nonfunctional receptors or receptor redundancy. A strikingly advantageous testis model was described for FSH studies consisting of only Sertoli cell tubules from rats irradiated in utero. Morphologic characteristics of Sertoli cells appeared normal, and the cells bound FSH at the same levels as normal tubule preparations. The effects of FSH on cAMP in the Sertoli-cell only (SCO) animals were similar to the controls confirming FSH action on the Sertoli cells.

Dr. Braun reported the existence of two apparently different adenyl cyclase activities in the testis which correlated with different cell populations. The two enzyme activities differed with respect to their metal cofactors and subcellular distribution. The Mn^{++}-dependent enzyme is the soluble cell fraction, whereas the Mg^{++}-dependent enzyme is a particulate enzyme. When the cyclase activity was measured in developing rats at various days of age, the Mn^{++}-dependent enzyme titer began to rise from undetectable levels from day 12 onward, while the Mg^{++}-dependent enzyme activity decreased to low levels beyond day 15. The mature sperm were thought to contain the Mn^{++}-activated type of enzyme.

The transport of androgens out of the testis via the testicular fluid has become an important area of study since the detection of a specific androgen-binding protein (ABP) in this fluid. The titer of ABP androgen complexes decreases along the length of the epididymis, suggesting a role for ABP in the delivery of androgen to the epididymis. The central theme for ABP studies at the symposium concerned the role of ABP as a likely candidate for an FSH-specific end-point protein, synthesized in the Sertoli cells in response to this hormone.

Dr. French described studies by his group using electrophoretic methods to quantitate ABP. The protein resembles plasma steroid-binding globulins in its general physical characteristics, and binds dihydrotestosterone better than testosterone. The testis levels of ABP rise when the afferent ducts are ligated, confirming its synthesis in the testis. Autoradiographic studies showed ABP was secreted into the tubular lumen. Hypophysectomy caused ABP levels to fall, which could be restored by FSH but not by LH. Destruction; of the germinal epithelium with X-rays caused no loss of ABP, indicating a nongerminal cell source for this protein. The ABP is distinctly separate from intracellular androgen receptor proteins of the testis and epididymis. The two types of binding protein were distinguishable by both physical means on electrophoresis and also by nuclear uptake studies, in which receptor enters nuclei but ABP does not. Cytoplasmic receptor levels are not affected by FSH or hypophysectomy.

Dr. Sanborn's studies of androgen binding in testis also showed there were two classes of binding sites. One class rapidly dissociated with a half-life on the order of minutes. This class was maintained by FSH and represented the androgen-binding proteins isolated by Dr. French. A second class of sites bound testosterone with a very long half-life.

Dr. Fritz's studies were also pointed toward identifying the cell source of ABP and its possible control by FSH. Hypophysectomy for 7 days was used to lower endogenous androgen titers, allowing resolution of two binding components. The rapidly equilibrating ABP fraction was not detectable after 30 days of hypophysectomy, but levels returned to normal after 3 days of FSH administration. A mouse strain having only Sertoli cells was studied and found to contain 80% of the normal level of ABP, again confirming the Sertoli cell as an FSH target cell which makes ABP as a product.

Dr. van der Molen's laboratory has characterized an estrogen receptor protein in the testis. Although there is at present no recognized function for this protein, he pointed out that about 20% of the male rat estrogen is synthesized in the testis and is localized in the interstitial tissues. The estrogen receptor is very similar to the estrogen receptor protein located in the rat uterus. Its size, K_d and steroid specificity all compare closely to this more commonly studied material. The behavior of the receptor was studied by observation of nuclear uptake of labeled steroid in vivo, suggesting that this complex behaves in similar fashion to other cytoplasmic receptors.

The rapid progress occurring in this field over the past three years was clearly evident and can only remain as a tribute to the scientists involved. Nevertheless, there is even more to be accomplished over the next five years when, undoubtedly, the intracellular events which culminate in altered target cell function will be finally elucidated.

INDEX
(Listed by Chapter Number)

A

Acetylation   5
N-Acetylglucosamine   7
Actinomycin D   1,20
Adenosine triphosphate (ATP)   3,15,20
Adenylate cyclase   1,8,13,14,15,19,22
Adipose tissue   8
Adrenal   4,8,21
Adrenocorticotrophic hormone (ACTH)   1,4,8,10
Affinity chromatography   3
Agar electrophoresis   21
Aging   3,18
Agonist   1,3
Alkylation   3
Amino acid sequence   5,7
Androgen   1,2,3,4,7,8,9,10,16,17,18,19,20,21,22
Androgen binding protein (ABP)   9,16,17,18,19,20,21,22
Antagonist   1
Antiserum   11
Asialo-agalacto human chorionic gonadotropin   1,7
Association constant (K a)   1,2,3,8,10,16,18,21
Autoradiography   10,13,16

B

Binding capacity   1,2,3,8,10,16,19
Binding protein   9,16,17,18,19,20
Binding sites   1,2,3,4,5,6,7,8,10,11,13,16,19
Binding studies   1,3,7,8,9,10,17
Bioassay   1,2,3,5,6,7
Biological activity   1,3,22
Blood coagulation factors   3
Blood testis barrier   8,9
Blue Dextran   3

C

Calcium   1,3
Carbamylation   5,22
Catalytic subunit   8
Cesium chloride isopycnic gradients   3
Cellulose adsorption chromatography   1,2,3
Charcoal   9,16,18,19,21
Chloramine T   1,3,7,10,11,12

U

V

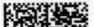